Polycystic Ovary Syndrome

T0172779

Polycystic Ovary Syndrome

A Guide to Clinical Management

Adam H Balen MB BS MD FRCOG
Professor of Reproductive Medicine and Surgery
Department of Reproductive Medicine
Leeds General Infirmary
Leeds
UK

Gerard S Conway MB BS MD FRCP
Consultant Endocrinologist
Department of Endocrinology
The Middlesex Hospital
London
UK

Roy Homburg MB BS
Professor of Reproductive Medicine
Department of Obstetrics and Gynecology
Reproductive Medicine, Department. Ob/Gyn
Vrije Universiteit Medisch Centrum
1007 MB Amsterdam
The Netherlands

Richard S Legro MD
Professor of Obstetrics and Gynecology
Department of Obstetrics and Gynecology
Penn State College of Medicine
Hershey, PA 17033
USA

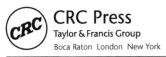

CRC Press

Taylor & Francis Group
Boca Raton London New York

CRC Press is an imprint of the
Taylor & Francis Group, an **informa** business

CRC Press
Taylor & Francis Group
6000 Broken Sound Parkway NW, Suite 300
Boca Raton, FL 33487-2742

First issued in paperback 2019

© 2010 by Taylor & Francis Group, LLC
CRC Press is an imprint of Taylor & Francis Group, an Informa business

No claim to original U.S. Government works

ISBN-13: 978-1-84214-211-0 (hbk)
ISBN-13: 978-0-367-39286-4 (pbk)

This book contains information obtained from authentic and highly regarded sources. While all reasonable efforts have been made to publish reliable data and information, neither the author[s] nor the publisher can accept any legal responsibility or liability for any errors or omissions that may be made. The publishers wish to make clear that any views or opinions expressed in this book by individual editors, authors or contributors are personal to them and do not necessarily reflect the views/opinions of the publishers. The information or guidance contained in this book is intended for use by medical, scientific or health-care professionals and is provided strictly as a supplement to the medical or other professional's own judgement, their knowledge of the patient's medical history, relevant manufacturer's instructions and the appropriate best practice guidelines. Because of the rapid advances in medical science, any information or advice on dosages, procedures or diagnoses should be independently verified. The reader is strongly urged to consult the relevant national drug formulary and the drug companies' and device or material manufacturers' printed instructions, and their websites, before administering or utilizing any of the drugs, devices or materials mentioned in this book. This book does not indicate whether a particular treatment is appropriate or suitable for a particular individual. Ultimately it is the sole responsibility of the medical professional to make his or her own professional judgements, so as to advise and treat patients appropriately. The authors and publishers have also attempted to trace the copyright holders of all material reproduced in this publication and apologize to copyright holders if permission to publish in this form has not been obtained. If any copyright material has not been acknowledged please write and let us know so we may rectify in any future reprint.

Except as permitted under U.S. Copyright Law, no part of this book may be reprinted, reproduced, transmitted, or utilized in any form by any electronic, mechanical, or other means, now known or hereafter invented, including photocopying, microfilming, and recording, or in any information storage or retrieval system, without written permission from the publishers.

For permission to photocopy or use material electronically from this work, please access www.copyright.com (http://www.copyright.com/) or contact the Copyright Clearance Center, Inc. (CCC), 222 Rosewood Drive, Danvers, MA 01923, 978-750-8400. CCC is a not-for-profit organization that provides licenses and registration for a variety of users. For organizations that have been granted a photocopy license by the CCC, a separate system of payment has been arranged.

Trademark Notice: Product or corporate names may be trademarks or registered trademarks, and are used only for identification and explanation without intent to infringe.

A CIP record for this book is available from the British Library.

Library of Congress Cataloging-in-Publication Data available on application

Visit the Taylor & Francis Web site at
http://www.taylorandfrancis.com

and the CRC Press Web site at
http://www.crcpress.com

Contents

Foreword

Two advances have transformed our understanding of polycystic ovary syndrome. The first is the development of pelvic ultrasound as a simple, reliable and non-invasive method of identifying the polycystic ovary. While there may be debate over precise morphological details, there is general agreement that ultrasound has transformed our ideas of the prevalence of polycystic ovaries, their association with other conditions and their etiology. The authors of this book have made significant contributions to morphological characterization and each has practical experience of the value of high-quality ultrasonography in both research and in diagnosis and management.

The second important advance is the recognition that transformation of the symptomless woman with ovaries that are polycystic into a case of polycystic ovary syndrome is commonly mediated through insulin resistance with compensatory hypersecretion of insulin. The causes of insulin resistance are several; in practical terms the most widespread is obesity. The current epidemic of obesity, particularly, but not exclusively, in North American and the UK, means that the number of clinically apparent cases of the syndrome will increase and begin to approach the number of cases detected only by scan. Again the authors of this text have made significant contributions to our understanding of the causes and consequences of insulin resistance in polycystic ovary syndrome.

This book provides its reader with an up-to-date and accessible text about a syndrome which is very common, has very important consequences on reproductive and general health, and whose prevalence will almost certainly increase in the coming decades. I strongly commend it to you.

Professor Howard S Jacobs
Emeritus Professor of Reproductive Endocrinology
The Middlesex Hospital and University College Hospital, London

Preface

Polycystic ovary syndrome (PCOS) excites immense interest and debate. PCOS is a condition with different manifestations and so may present to a number of different medical specialists, from the general practitioner to gynecologists, infertility specialists, endocrinologists, dermatologists or to those who deal with metabolic and cardiovascular disease. Not only may the presentation vary but also the nature of the condition in an individual may change over time. As we have begun to understand more about the origins of PCOS, its pathophysiology and genetics, we have seen an exponential rise in the number of publications in this exciting area of medicine.

The management of PCOS is not without controversy – from making the diagnosis to the appropriate forms of therapy, and there are some differences around the world. We have therefore provided an overview of PCOS with a synthesis of our current understanding of its diagnosis and management. We hope that we have offered a pragmatic approach to treatment from the viewpoint of four busy practitioners and researchers in the fields of endocrinology, gynecology and reproductive medicine – and also from a transglobal perspective!

Adam Balen
Gerry Conway
Roy Homburg
Rick Legro
April 2005

Chapter 1
Introduction and overview

Many believe polycystic ovary syndrome (PCOS) to be a condition of our time. Certainly PCOS is the most common endocrine disturbance to affect women and it appears that its prevalence is on the increase. There is considerable heterogeneity of symptoms and signs among women with PCOS, and for an individual these may change over time. The extreme end of the spectrum, once known as the Stein–Leventhal syndrome, encompasses the combination of hyperandrogenism (hirsutism, acne, alopecia and elevated serum testosterone concentrations), severe menstrual disturbance (amenorrhea or oligomenorrhea) and obesity. We now appreciate that polycystic ovaries may exist without clinical signs of the syndrome. PCOS is familial, and various aspects of the syndrome may be differentially inherited. There are a number of interlinking factors that affect expression of PCOS. A gain in weight is associated with a worsening of symptoms while weight loss will ameliorate the endocrine and metabolic profile and symptomatology. Normal ovarian function relies upon the selection of a follicle, which responds to an appropriate signal (follicle stimulating hormone) in order to grow, become 'dominant' and ovulate. This mechanism is disturbed in women with PCOS, resulting in multiple small cysts, most of which contain potentially viable oocytes but within dysfunctional follicles.

In recent times there has been a significant change in lifestyle in many parts of the world, with most people experiencing a more sedentary existence combined with an abundance of food. This has resulted in the modern epidemic of obesity and consequent hyperinsulinemia – a situation which in women may precipitate expression of PCOS, while in men presentation is often with cardiovascular disease and type 2 diabetes in later life. Elevated serum concentrations of insulin are more common in both lean and obese women with PCOS than in weight-matched controls. Indeed it is hyperinsulinemia that appears to be the key to the pathogenesis of the syndrome, as insulin stimulates androgen secretion by the ovarian stroma and appears to affect the normal development of ovarian follicles, both by the adverse effects of androgens on follicular growth, and possibly also by suppressing apoptosis and permitting the survival of follicles otherwise destined to disappear.

Women with polycystic ovaries may experience a range of the clinical and biochemical features that define PCOS. These features include menstrual cycle disturbances, obesity, hirsutism, acne, and abnormalities of biochemical profiles including elevated serum concentrations of luteinizing hormone (LH), testosterone, androstenedione, and insulin. Presentation of the syndrome is so varied that one, all, or any combination of the above features may be present in association with an ultrasound picture of polycystic ovaries.

In this book we aim to provide a practical appraisal of our current understanding of PCOS. We shall discuss in detail the diagnosis of PCOS, with reference to ultrasonography and endocrine assessment (Chapter 2). We shall expand upon the assessment of hyperinsulinemia and its short-term and long-term health consequences (Chapters 4, 6, 7 and 8). Women who are obese, and also many slim women with PCOS, will have insulin resistance and elevated serum concentrations of insulin (usually <30 mU/l fasting). We suggest that a 75 g oral glucose tolerance test (GTT) be performed in women with PCOS and a body mass index (BMI) >30 kg/m^2, with an assessment of the fasting and two-hour glucose concentration. It has been suggested that South Asian women should have an assessment of glucose tolerance if their BMI is greater than 25 kg/m^2 because of the greater risk of insulin resistance at a lower BMI than seen in the Caucasian population.

The epidemiology of PCOS has received increasing attention in recent times, with respect both to prevalence in the general population and racial differences (Chapter 3). The highest reported prevalence of PCO has been 52% amongst South Asian immigrants in Britain, of whom 49.1% had menstrual irregularity.[1] Rodin and coworkers (1998) demonstrated that South Asian women with PCO had a comparable degree of insulin resistance to controls with established type 2 diabetes mellitus.[1] Generally, there has been a paucity of data on the prevalence of PCOS among women of South Asian origin, both among migrant and native groups. Type 2 diabetes and insulin resistance have a high prevalence among indigenous populations in South Asia, with a rising prevalence among women. Insulin resistance and hyperinsulinemia are common antecedents of type 2 diabetes, with a high prevalence in South Asians. Type 2 diabetes also has a familial basis, inherited as a complex genetic trait that interacts with environmental factors, chiefly nutrition, commencing from fetal life. We have already found that South Asians with anovular PCOS have greater insulin resistance and more severe symptoms of the syndrome than anovular Caucasians with PCOS.[2] Furthermore, we have found that women from South Asia living in the UK appear to express symptoms at an earlier age than their Caucasian British counterparts.

Obesity and metabolic abnormalities are recognized risk factors for the development of ischemic heart disease (IHD) in the general population, and these are also recognized features of PCOS. The questions are whether women with PCOS are at an increased risk of IHD, and whether this will occur at an earlier age than in women with normal ovaries. The basis for the idea that women with PCOS are at greater risk for cardiovascular disease is that these women are more insulin resistant than weight-matched controls and that the metabolic disturbances associated with insulin resistance are known to increase cardiovascular risk in other populations (Chapter 8).

Insulin resistance is defined as a diminution in the biological responses to a given level of insulin. In the presence of an adequate pancreatic reserve, normal circulating glucose levels are maintained at higher serum insulin concentrations. In the general population, cardiovascular risk factors include insulin resistance, obesity, glucose intolerance, hypertension, and dyslipidemia.

Insulin sensitivity varies depending upon menstrual pattern. Women with PCOS who are oligomenorrheic are more likely to be insulin resistant than those with regular cycles – irrespective of their BMI. Insulin resistance is restricted to the extra-splanchnic actions of insulin on glucose dispersal. The liver is not affected (hence the fall in sex hormone binding globulin (SHBG) and high-density lipoprotein (HDL)), neither is the ovary (hence the menstrual problems and hypersecretion of androgens) nor the skin (hence the development of acanthosis nigricans). The insulin resistance causes compensatory hypersecretion of insulin, particularly in response to glucose, so euglycemia is usually maintained at the expense of hyperinsulinemia.

Simple obesity is associated with greater deposition of gluteo-femoral fat while central obesity involves greater truncal abdominal fat distribution. Obesity is observed in 35–60% of women with PCOS. Hyperandrogenism is associated with a preponderance of fat localized to truncal abdominal sites. Women with PCOS have a greater truncal abdominal fat distribution as demonstrated by a higher waist:hip ratio. The central distribution of fat is independent of BMI and associated with higher plasma insulin and triglyceride concentrations, and reduced HDL cholesterol concentrations. Thus, examining the surrogate risk factors for cardiovascular disease, there is evidence that insulin resistance, central obesity and hyperandrogenemia are features of PCOS and have an adverse effect on lipid metabolism. Women with PCOS have been shown to have dyslipidemia, with reduced HDL cholesterol and elevated serum triglyceride concentrations, along with elevated serum plasminogen activator inhibitor-I concentrations. The evidence is thus mounting that women with PCOS may have an increased risk of developing cardiovascular disease and diabetes later in life, which has important implications in their management. However, Pierpoint and coworkers reported the mortality rate in 1,028 women diagnosed as having PCOS between 1930 and 1979.[3] The standard mortality rate both overall and for cardiovascular disease was not higher in the women with PCOS compared with the national mortality rates in women, although the observed proportion of women with diabetes as a contributory or underlying factor leading to death was significantly higher than expected (odds ratio 3.6, 95% confidence interval (CI) 1.5–8.4). Thus, despite surrogate markers for cardiovascular disease, in this study no increased rate of death from cardiovascular disease could be demonstrated. An overview of the epidemiology of insulin resistance in PCOS is provided in Chapter 8.

Other long-term consequences of PCOS arise from chronic exposure to increased serum concentrations of estrogen, often unopposed by the post-ovulatory secretion of progesterone by the corpus luteum. Patients with PCOS are therefore not estrogen deficient and those with amenorrhea are at risk not of osteoporosis but rather of endometrial hyperplasia and adenocarcinoma and there may be an association also with breast cancer (Chapter 9). Cycle control and regular withdrawal bleeding is achieved with the oral contraceptive pill, which has the additional beneficial effect of suppressing serum testosterone concentrations and hence improving hirsutism and acne. Dianette® and Yasmin®, containing the anti-androgens cyproterone acetate and drosperinone respectively, are commonly recommended.

The symptoms of PCOS may cause significant distress and are dealt with in turn (hirsutism – Chapter 10; acne – Chapter 11; menstrual disturbance – Chapter 12 and infertility – Chapter 13). Little attention has been paid to the effect that PCOS has on the quality of life of the woman. The psychological stress experienced by sufferers of obesity, menstrual disturbance, infertility and hirsutism has been studied separately, yet the overall effects of PCOS and the changing spectrum of the condition necessitates especial attention (Chapter 6). Treatment options for hirsutism include cosmetic and medical therapies (Chapter 10). As drug therapies may take six to nine months or longer before any improvement of hirsutism is perceived, physical treatments including electrolysis, laser therapy, waxing and bleaching may be helpful while waiting for medical treatments to work.

The management of the PCOS is symptom orientated. Whilst obesity worsens the symptoms, the metabolic scenario can conspire against weight loss. Diet and exercise are key to symptom control and weight loss improves the endocrine profile, and the likelihood of ovulation and a healthy pregnancy. Much has been written about diet and PCOS. The right diet for an individual is one that is practical, sustainable and compatible with her lifestyle. It is sensible to keep carbohydrate content down and to avoid fatty foods (Chapter 7). It is often helpful to refer to a dietitian. Anti-obesity drugs may help with weight loss. Metformin may lead to improvements with insulin resistance and may aid some women with weight loss, combined with a healthy diet and exercise program.

For women with infertility, ovulation can be induced with the anti-estrogens, clomifene citrate or tamoxifen. While clomifene is successful in inducing ovulation in over 80% of women, pregnancy only occurs in about 40%. Clomifene citrate should only be prescribed in a setting where ultrasound monitoring is available (and performed) in order to minimize the 10% risk of multiple pregnancy and to ensure that ovulation is taking place (Chapter 13). Recently attention has turned to the use of aromatase inhibitors and further research is ongoing. The therapeutic options for patients with anovulatory infertility who are resistant to anti-estrogens are either parenteral gonadotrophin therapy, or laparoscopic ovarian diathermy. Because the polycystic ovary is very sensitive to stimulation by exogenous hormones, it is very important to start with very low doses of gonadotrophins and follicular development must be carefully monitored by ultrasound scans. The advent of transvaginal ultrasonography has enabled the multiple pregnancy rate to be reduced to approximately 5% because of its higher resolution and clearer view of the developing follicles. Cumulative conception and livebirth rates after 6 months may be 62% and 54%, respectively, and after 12 months 73% and 62%, respectively.[4] Close monitoring should enable treatment to be suspended if three or more mature follicles develop, as the risk of multiple pregnancy obviously increases.

Women with PCOS are also at increased risk of developing ovarian hyperstimulation syndrome (OHSS). This occurs if too many follicles (>10 mm) are stimulated, and results in abdominal distension, discomfort, nausea, vomiting and sometimes difficulty in breathing. The mechanism for OHSS is thought to be secondary to activation of the ovarian renin–angiotensin pathway and excessive secretion of vascular endothelial growth factor (VEGF). The ascites, pleural and pericardial effusions exacerbate this serious condition and the resultant hemoconcentration can lead to thromboembolism. The situation worsens if a pregnancy has resulted from the treatment, as human chorionic gonadotropin (hCG) from the placenta further stimulates the ovaries. Hospitalization is sometimes necessary in order for intravenous fluids and heparin to be given to prevent dehydration and thromboembolism. Although OHSS is rare it is potentially fatal and should be avoidable with appropriate monitoring of gonadotropin therapy.

Ovarian diathermy is free of the risks of multiple pregnancy and ovarian hyperstimulation, and does not require intensive ultrasound monitoring. Laparoscopic ovarian diathermy has taken the place of wedge resection of the ovaries (which resulted in extensive peri-ovarian and tubal adhesions), and it appears to be as effective as routine gonadotrophin therapy in the treatment of clomifene-insensitive PCOS.

A number of pharmacological agents have been used to amplify the physiological effect of weight loss, notably insulin-lowering agents such as metformin. This biguanide inhibits the production of hepatic glucose and enhances the sensitivity of peripheral tissue to insulin, thereby decreasing insulin secretion. It has been shown that metformin ameliorates hyperandrogenism and abnormalities of gonadotropin secretion in women with PCOS and can restore menstrual cyclicity and fertility.[5]

In summary, PCOS is a heterogeneous, familial condition. Ovarian dysfunction leads to the main signs and symptoms and the ovary is influenced by external factors in particular the gonadotropins, insulin and other growth factors, which are dependent upon both genetic and environmental influences. There are long-term risks of developing diabetes and possibly cardiovascular disease. Therapy to date has been symptomatic but by our improved understanding of the pathogenesis, treatment options are becoming available that strike more at the heart of the syndrome.

Key points

- PCOS is the most common endocrine disorder in women (prevalence 15–20%).
- PCOS is a heterogeneous condition. Diagnosis is made by the ultrasound detection of polycystic ovaries and one or more of a combination of symptoms and signs (hyperandrogenism (acne, hirsutism, alopecia), obesity, menstrual cycle disturbance (oligo-/amenorrhea)) and biochemical abnormalities (hypersecretion of testosterone, luteinizing hormone and insulin).
- Management is symptom orientated.
- If obese, weight loss improves symptoms and endocrinology and should be encouraged. A glucose tolerance test should be performed if the BMI is >30 kg/m².
- Menstrual cycle control is achieved by cyclical oral contraceptives or progestogens.
- Ovulation induction may be difficult and require progression through various treatments which should be monitored carefully to prevent multiple pregnancy.
- Hyperandrogenism is usually managed with Dianette®, containing ethinylestradiol in combination with cyproterone acetate. A new combined oral contraceptive pill, Yasmin® may also be of benefit. Alternatives include spironolactone. Flutamide and finasteride are not routinely prescribed because of potential adverse effects. Reliable contraception is required.
- Insulin-sensitizing agents (e.g. metformin) are showing early promise but require further long-term evaluation and should only be prescribed by endocrinologists/reproductive endocrinologists.

Indications for referral to a reproductive medicine specialist
- Serum testosterone >5 nmol/l (to exclude other causes of androgen excess, e.g. tumors, late onset congenital adrenal hyperplasia, Cushing's syndrome)
- Infertility
- Rapid onset hirsutism (to exclude androgen-secreting tumors)
- Glucose intolerance/diabetes
- Amenorrhea of more than 6 months – for pelvic ultrasound scan to exclude endometrial hyperplasia
- Refractory symptoms

References

1. Rodin DA, Bano G, Bland JM, Taylor K, Nussey SS. Polycystic ovaries and associated metabolic abnormalities in Indian subcontinent Asian women. Clin Endocrinol (Oxf) 1998; 49(1):91–99.

2. Wijeyaratne CN, Balen AH, Barth J, Belchetz PE. Clinical manifestations and insulin resistance (IR) in polycystic ovary syndrome (PCOS) among South Asians and Caucasians: is there a difference? Clin Endocrinol (Oxf) 2002; 57:343–350.

3. Pierpoint T, McKeigue PM, Isaacs AJ, Wild SH, Jacobs HS. Mortality of women with polycystic ovary syndrome at long-term follow-up. J Clin Epidemiol 1998; 51:581–586.

4. Balen AH, Conway GS, Kaltsas G, Techatraisak K, Manning PJ, West C, Jacobs HS. Polycystic ovary syndrome: The spectrum of the disorder in 1741 patients. Hum Reprod 1995; 10:2107–2111.

5. Lord JM, Flight IHK, Norman RJ. Metformin in polycystic ovary syndrome: systematic review and meta-analysis. Br Med J 2003; 327:951–955.

Chapter 2
Defining the polycystic ovary syndrome

Introduction

Polycystic ovary syndrome (PCOS) is a heterogeneous collection of signs and symptoms that, when gathered together, form a spectrum of a disorder with a mild presentation in some, and a severe disturbance of reproductive, endocrine and metabolic function in others. The pathophysiology of PCOS appears to be multifactorial and polygenic. The definition of the syndrome has been much debated. Key features include menstrual cycle disturbance, hyperandrogenism and obesity. There are many extra-ovarian aspects to the pathophysiology of PCOS, yet ovarian dysfunction is central. At a recent joint European Society of Human Reproduction and Embryology/American Society for Reproductive Medicine (ESHRE/ASRM) consensus meeting, a refined definition of PCOS was agreed: namely the presence of two out of the following three criteria:

1. oligo- and/or anovulation
2. hyperandrogenism (clinical and/or biochemical)
3. polycystic ovaries,
   with the exclusion of other etiologies.[1]

The morphology of the polycystic ovary has been redefined as an ovary with 12 or more follicles measuring 2–9 mm in diameter and/or increased ovarian volume (>10 cm³)[2] (see also Appendix 1).

There is considerable heterogeneity of symptoms and signs amongst women with PCOS and for an individual these may change over time.[3] PCOS is familial, and various aspects of the syndrome may be differentially inherited. Polycystic ovaries can exist without clinical signs of the syndrome, which may then become expressed over time. There are a number of inter-linking factors that affect expression of PCOS. A gain in weight is associated with a worsening of symptoms, while weight loss may ameliorate the endocrine and metabolic profile and symptomatology.[4]

Genetic studies have identified a link between PCOS and disordered insulin metabolism, and indicate that the syndrome may be the presentation of a complex genetic trait disorder.[5] The features of obesity, hyperinsulinemia, and hyperandrogenemia which are commonly seen in PCOS are also known to be factors that confer an increased risk of cardiovascular disease and non-insulin dependent diabetes mellitus (NIDDM).[6] There are studies which indicate that women with PCOS have an increased risk for these diseases which pose long-term risks for health, and this evidence has prompted debate as to the need for screening women for polycystic ovaries.

Various factors influence ovarian function, and fertility is adversely affected by an individual being overweight or having elevated serum concentrations of luteinizing hormone (LH). Strategies to induce ovulation include weight loss, oral anti-estrogens (principally clomifene citrate), parenteral gonadotropin therapy and laparoscopic ovarian surgery. There have been no adequately powered randomized studies to determine which of these therapies provides the best overall chance of an ongoing pregnancy. Women with PCOS are at risk of ovarian hyperstimulation syndrome (OHSS) and so ovulation induction has to be carefully monitored with serial ultrasound scans. The realization of an association between hyperinsulinemia and PCOS has resulted in the use of insulin-sensitizing agents, such as metformin, which appear to ameliorate the biochemical profile and improve reproductive function.

Elevated serum concentrations of insulin are more common in both lean and obese women with PCOS than in weight-matched controls. Indeed it is hyperinsulinemia that appears to be the key to the pathogenesis of the syndrome as insulin stimulates androgen secretion by the ovarian stroma and appears to affect the normal development of ovarian follicles, both by the adverse effects of androgens on follicular growth and possibly also by suppressing apoptosis and permitting the survival of follicles otherwise destined to disappear.[7] The prevalence of diabetes in obese women with PCOS is approximately 11% and so a measurement of impaired glucose tolerance is important and long-term screening advisable.

What is polycystic ovary syndrome?

Polycystic ovaries are commonly detected by ultrasound or other forms of pelvic imaging, with estimates of the prevalence in the general population being in the order of 20–33%.[8,9] However, not all women with polycystic ovaries demonstrate the clinical and biochemical features that define PCOS. While it is now clear that ultrasound provides an excellent technique for the detection of polycystic ovarian morphology, identification of polycystic ovaries by ultrasound does not automatically confer a diagnosis of PCOS.

Despite the recent ESHRE/ASRM consensus meeting, controversy still exists over a precise definition of the 'syndrome' and whether or not the diagnosis should require confirmation of polycystic ovarian morphology. The generally accepted view in Europe and much of the world is that a spectrum exists, ranging from women with polycystic ovarian morphology and no overt abnormality at one end, to those with polycystic ovaries associated with severe clinical and biochemical disorders at the other end. Using a combination of clinical, ultrasonographic, and biochemical criteria, the diagnosis of PCOS is usually reserved for those women who exhibit an ultrasound picture of polycystic ovaries, and who display one or more of the clinical symptoms (menstrual cycle disturbances, hyperandrogenism), and/or one or more of the recognized biochemical disturbances (elevated LH, testosterone, androstenedione, or insulin). The 1990

National Institute of Health Conference on PCOS, however, recommended that diagnostic criteria should include evidence of hyperandrogenism and ovulatory dysfunction, in the absence of non-classic adrenal hyperplasia, and that evidence of polycystic ovarian morphology was not essential.[10] It has been considered necessary to redefine PCOS and include within it an appropriate definition of the polycystic ovary.[11,12]

Thus the 2003 ESHRE/ASRM consensus definition of PCOS requires the presence of two out of the following three criteria:

1. oligo- and/or anovulation
2. hyperandrogenism (clinical and/or biochemical)
3. polycystic ovaries,
   with the exclusion of other etiologies.[1]

Menstrual disturbances and infertility will be considered in detail in Chapters 12 and 13 and the consequences of hyperandrogenism will be discussed in Chapters 10 and 11. In this chapter we shall deal principally with defining hyperandrogenism and the morphological aspects of the polycystic ovary.

Hyperandrogenism

Hyperandrogenism may be determined by clinical or biochemical parameters. The clinical manifestations of androgen excess are hirsutism, alopecia and acne. The presence of hirsutism is the key feature but this is a relatively subjective diagnosis and few physicians in clinical practice actually use standardized scoring methods.[1,13] Furthermore, there are significant racial differences, with hirsutism being significantly less prevalent in hyperandrogenic women of Eastern Asian origin,[14] or in adolescence,[15] while being more prevalent in women from Southern Asia (i.e. the Indian subcontinent) and Mediterranean or Middle Eastern countries.[16]

The presence of acne after adolescence is thought also to be a relatively good indicator of hyperandrogenism,[1] although studies are somewhat conflicting regarding the exact prevalence of androgen excess in these patients.[17]

Most patients with PCOS have evidence of biochemical hyperandrogenemia, and circulating androgen levels may also represent an inherited marker for androgen excess.[18] However, it has been shown that some patients with PCOS may not demonstrate an overt abnormality in circulating androgens.[3,19–22]

A significant problem is the limitations of laboratory assay methodology. Many assays are inaccurate,[23–25] normative ranges have not been well-established using well-characterized control populations, and age and body mass index (BMI) have not been considered when establishing normative values for androgen levels.[26,27]

Testosterone is bound both to sex hormone binding globulin (SHBG) and albumin. The measurement of total testosterone is probably all that is required in order to exclude the presence of an androgen-secreting tumor.[3] In other words the value of measuring testosterone is primarily to help to exclude other causes of androgen excess. The measurement of free testosterone (T) or the free T (free androgen) index (FAI) may also be used for assessing for hyperandrogenemia.[28,29] Methods for the assessment of T include equilibrium dialysis,[24,25] calculation of T from the measurement of SHBG and total T, or ammonium sulfate precipitation.[30]

A few patients with PCOS may have isolated elevations in dihydroepiandrosteronesulfate (DHEAS). Furthermore androstenedione may be more elevated in patients with 21–hydroxylase-deficient non-classic adrenal hyperplasia than those with PCOS,[22] although the paucity of normative and clinical data with DHEAS and androstenedione preclude their routine measurement.[1]

terone, and androstenedione, in association with low or normal levels of follicle stimulating hormone (FSH) and abnormalities of estrogen secretion, described an endocrine profile which many believed to be diagnostic of PCOS.[32] Well recognized clinical presentations included menstrual cycle disturbances (oligo-/amenorrhea), obesity, and hyperandrogenism manifesting as hirsutism, acne, or androgen-dependent alopecia. These definitions proved inconsistent, however, as clinical features were noted to vary considerably between women, and indeed some women with histological evidence of polycystic ovaries consistently failed to display any of the common symptoms. Likewise, the biochemical features associated with PCOS were not consistent in all women. Thus consensus on a single biochemical or clinical definition for PCOS was thwarted by the heterogeneity of presentation of the disorder.

Numerous descriptions have been made of the morphology of the polycystic ovary and these have been refined over time, alongside advances in imaging technology. The first histological description of the polycystic ovary and features of the condition was made in 1721 by Vallisneri. In more recent times it was Stein and Leventhal who described the features of seven hirsute, amenorrheic women based on the characteristic ovarian morphology from histological specimens taken at wedge resection of the ovaries.[31] The histology of the polycystic ovary was of an ovary with prominent theca, fibrotic thickening of the tunica albuginea and multiple cystic follicles (Figure 2.1).[31] The number of antral follicles (2–6 mm in diameter)

The polycystic ovary

Historical and histopathological considerations

Historically the detection of the polycystic ovary required visualization of the ovaries at laparotomy and histological confirmation following biopsy.[31] As further studies identified the association of certain endocrine abnormalities in women with histological evidence of polycystic ovaries, biochemical criteria became the mainstay for diagnosis. Raised serum levels of LH, testos-

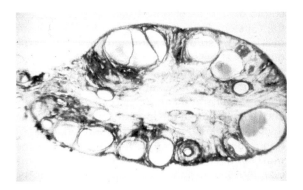

Figure 2.1

Histological cross section of a polycystic ovary.

was described as 'excessive' by Goldzieher and Green but not quantified.[33]

For many years wedge resection was the only treatment for PCOS and histological assessment of the ovaries was therefore routine practice. Wedge resection is, however, an outdated operation, so polycystic ovaries are no longer readily available for detailed histological examination. The histopathological criteria have been defined as the observation of: atretic follicles and/or degenerating granulosa cells, hypertrophy and luteinization of the inner theca cell layer, and thickened ovarian tunica. Good correlation has been shown between ultrasound diagnoses of polycystic morphology, and the histopathological criteria for polycystic ovaries, by studies examining ovarian tissue obtained at hysterectomy or after wedge resection.[34,35] The literature on correlations between ultrasound and histology is sparse, as histological assessment of the ovary became obsolete before ultrasound became common practice. The histological data of Hughesdon (1982), indicated a two- to three-fold increase of the follicle number in PCOS, from the stage of primary follicles up to tertiary follicles, and identified the cystic structures as follicles as opposed to pathological cysts.[36]

Ultrasound descriptions of the polycystic ovary

The advent of high-resolution ultrasound scanning provided a non-invasive technique for the assessment of ovarian size and morphology. Good correlation has been shown between ultrasound diagnoses of polycystic morphology, and the histopathological criteria for polycystic ovaries by studies examining ovarian tissue obtained at hysterectomy or after wedge resection.[34,35] The histopathological criteria have been defined as the observation of: atretic follicles and/or degenerating granulosa cells, hypertrophy and luteinization of the inner theca cell layer, and thickened ovarian tunica. Transabdominal and/or transvaginal ultrasound have since become the most commonly used diagnostic methods for the identification of polycystic ovaries. Although the ultrasound criteria for the diagnosis of polycystic ovaries have not been universally agreed, the characteristic features are accepted as being an

increase in the number of follicles and the amount of stroma as compared with normal ovaries.

Swanson and coworkers were the first to use high-resolution real-time ultrasound (static B-scanner 3.5 MHz, transabdominal) to describe polycystic ovaries.[37] Prior to this it was thought that the tiny cysts of the polycystic ovary could not be detected by ultrasound. The cysts were noted to be 2–6 mm in diameter, but the number of cysts was neither recorded nor defined. Stromal characteristics were not described. Ovarian volume was calculated using a simplified formula for a prolate ellipse (1/2 × length × width × thickness) and found on average to be 12.5 cm³ (range 6–30 cm³).[37] This formula was also used by Hann and coworkers who reported considerable variety in ultrasound characteristics in women with PCOS.[38] They took the upper limit of ovarian volume to be 5.7 cm³ based on data from Sample et al.[39] The cysts were taken to be <8 mm but a prerequisite number was not defined.

The early studies were hampered by the limitations of static B-scanners which were superseded by high-resolution real-time sector scanners in the early 1980s.[40,41] Ultrasound was used to describe the ovarian appearance in women classified as having PCOS (by symptoms and serum endocrinology), rather than to make the diagnosis. Orsini et al. described ovaries as either being predominantly solid if fewer than four small (<9 mm) cystic structures were detected in the ovary, or predominantly cystic if multiple small (neither quantified) cystic structures or at least one large (> 10 mm) cyst were present.[42] Patients with PCOS usually had cysts of between 4 and 10 mm but occasionally cysts of 15 mm were seen – presumably indicative of follicular recruitment.

Ovarian volume was calculated using the formula for a prolate ellipsoid (0.5233 × maximal longitudinal, anteroposterior and transverse diameters).[39] Women with PCOS were compared with normal controls and were found to have significantly greater ovarian volume (14.04 ± 7.36 cm³ vs 7.94 ± 2.34 cm³) and larger uterine volumes. There was no record of timing of the scan in relation to the menstrual cycle in either PCOS or control subjects. The ratio of ovarian:uterine volume was assessed, as previously it had been suggested that in women with PCOS this was never higher than 1.0.[43] Orsini and colleagues found a wide range of ovarian: uterine volumes and this diagnostic criterion was subsequently abandoned.[42]

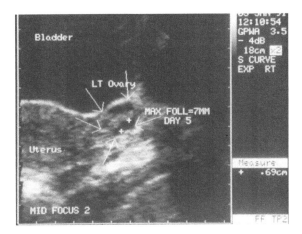

Figure 2.2

Transabdominal ultrasound scan of a normal ovary.

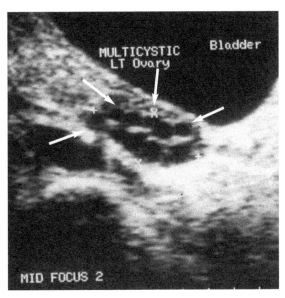

Figure 2.4

Transabdominal ultrasound scan of a multicystic ovary.

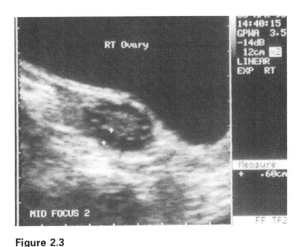

Figure 2.3

Transabdominal ultrasound scan of a polycystic ovary.

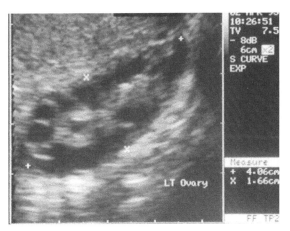

Figure 2.5

Transvaginal ultrasound scan of a polycystic ovary.

Ultrasound scans of normal and both polycystic and multicystic ovaries are shown in Figures 2.2 to 2.5.

The transabdominal ultrasound criteria of Adams et al defined a polycystic ovary as one which contains, in one plane, at least 10 follicles (usually between 2 and 8 mm in diameter) arranged peripherally around a dense core of ovarian stroma or scattered throughout an increased amount of stroma.[44] When scattered through the stroma, it was suggested that the cysts were usually 2–4 mm in diameter.[45] Volume was again calculated using the formula described by Sample and colleagues.[39] Polycystic ovaries were found to have a higher volume (14.6 ± 1.1 cm³) than both multicystic (8.0 ±

0.8 cm^3) and normal ovaries (6.4 ± 0.4 cm^3).[45] Uterine cross-sectional area was also greater in women with PCOS than those with multicystic or normal ovaries (26.0 ± 1.4 vs 13.1 ± 0.9 vs 22.4 ± 1.0 cm^3), which is a reflection of the degree of estrogenization.

The criteria of Adams and colleagues have been adopted by many subsequent studies which have used ultrasound scanning to detect polycystic ovaries.[3,8,46–51] In common with many authors, Abdel Gadir et al, found that the visualization of polycystic ovaries supported the diagnosis of the syndrome in women with signs and symptoms, rather than being key in making the diagnosis.[49] The subjective appearance of polycystic ovaries may be useful, for example, in women taking the combined oral contraceptive pill, in whom the volume will be suppressed but the appearance may still be polycystic.[52]

Multicystic and polycystic ovaries

The multicystic ovary is one in which there are multiple (≥6) cysts, usually 4–10 mm in diameter with normal stromal echogenicity (see Figure 2.4).[45] This is the characteristic appearance during puberty and in women recovering from hypothalamic amenorrhea – both situations being associated with follicular growth without consistent recruitment of a dominant follicle.[53,54] There may be confusion among inexperienced ultrasonographers, radiologists and gynecologists, hence the need for careful consideration of the clinical picture and endocrinology.

Polycystic ovaries are evident in adolescent girls as a distinct entity from multicystic ovaries.[55] Indeed it appears that PCOS manifests for the first time during the adolescent years, which is a critical time for future ovarian and metabolic function.[56,57]

Transvaginal ultrasound

Transabdominal ultrasound has been largely superseded by transvaginal scanning because of greater resolution and in many cases patient preference – as the need for a full bladder is avoided, which saves time and may be more comfortable.[58] Whilst this may be the case in the context of infertility clinics, where women are used to having repeated scans, it was found that 20% of women who were undergoing routine screening declined a transvaginal scan after having first had a transabdominal scan.[51] In this study there was no significant difference in the detection of polycystic ovaries and the same criteria for the number of cysts were felt to be appropriate for both types of scan. There was, however, only a 78% agreement between transabdominal and transvaginal ultrasound for polycystic ovaries, although this was 92% for normal ovaries.[51]

A recent study that set out to assess variability in the detection of polycystic and normal ovaries demonstrated intra-observer agreement of 69.4% and inter-observer agreement of 51%.[59] Polycystic ovaries were defined as the presence of ≥10 cysts (2–8 mm diameter), ovarian volume ≥12 cm^3 and bright echogenic stroma. Thus there was significant intra-observer and inter-observer variability using these criteria. This suggests either that the criteria are too subjective, or that their measurement is too insensitive. Amer and colleagues concluded that the use of three-dimensional ultrasound might provide a more reliable and reproducible diagnostic tool, although they did not perform a similar evaluation of observer variability.[59]

It has been argued by others that transvaginal ultrasound is a more sensitive method for the detection of polycystic ovaries, and that the transvaginal definition of a polycystic ovary should require the presence of at least 15 follicles (2–10 mm in diameter) in a single plane.[60] Fox and coworkers found that polycystic ovaries were not detected in 30% of women with PCOS when a 3.5 MHz transabdominal transducer was used, and found a 7.5 MHz transvaginal probe to be more reliable.[60]

Ardaens et al compared transabdominal (3.5 MHz) with transvaginal (6.5 MHz) ultrasound, and reported that the latter was more consistent in achieving the diagnosis of polycystic ovaries in women with PCOS.[61] Increased stromal echogenicity assessed transvaginally appeared to be exclusively associated with PCOS, although this was a subjective appearance rather than a quantifiable measurement.[61]

Pache and colleagues performed a series of studies to distinguish between normal and polycystic ovaries and to determine the key features of the polycystic ovary.[62–65] First PCOS was defined (on the basis of elevated testosterone or LH) and transvaginal ultrasound (5 MHz) was used to compare those with the syndrome to a control group.[64] Women with amenorrhea had similar ultrasound features to those with oligomenorrhea. Control ovaries never had a volume of more than 8.0 cm³ or more than 11 follicles. The mean number of follicles was 10 in polycystic ovaries and five in normal ovaries. Median values for mean ovarian volume were 5.9 cm³ in controls and 9.8 cm³ in PCOS (p <0.001); mean follicular size and number were 5.1 vs 3.8 and 5.0 vs 9.8 for controls and PCOS respectively. Stromal echogenicity was also significantly increased in the PCOS patients, based on a semi-quantitative assessment (see below).[64] The greatest power of discrimination between normal and polycystic ovaries was provided by a combined measurement of follicular size and ovarian volume (sensitivity 92%, specificity 97%).

Pache and coworkers went on to correlate ultrasound parameters with serum endocrinology and found that the degree of insulin resistance correlated with ovarian volume and stromal echogenicity.[65] Serum LH and testosterone concentrations also correlated with ovarian volume, stromal echogenicity, and follicle number. A later study from the same group defined normal ovarian morphology in a control group of 48 normally cycling women, and compared both ultrasound and endocrine parameters with those in patients with normogonadotrophic oligomenorrhea or amenorrhea.[66] In the normal ovaries, the mean number of follicles per ovary was 7.0 ± 1.7 and none had more than nine follicles or an ovarian volume of greater than 10.7 cm³. Polycystic ovaries were therefore considered to have ≥10 follicles and a volume of ≥10.8 cm³. Sonographic parameters did not correlate well with endocrinology. The best predictor for hyperandrogenism was increased mean ovarian volume (sensitivity 57%; specificity 67%); follicle number also correlated well with both serum testosterone and LH concentrations.[66] Considerable overlap was found between all other sonographic and endocrine parameters in the women with normal and polycystic ovaries.

Jonard et al studied 214 women with PCOS (oligo-/amenorrhea, elevated serum LH and/or testosterone, and/or ovarian area >5.5 cm²) and 112 women with normal ovaries to determine the importance of follicle number per ovary (FNPO).[67]

A 7 MHz transvaginal ultrasound scan was performed and three different categories of follicle size analyzed separately (2–5, 6–9 and 2–9 mm). Size range of the follicles has been considered important by some, with polycystic ovaries tending to have smaller follicles than normal or multicystic ovaries.[36,65] The mean FNPO was similar between normal and polycystic ovaries in the 6–9 mm range but significantly higher in the polycystic ovaries in both the 2–5 and 2–9 mm ranges.[67] Within the 2–5 mm range, there were significant positive correlations with serum testosterone, androstenedione and LH concentrations. There was an inverse correlation within the 6–9 mm range between FNPO and testosterone, BMI, and fasting insulin concentrations, and a positive correlation with inhibin B concentrations. The mean FNPO in the 2–5 mm range was significantly greater in the polycystic ovaries than the controls, while it was similar in the 6–9 mm range. A FNPO of ≥12 follicles of 2–9 mm diameter gave the best threshold for the diagnosis of PCOS (sensitivity 75%; specificity 99%).[67] The authors suggest that intra-ovarian hyperandrogenism promotes excessive early follicular growth up to 2–5 mm, with more follicles able to enter the growing cohort which then become arrested at the 6–9 mm size. A new definition of the polycystic ovary is proposed: increased ovarian area (>5.5 cm²) or volume (>11 cm³) and/or the presence of ≥12 follicles of 2–9 mm diameter (as a mean of both ovaries) (Table 2.1).[67]

Table 2.1 Receiver operating characteristic (ROC) curve data for the assessment of polycystic ovaries[67]

FNPO	Area under the curve	Threshold	Sensitivity (%)	Specificity (%)
2–5 mm	0.924	10	65	97
		12	57	99
		15	42	100
6–9 mm	0.502	3	42	69
		4	32.5	80
		5	24	89
2–9 mm	0.937	10	86	90
		12	75	99
		15	58	100

FNPO = follicle number per ovary

Polycystic ovaries can also be detected in post-menopausal women and while, not surprisingly, they are smaller than in pre-menopausal women with polycystic ovaries, they are still larger (6.4 cm³ vs 3.7 cm³) with more follicles (9.0 vs 1.7) than normal post-menopausal ovaries.[68]

Stromal echogenicity

The increased echodensity of the polycystic ovary is a key histological feature (Hughesdon 1982) but is a subjective assessment that may vary depending upon the setting of the ultrasound machine and the patient's body habitus. In a study by Ardaens and coworkers,[61] subjectively increased stromal hyperechogenicity assessed transvaginally appeared to be exclusively associated with PCOS.

Normal stromal echogenicity is said to be less than that of the myometrium, which is a simple guide that will take into account the setting of the ultrasound machine. Stromal echogenicity has been described in a semi-quantitative manner with a score for normal (=1), moderately increased (=2) or frankly increased (=3).[62,63] In this study, the total follicle number of both ovaries combined correlated significantly with stromal echogenicity. Follicle number also correlated significantly with free androgen index (FAI). A further study comparing women with PCOS with controls found that the sensitivity and specificity of ovarian stromal echogenicity in the diagnosis of polycystic ovaries were 94% and 90% respectively.[64]

Dewailly and coworkers designed a computer-assisted method for standardizing the assessment of stromal hypertrophy.[69] Patients with hyperandrogenism, of whom 68% had menstrual cycle disturbances, were compared with a control group and a group with hypothalamic amenorrhea. Transvaginal ultrasound (5 MHz) was used and polycystic ovaries defined as the presence of 'abnormal ovarian stroma and/or the presence of at least 10 round areas of reduced echogenicity <8 mm in size on a single ovarian section and/or an increased cross-sectional ovarian area (>10 cm²).[61,69] The computerized technique for reading the scans involved a longitudinal section in the middle part of the ovary and a calculation of stromal area and the area of the cysts. Of 57 women with hyperandrogenism, 65% had polycystic ovaries visualized on ultrasound and elevated serum testosterone and LH concentrations were found in 50% and 45% respectively. There was no correlation between LH and androstenedione (A) concentrations. Stromal area, however, correlated significantly with A and 17-hydroxyprogesterone, but not testosterone, LH or insulin concentrations; cyst area did not correlate with endocrine parameters.[69] Thus it was suggested that the analysis of ovarian stromal area is better than quantification of the cysts in polycystic ovaries.

Three-dimensional ultrasound has been shown to be a good tool for the accurate measurement of ovarian volume and more precise than two-dimensional ultrasound.[70] Three groups of patients were defined:

1. those with normal ovaries
2. those with asymptomatic polycystic ovaries
3. those with polycystic ovary syndrome.[71]

The ovarian and stromal volumes were similar in groups 2 and 3 and both greater than group 1. Stromal volume was positively correlated with serum androstenedione concentrations in group 3 only.[71] The mean total volume of the cysts was similar in all groups, indicating that increased stromal volume is the main cause of ovarian enlargement in polycystic ovaries. Dewailly and coworkers had also previously found a correlation between stromal area and androstenedione concentrations.[69] Neither Dewailly et al nor Kyei-Mensah et al found a correlation of stromal area or volume with serum testosterone concentrations,[69,71] unlike the study of Balen and coworkers which also showed a positive correlation between ovarian volume and serum LH concentrations.[3]

Echogenicity has been quantified by Al-Took et al[72] as the sum of the product of each intensity level (ranging from 0–63 on the scanner) and the number of pixels for that intensity level divided by the total number of pixels in the measured area: Mean = $(\sum x_i.f_i)/n$, where n = total number of pixels in the measured area, x = intensity level (from 0–63) and f = number of pixels corresponding with the level. The stromal index was calculated by dividing the mean stromal echogenicity by the mean echogenicity of the entire ovary, in order to correct for cases in which the gain was adjusted to optimize image definition.[72] Using these measurements, the stromal index did not predict responsiveness to clomifene citrate and neither did the stromal index differ after ovarian drilling.[72]

Another approach used a 7.5 MHz transvaginal probe with histogram measurement of echogenicity.[73] The mean echogenicity was defined as the sum of the product of each intensity level (from 0–63) using the same formula as Al-Took et al.[72] (see above). Women with PCOS had greater total ovarian volume, stromal volume and peak stromal blood flow compared with women with normal ovaries, yet mean stromal echogenicity was similar. The stromal index (mean stromal echogenicity:mean echogenicity of the entire ovary) was higher in PCOS, due to the finding of a reduced mean echogenicity of the entire ovary.[73] The inference was that the subjective impression of increased stromal echogenicity was due to increased stromal volume alongside reduced echogenicity of the multiple cysts. Moreover, the increased stromal blood flow was suggested to be a more relevant predictor of ovarian function.[73]

A large study of 80 oligo-/amenorrhoeic women with PCOS was compared with a control group of 30 using a 6.5 MHz transvaginal probe.[74] Based on mean ± 2 standard deviation (SD) data from the control group the cut-off values were calculated for ovarian volume (13.21 cm^3), ovarian total area (7.00 cm^2), ovarian stromal area (1.95 cm^2), and stromal/area ratio (0.34). The sensitivity of these parameters for the diagnosis of PCOS was 21%, 4%, 62% and 100% respectively, suggesting that a stromal/area ratio >0.34 is diagnostic of PCOS.[74]

Three-dimensional ultrasound, Doppler and magnetic resonance imaging

The recent innovation of three-dimensional ultrasound, and the use of color and pulsed Doppler ultrasound, are techniques that may further enhance the detection of polycystic ovaries, and which may be more commonly employed in time.[75,76] A number of studies of color Doppler measurement of uterine and ovarian vessel blood flow have demonstrated a low resistance index in the stroma of polycystic ovaries (i.e. increased flow), and correlations with endocrine changes.[77–79] Battaglia and coworkers reported a good correlation between serum androstenedione concentrations and the LH:FSH ratio,[80] with the number of small follicles and the LH:FSH ratio also correlating well with the stromal artery pulsatility index.

Three-dimensional ultrasound requires longer time for storage and data analysis, increased training and more expensive equipment. Yet good correlations have been found between stromal volume and serum androstenedione concentrations.[71] Stromal hypertrophy itself appears to be secondary

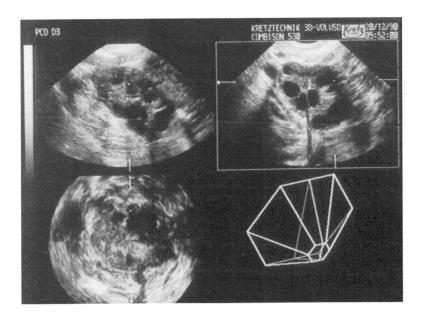

Figure 2.6

Three-dimensional transvaginal ultrasound scan of a polycystic ovary.

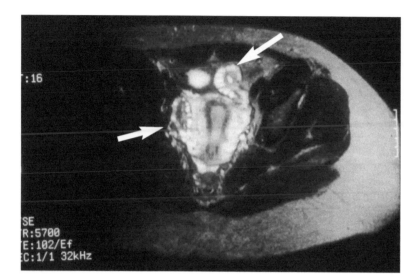

Figure 2.7

MRI scan of the pelvis demonstrating polycystic ovaries (arrows)

to increased blood flow.[76] A more recent study using three-dimensional ultrasound did not, however, find a correlation between ovarian stromal volume and endocrine parameters.[81] Total ovarian volume, follicular volume and follicle number did, however, correlate with serum FSH and LH but not testosterone concentrations (Figure 2.6).

The use of magnetic resonance imaging (MRI) for the visualization of the structure of pelvic organs has been claimed to have even greater sensitivity than ultrasound for the detection of polycystic ovaries (Figure 2.7).[82,83] However, the substantial cost and practical problems involved with this imaging technique limit its use as an easily accessible diagnostic tool for use in general clinical practice. The early reports of MRI were also made at a time when high-resolution transvaginal ultrasound was emerging as a valuable tool and time has confirmed the place of the latter and limited further interest in MRI.

It appears, therefore, that ovarian size (i.e. volume) combined with the number of pre-antral follicles are in combination the key and consistent features of polycystic ovaries.

Exclusion of related disorders

In order to establish the diagnosis of PCOS it is important to exclude other disorders with a similar clinical presentation, such as congenital adrenal hyperplasia, Cushing's syndrome and androgen-secreting tumors of the adrenal gland or ovary (Figures 2.8 and 2.9).[1] The measurement of total testosterone is usually sufficient in most populations. In some populations, however, 21–hydroxylase-deficient non-classic adrenal hyperplasia (NCAH) is more prevalent than in others and this can be excluded by measuring a basal morning 17-hydroxyprogesterone level, with cut-off values up to 20 nmol/L (3 ng/ml).[84]

The routine exclusion of thyroid dysfunction in patients deemed to be hyperandrogenic is of limited value, as the incidence of this disorder among women with hyperandrogenism is no higher than that in normal women of reproductive age (approximately 5% of the female population). The measurement of thyroid-stimulating hormone may, therefore, be a useful screening test , but certainly not obligatory in the diagnosis of PCOS.

If the patient presents with oligo-anovulation it is necessary to measure serum FSH, LH and estradiol (E_2) levels in order to exclude hypogonadotropic hypogonadism (low FSH, LH and E_2) or premature ovarian failure (high FSH, LH and low E_2). PCOS is part of the spectrum of normogonadotropic normo-estrogenic anovulation (WHO Group 2).[22,66] A measurement of prolactin should also be performed to exclude hyperprolactinemia, although women with PCOS as a sole diagnosis may sometimes have moderately elevated serum prolactin concentrations.[56]

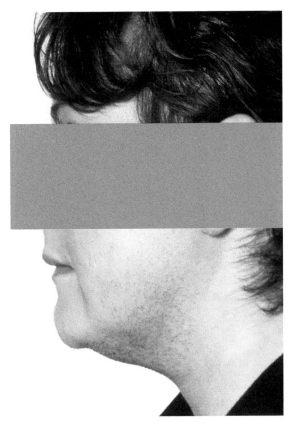

Figure 2.8

Case of a 32-year-old with recent onset hirsutism and a serum testosterone concentration of 25 nmol/l. Imaging revealed an adrenal tumor for which an adrenalectomy was required.

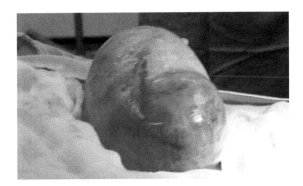

Figure 2.9

Case of a 62-year-old with hirsutism, deepening of the voice and clitoromegaly. Imaging revealed a 10 cm diameter ovarian cyst for which an oophorectomy was performed.

There may be clinical suspicions either of syndromes of severe insulin resistance (e.g. for the diagnosis of the hyperandrogenic insulin-resistant acanthosis nigricans or HAIRAN syndrome),[84] Cushings syndrome,[85] androgen-secreting neoplasms,[85,86] or the use of high-dose exogenous androgens,[63] and all of these should be excluded if clinically suspected.[1]

Glucose tolerance

Women who are obese, and also many slim women with PCOS, will have insulin resistance and elevated serum concentrations of insulin (usually <30 mU/l fasting). We suggest that a 75 g oral glucose tolerance test (GTT) be performed in women with PCOS and a BMI >30 kg/m², with an

Key points

- The consensus definition of the PCOS is the presence of two out of the following three criteria:
  1. oligo- and/or anovulation,
  2. hyperandrogenism (clinical and/or biochemical)
  3. polycystic ovaries
  with the exclusion of other etiologies.
- The morphology of the polycystic ovary, has been redefined as an ovary with 12 or more follicles measuring 2–9 mm in diameter and/or increased ovarian volume (>10 cm³).
- There is considerable heterogeneity of symptoms and signs and these may change over time.
- Elevated serum concentrations of insulin are more common in both lean and obese women with PCOS than weight-matched controls and hyperinsulinemia is key to the pathogenesis of PCOS.
- Polycystic ovaries are commonly detected by ultrasound with a prevalence in the general population of 20–33%, of whom approximately three-quarters will exhibit clinical features of the syndrome.
- Clinical hyperandrogenism is difficult to quantify and there are racial variations.
- Biochemical hyperandrogenism is assessed by a variety of assays, the methodology for which is fraught with problems.
- In order to establish the diagnosis of PCOS it is important to exclude other disorders with a similar clinical presentation, such as congenital adrenal hyperplasia, Cushing's syndrome and androgen-secreting tumors.

Table 2.2 The spectrum of clinical manifestations of polycystic ovary syndrome

Symptoms
- Hyperandrogenism (acne, hirsutism, alopecia – <u>not</u> virilization)
- Menstrual disturbance
- Infertility
- Obesity
- Sometimes asymptomatic, with polycystic ovaries on ultrasound scan

Serum endocrinology
- ↑ Fasting insulin (not routinely measured; insulin resistance or impaired glucose tolerance assessed by glucose tolerance test)
- ↑ Androgens (testosterone and androstenedione)
- ↑ LH, usually normal FSH
- ↓ SHBG, results in elevated 'free androgen index'
- ↑ estradiol, estrone (neither measured routinely as there is a very wide range of values)
- ↑ Prolactin

Possible late sequelae
- Diabetes mellitus
- Dyslipidemia
- Hypertension, cardiovascular disease
- Endometrial carcinoma
- Breast cancer (?)

Table 2.3 Investigations for polycystic ovary syndrome

Test	Normal range (may vary with local laboratory assays)	Additional points
Pelvic ultrasound	To assess ovarian morphology and endometrial thickness	Transabdominal scan usually satisfactory in women who are not sexually active (depends upon body habitus)
Testosterone (T)	0.5–3.5 nmol/l	A total testosterone is adequate for general screening. It is unnecessary to measure other androgens unless total testosterone is >5 nmol/l, in which case referral is indicated
SHBG Free androgen index (FAI): T × 100/SHBG	16–119 nmol/l <5	Insulin suppresses SHBG, resulting in a high FAI in the presence of a normal total T. The measurement of SHBG is not required in routine practice and will not affect management
Estradiol	Measurement is unhelpful for diagnosis	Estrogenization may be confirmed by endometrial assessment
LH FSH	2–10 IU/l 2–8 IU/l	FSH and LH are best measured during days 1–3 of a menstrual bleed. If oligo-/amenorrheic then random samples are taken
Prolactin TSH	<500 mU/l 0.5 – 5 IU/l	Measure if oligo-/amenorrheic
Fasting insulin	<30 mU/l	Not routinely measured; insulin resistance assessed by glucose tolerance test (Table 2.4)

Table 2.4 Definitions of glucose tolerance after a 75 g glucose tolerance test

	Diabetes mellitus	Impaired glucose tolerance	Impaired fasting glycemia
Fasting glucose (mmol/l)	≥7.0	<7.0	≥6.1 and <7.0
2-h glucose (mmol/l)	≥11.1	≥7.8 and <11.1	<7.8
Action	Refer to diabetic clinic	Dietary advice. Check fasting glucose annually	Dietary advice. Check fasting glucose annually

assessment of the fasting and two-hour glucose concentration. It has been suggested that South Asian women should have an assessment of glucose tolerance if their BMI is greater than 25 kg/m^2 because of the greater risk of insulin resistance at a lower BMI than seen in the Caucasian population (Table 2.4, see also Chapter 8).

Conclusion

PCOS is a true syndrome with varied manifestations in different populations and between different populations. With recent increases in understanding of the pathophysiology of PCOS and the recognition of the importance of ultrasound in defining the morphology of the polycystic ovary, the syndrome has now been defined as the presence of two out of the following three criteria: 1. oligo- and/or anovulation; 2. hyperandrogenism (clinical and/or biochemical); 3. polycystic ovaries, with the exclusion of other etiologies.[1] The following chapters will discuss the pathophysiology, manifestations and treatment of these features in greater detail.

References

1. The Rotterdam ESHRE/ASRM-sponsored PCOS consensus workshop group: Fauser B, Tarlatzis B, Chang J, Azziz R et al. Revised 2003 consensus on diagnostic criteria and long-term health risks related to polycystic ovary syndrome (PCOS). Hum Reprod 2004; 19:41–47.
2. Balen AH, Laven JSE, Tan SL, Dewailly D. Ultrasound assessment of the polycystic ovary: international consensus definitions. Hum Reprod Update 2003; 9:505–514.
3. Balen AH, Conway GS, Kaltsas G, Techatrasak K et al. Polycystic ovary syndrome: the spectrum of the disorder in 1741 patients. Hum Reprod 1995; 10:2107–2111.
4. Clarke AM, Ledger W, Galletly C, Tomlinson L, Blaney F, Wang X, Norman RJ. Weight loss results in significant improvement in pregnancy and ovulation rates in anovulatory obese women. Hum Reprod 1995; 10:2705–2712.
5. Franks S, Gharani N, McCarthy M. Candidate genes in polycystic ovary syndrome. Hum Reprod Update 2001; 7:405–410.
6. Rajkowha M, Glass MR, Rutherford AJ, Michelmore K, Balen AH. Polycystic ovary syndrome: a risk factor for cardiovascular disease? Br J Obstet Gynaecol 2000; 107:11–18.
7. Balen AH, The pathogenesis of polycystic ovary syndrome: the enigma unravels. Lancet 1999; 354:966–967.
8. Polson DW, Adams J, Wadsworth J, Franks S. Polycystic ovaries – a common finding in normal women. Lancet 1988; 1:870–872.
9. Michelmore KF, Balen AH, Dunger DB, Vessey MP. Polycystic ovaries and associated clinical and biochemical features in young women. Clin Endocrinol (Oxf) 1999; 51:779–786.
10. Zawadzki JA, Dunaif A. Diagnostic criteria for polycystic ovary syndrome: towards a rational approach. In: Dunaif A, Givens JR, Haseltine FP, Merriam GR, eds. Polycystic ovary syndrome. Boston: Blackwell Scientific, 1992:377–384.
11. Balen AH, Michelmore K. What is polycystic ovary syndrome? Are national views important? Human Reprod 2002; 17: 2219–2227.
12. Homburg R. What is polycystic ovary syndrome? A proposal for a consensus on the definition and diagnosis of PCOS. Human Reprod 2002; 17: 2495–2499.
13. Diamanti-Kandarakis E, Koulie CR, Bergiele AT, Filandra FA et al. A survey of the polycystic ovary syndrome in the Greek Island of Lesbos: a hormonal and metabolic profile. J Clin Endocrinol Metab 1999; 84:4006–4011.
14. Carmina E, Koyama T, Chang L, Stanczyk FZ, Lobo

RA. Does ethnicity influence the prevalence of adrenal hyperandrogenism in insulin resistance in the polycystic ovary syndrome? Am J Obstet Gynecol 1992; 167:1807–1812.

15. Ruutiainen K, Erkkola R, Gronroos MA, Irjala K. Influence of body mass index and age on the grade of hair growth in hirsute women of reproductive ages. Fertil Steril 1998; 50:260–265.

16. Wijeyaratne CN, Balen AH, Barth J, Belchetz PE. Clinical manifestations and insulin resistance (IR) in polycystic ovary syndrome (PCOS) among south asians and caucasians: is there a difference? Clin Endocrin 2002; 57:343–350.

17. Slayden SM, Moran C, Sams WM, Jr, Boots LR, Azziz R. Hyperandrogenemia in patients presenting with acne. Fertil Steril 2001; 75:889–892.

18. Legro RS, Driscoll D, Strauss JF 3rd, Fox J, Dunaif A. Evidence for a genetic basis for hyperandrogenemia in polycystic ovary syndrome. Proc Natl Acad Sci USA 1998; 95:14956–14960.

19. Knochenhauer ES, Key TJ, Kahsar-Miller M, Waggoner W, Boots LR, Azziz R. Prevalence of the polycystic ovary syndrome in unselected black and white women in the Southeastern United States: A prospective study. J Clin Endocrinol Metab 1988; 83:3078–3082.

20. Pugeat M, Nicolas MH, Craves JC, Alvarado-Dubost C, Fimbel S, Cechaud H, Lejeune H. Androgens in polycystic ovarian syndrome. Ann NY Acad Sci 1993; 687:124–135.

21. Asuncion M, Calvo RM, San Millan JL, Sancho J, Avila S, Escobar-Morreale HF. A prospective study of the prevalence of the polycystic ovary syndrome in unselected Caucasian women from Spain. J Clin Endocrinol Metab 2000; 85:2434–2438.

22. Laven JS, Imani B, Eijkemans MJ, Fauser BC. New approaches to PCOS and other forms of anovulation. Obstet Gynecol Surv 2002; 57:755–767.

23. Boots LR, Potter S, Potter HD, Azziz R. Measurement of total serum testosterone levels using commercially available kits: High degree of between-kit variability. Fertil Steril 1998; 69:286–292.

24. Rosner W. Errors in the measurement of plasma free testosterone. J Clin Endocrinol Metab 1997; 82:2014–2015.

25. Vermeulen A, Verdonck L, Kaufman JM. A critical evaluation of simple methods for the estimation of free testosterone in serum. J Clin Endocrinol Metab 1999; 84:3666–3672.

26. Bili H, Laven J, Imani B, Eijkemans MJ, Fauser BC. Age related differences in features associated with PCOS in normogonadotrophic oligo-amenorrheic infertile women of reproductive years. Eur J Endocrinol 2001; 145:749–755.

27. Moran C, Knochenhauer E, Boots LR, Azziz R. Adrenal androgen excess in hyperandrogenism:

Relation to age and body mass. Fertil Steril 1999; 71:671–674.

28. Cibula D, Hill M, Starka L. The best correlation of the new index of hyperandrogenism with the grade of increased hair. Eur J Endocrinol 2000; 143:405–408.

29. Imani B, Eijkemans MJ, de Jong FH, Payne NN et al. Free androgen index and leptin are the most prominent endocrine predictors of ovarian response during clomiphene citrate induction of ovulation in normogonadotropic oligoamenorrheic infertility. J Clin Endocrinol Metab 2000; 85:676–682.

30. Tremblay RR, Dube JY. Plasma concentration of free and non-TeBG bound testosterone in women on oral contraceptives. Contraception 1974; 10:599–605.

31. Stein IF, Leventhal ML. Amenorrhea associated with bilateral polycystic ovaries. Am J Obstet Gynecol 1935; 29:181–191.

32. Franks S. Polycystic ovary syndrome. N Engl J Med 1995; 333:853–861.

33. Goldzieher MW, Green JA. The polycystic ovary. I. Clinical and histologic features. J Clin Endocrinol Metab 1962; 22:325–338.

34. Saxton DW, Farquhar CM, Rae T, Beard RW, Anderson MC, Wadsworth J. Accuracy of ultrasound measurements of female pelvic organs. Br J Obstet Gynaecol 1990; 97:695–699.

35. Takahashi K, Eda Y, Abu Musa A, Okada S et al. Transvaginal ultrasound imaging, histopathology and endocrinopathy in patients with polycystic ovarian syndrome. Hum Reprod 1994; 9:1231–1236.

36. Hughesdon PE. Morphology and morphogenesis of the Stein–Leventhal ovary and of so-called 'hyperthecosis'. Obstet Gynecol Survey 1982; 37:59–77.

37. Swanson M, Sauerbrei EE, Cooperberg PL. Medical implications of ultrasonically detected polycystic ovaries. J Clin Ultrasound 1981; 9:219–222.

38. Hann LE, Hall DA, McArdle CR, Seibel M. Polycystic ovarian disease: sonographic spectrum. Radiology 1984; 150:531–534.

39. Sample WF, Lippe BM, Gyepes MT. Grey-scale ultrasonography of the normal female pelvis. Radiology 1977; 125:477–483.

40. Campbell S, Goessens L, Goswamy R, Whitehead M. Real-time ultrasonography for determination of ovarian morphology and volume. Lancet 1982; 1:425–428.

41. Orsini LF, Rizzo N, Calderoni P, Pilu G, Bovicelli L. Ultrasound monitoring of ovarian follicular development: a comparison of real-time and static scanning techniques. J Clin Ultrasound 1983; 11:207–211.

42. Orsini LF, Venturoli S, Lorusso R, Pluchinotta V et al. Ultrasonic findings in polycystic ovarian disease. Fertil Steril 1985; 43:709–714.

43. Parisi L, Tramonti M, Casciano S, Zurli A, Gazzarini O. The role of ultrasound in the study of polycystic ovarian disease. J Clin Ultrasound 1982; 10:167–172.

44. Adams J, Polson DW, Franks S. Prevalence of polycystic ovaries in women with anovulation and idiopathic hirsutism. Br Med J 1986; 293:355–359.

45. Adams J, Polson DW, Abdulwahid N, Morris DV et al. Multifollicular ovaries: clinical and endocrine features and response to pulsatile gonadotropin releasing hormone. Lancet 1985; 2:1375–1379.

46. Conway GS, Honour JW, Jacobs HS. Heterogeneity of the polycystic ovary syndrome: clinical, endocrine and ultrasound features in 556 patients. Clin Endocrinol (Oxf) 1989; 30:459–470.

47. Kiddy DS, Sharp PS, White DM, Scanlon MF et al. Differences in clinical and endocrine features between obese and non-obese subjects with polycystic ovary syndrome: an analysis of 263 consecutive cases. Clin Endocrinol (Oxf) 1990; 32:213–220.

48. Fox R, Corrigan E, Thomas PA, Hull MG. The diagnosis of polycystic ovaries in women with oligo-amenorrhoea: predictive power of endocrine tests. Clin Endocrinol (Oxf) 1991; 34:127–131.

49. Abdel Gadir A, Khatim MS, Mowafi RS, Alnaser HM et al. Implications of ultrasonically diagnosed polycystic ovaries. I, Correlations with basal hormonal profiles. Hum Reprod 1992; 7:453–457.

50. Clayton RN, Ogden V, Hodgkinson J, Worswick et al. How common are polycystic ovaries in normal women and what is their significance for the fertility of the population? [see comments]. Clin Endocrinol (Oxf) 1992; 37:127–134.

51. Farquhar CM, Birdsall M, Manning P, Mitchell JM, France JT. The prevalence of polycystic ovaries on ultrasound scanning in a population of randomly selected women. Aust NZ J Obstet Gynaecol 1994; 34:67–72.

52. Franks S, Adams J, Mason HD, Polson DW. Ovulatory disorders in women with polycystic ovary syndrome. Clin Obstet Gynecol 1985; 12:605–632.

53. Venturoli S, Porcu E, Fabbri R, Paradisi R et al. Ovaries and menstrual cycles in adolescence. Gynecol Obstet Invest 1983; 17:219–223.

54. Stanhope R, Adams J, Jacobs HS, Brook CG. Ovarian ultrasound assessment in normal children, idiopathic precocious puberty, and during low dose pulsatile gonadotrophin releasing hormone treatment of hypogonadotrophic hypogonadism. Arch Dis Child 1985; 60:116–119.

55. Herter LD, Magalhaes JA, Spritzer PM. Relevance of the determination of ovarian volume in adolescent girls with menstrual disorders. J Clin Ultrasound 1996; 24:243–248.

56. Balen AH, Dunger D. Pubertal maturation of the internal genitalia. Ultrasound Obstet Gynaecol 1995; 6:164–165.

57. Gulekli B, Turhan NO, Senoz S, Kukner S, Oral H, Gokmen O. Endocrinological, ultrasonographic and clinical findings in adolescent and adult polycystic ovary patients: a comparative study. Gynecol Endocrinol 1993; 7:273–277.

58. Goldstein G. Incorporating endovaginal ultrasonographyt into the overall gynaecologic examination. Am J Obstet Gynecol 1990; 160:625–632.

59. Amer SAKS, Li TC, Bygrave C, Sprigg A, Saravelos H, Cooke ID. An evaluation of the inter-observer and intra-observer variability of the ultrasound diagnosis of polycystic ovaries. Hum Reprod 2002; 17:1616–1622.

60. Fox R, Corrigan E, Thomas PA, Hull MG. The diagnosis of polycystic ovaries in women with oligo-amenorrhoea: predictive power of endocrine tests. Clin Endocrinol (Oxf) 1991; 34:127–131.

61. Ardaens Y, Robert Y, Lemaitre L, Fossati P, Dewailly D. Polycystic ovarian disease: contribution of vaginal endosonography and reassessment of ultrasonic diagnosis. Fertil Steril 1991; 55:1062–1068.

62. Pache TD, Hop WC, Wladimiroff JW, Schipper J, Fauser BCJM. Transvaginal sonography and abnormal ovarian appearance in menstrual cycle disturbances. Ultrasound Med Biol 1991; 17:589–593.

63. Pache TD, Chadha S, Gooren LJ, Hop WC et al. Ovarian morphology in long-term androgen-treated female-to-male transsexuals. A human model for the study of PCOS? Histopathol 1991; 19:445–452.

64. Pache TD, Wladimiroff JW, Hop WC, Fauser BCJM. How to discriminate between normal and polycystic ovaries: Transvaginal ultrasound study. Radiology 1992; 183:421–423.

65. Pache TD, de Jong FH, Hop WC, Fauser BCJM. Association between ovarian changes assessed by transvaginal sonogrophy and clinical and endocrine signs of the polycystic ovary syndrome. Fertil Steril 1993; 59:544–549.

66. van Santbrink EJP, Hop WC, Fauser BCJM. Classification of normogonadotropic infertility: polycystic ovaries diagnosed by ultrasound versus endocrine characteristics of polycystic ovary syndrome. Fertil Steril 1997; 67:452–458.

67. Jonard S, Robert Y, Cortet-Rudelli C, Decanter C, Dewailly D. Ultrasound examination of polycystic ovaries: is it worth counting the follicles? Hum Reprod 2003; 18:598–603.

68. Birdsall MA, Farquhar CM. Polycystic ovaries in pre and post-menopausal women. Clin Endocrinol (Oxf) 1996; 44:269–276.

69. Dewailly D, Robert Y, Helin I, Ardaens Y et al. Ovarian stromal hypertrophy in hgyperandrogenic women. Clin Endocrinol (Oxf) 1994; 41:557–562.

70. Kyei-Mensah A, Maconochie N, Zaidi J, Pittrof R et al. Transvaginal three-dimensional ultrasound:

reproducibility of ovarian and endometrial volume measurements. Fertil Steril 1996; 66:718–722.

71. Kyei-Mensah A, Tan SL, Zaidi J, Jacobs HS. Relationship of ovarian stromal volume to serum androgen concentrations in patients with polycystic ovary syndrome. Hum Reprod 1998; 13:1437–1441.

72. Al-Took S, Watkin K, Tulandi T, Tan SL. Ovarian stromal echogenicity in women with clomiphene citrate-sensitive and clomiphene citrate-resistant polycystic ovary syndrome. Fertil Steril 1999; 71:952–954.

73. Buckett WM, Bouzayen R, Watkin KL, Tulandi T, Tan SL. Ovarian stromal echogenicity in women with normal and polycystic ovaries. Hum Reprod 1999; 14:618–621.

74. Fulghesu AM, Ciampelli M, Belosi C, Apa R et al. A new ultrasound criterion for the diagnosis of polycystic ovary syndrome: the ovarian stroma:total area ratio. Fertil Steril 2001; 76:326–331.

75. Kyei-Mensah A, Tan SL, Zaidi J, Jacobs HS. Relationship of ovarian stromal volume to serum androgen concentrations in patients with polycystic ovary syndrome. Human Reprod 1998; 13:1437–1441.

76. Zaidi J, Campbell S, Pittrof R, Kyei-Mensah A, Jacobs HS, Tan SL. Ovarian stromal blood flow in women with polycystic ovaries-a possible new marker for diagnosis? Hum Reprod 1995; 10: 1992–1996.

77. Battaglia C, Artini PG, D'Ambrogio G, Genazzani AD, Genazzani AR. The role of colour Doppler imaging in the diagnosis of polycystic ovary syndrome. Am J Obstet Gynecol 1995; 172:108–113.

78. Loverro G, Vicino M, Lorusso F, Vimercati A, Greco P, Selvaggi L. Polycystic ovary syndrome: relation-ship between insulin sensitivity, sex hormone levels and ovarian stromal blood flow. Gynecol Endocrinol 2001; 15:142–149.

79. Pan H-A, Wu M-H, Cheng Y-C, Li C-H, Chang F-M. Quantification of Doppler signal in polycystic ovary syndrome using 3-D power Doppler ultrasonogra-phy: a possible new marker for diagnosis. Hum Reprod 2002; 17:201–206.

80. Battaglia C, Genazzani AD, Salvatori M, Giulini S et al. Doppler, ultrasonographic and endocrinological environment with regard to the number of small subcapsular foillicles in polycystic ovary syndrome. Gynecol Endocrinol 1999; 13:123–129.

81. Nardo LG, Buckett WM, White D, Digesu AG et al. Three-dimensional assessment of ultrasound features in women with clomiphene citrate-resis-tant polycystic ovary syndrome: ovarian stromal volume does not correlate with biochemical indices. Hum Reprod 2002; 17:1052–1055.

82. Faure N, Prat X, Bastide A, Lemay A. Assessment of ovaries by magnetic resonance imaging in patients presenting with polycystic ovarian syndrome. Hum Reprod 1989; 4:468–472.

83. Mitchell DG, Gefter WB, Spritzer CE, Blasco L et al. Polycystic ovaries: MRI imaging. Radiology 1986; 160:425–429.

84. Moller DE, Cohen O, Yamaguchi Y et al. Prevalence of mutations in the insulin receptor gene in subjects with features of the type A syndrome of insulin resistance. Diabetes 1994; 43:247–255.

85. Kreisberg RA. Clinical problem-solving. Half a loaf. N Engl J Med 1994; 330:1295–1299.

86. Waggoner W, Boots LR, Azziz R. Total testosterone and DHEAS levels predictors of androgen-secreting neoplasms: a populational study. Gynecol Endocrinol 1999; 13:394–400.

Chapter 3

Epidemiology of polycystic ovary syndrome

Introduction

When considering the epidemiology of polycystic ovary syndrome (PCOS) it is necessary to look at the components that define the syndrome, namely at least two of the following: menstrual disturbance (oligo-anovulation), hyperandrogenism, and polycystic ovaries and then explore their prevalence in different populations, whether defined by age, ethnicity or other factors, such as body weight (viz hyperinsulinism). It is well recognized that PCOS is a heterogeneous condition, and several large series exist that describe populations of patients with the condition.

The heterogeneity of PCOS

A few years ago we reported what we believe to be the largest published series of women with polycystic ovaries detected by ultrasound scan.[1] All of the 1871 patients had at least one symptom of PCOS combined with the presence of polycystic ovaries. Thirty eight per cent of the women were overweight (body mass index (BMI) >25 kg/m^2). Obesity was significantly associated with an increased risk of hirsutism, menstrual cycle disturbance and an elevated serum testosterone concentration. Obesity was also associated with an increased rate of infertility and menstrual cycle disturbance. Twenty six per cent of patients with primary infertility and 14% of patients with secondary infertility had a BMI of more than 30 kg/m^2. Approximately 30% of the patients had a regular menstrual cycle, 50% had oligomenorrhea and 20% amenorrhea. In this study, the classical endocrine features of raised serum luteinizing hormone (LH) and testosterone concentrations were found in only 39.8% and 28.9% of patients respectively.[1]

Many other groups have similarly reported heterogeneity in their populations with PCOS. Franks' series,[2] also from England, related to 300 women recruited from a specialist endocrine clinic. Some years earlier, Goldzieher and coworkers compiled a comprehensive review of 1079 cases of surgically proven polycystic ovaries.[3] The features of these series are represented in Tables 3.1 and 3.2.

Although the frequencies of clinical symptoms and signs in these women were similar, it is difficult to know if the criteria for hirsutism, acne and alopecia were comparable between the studies. The differences noted in the prevalence of menstrual cycle disturbance and infertility probably reflect selection bias created by the specialist nature of the clinics from which the women for these studies were recruited. Of particular note is that the women included in the Goldzieher review demonstrated symptomatology which at that time was considered significant enough to warrant surgical intervention,[3] and thus the recorded frequencies of amenorrhea and infertility would be expected to be higher. The prevalence of obesity was consistently high in all of these studies and obese women with polycystic ovaries were found to be more likely to be hirsute and to have menstrual cycle irregularities than lean women with polycystic ovaries.[1,2] The frequencies noted in these studies will be compared with studies where recruitment was based on more 'normal' populations of women (see below).

Table 3.1 Clinical symptoms and signs in women with polycystic ovary syndrome

	Percentage frequency of symptom or sign			
	Balen et al. (1995)[1] n = 1741 %	Franks (1989)[2] n = 300 %	Goldzieher et al. (1981)[3] n = 1079 %	No. of cases[a]
Menstrual cycle disturbance:				
• oligomenorrhea	47.0	52	29[b]	547
• amenorrhea	19.2	28	51	640
Hirsutism	66.2	64	69	819
Obesity	38.4	35	41	600
Acne	34.7	27	–	–
Alopecia	6.0	3	–	–
Acanthosis nigricans	2.5	<1	–	–
Infertility (primary/secondary)	20.0	42	74	596

– Denotes feature not recorded.

[a]In the Goldzieher study, clinical details were not available for the entire 1079 women, thus the number of cases that were used to determine the frequency of each symptom is stated.

[b]In this series, any abnormal pattern of uterine bleeding was included.

Table 3.2 Biochemical features of women with polycystic ovary syndrome

	Percentage frequency	
	Balen et al (1995)[1] n = 1741 %	Franks (1989)[2] n = 300 %
Elevated serum LH	39.8	51
Elevated serum testosterone	28.9	50
Elevated serum prolactin	11.8	7

The biochemical features of these women with PCOS are not easily compared, as the criteria for elevated serum concentrations of LH, testosterone and prolactin and their methods of measurement were not consistent between the studies. However, raised levels of LH and testosterone are clearly shown to be common, though not universal features of PCOS, while elevated prolactin concentrations are less commonly noted.

In the Franks study,[2] and in an earlier study by Conway et al which concerned an early subset from the same database used in Balen's study,[1,4] the results of the women with PCOS were compared with those obtained from 'reference' groups of 'normal' women who were described as having normal menstrual cycles and normal ovaries on ultrasound. Conway et al demonstrated a higher mean ovarian volume in the women with ultrasound diagnosed polycystic ovaries compared with the control group.[4] In addition, Franks, with a larger number of controls, demonstrated a significantly larger uterine area, and a nearly double mean ovarian volume in the PCOS group.[2]

Each study attempted to identify direct associations between biochemical and clinical features within the women with PCOS. Franks found BMI to be positively associated with hirsutism and menstrual cycle disturbances.[2] Balen and coworkers described highly significant correlations between BMI and hirsutism, menstrual cycle disturbances and infertility, and elevated levels of serum testosterone.[1] The BMI was also found to correlate with ovarian volume and uterine cross-sectional area. It is probable that the much larger population observed by Balen and colleagues allowed for the detection of some associations that may not have been noted due to the smaller sample size in Franks' earlier study.[1,2] Alternatively the discrepancies between the studies may reflect the population biases of each study.

High serum LH concentrations were found to be associated with infertility or menstrual cycle disturbances in both of the studies. In the study by Balen et al.,[1] high serum testosterone levels were associated with an increased risk of hirsutism, infertility, and cycle disturbances. Ovarian volume was significantly correlated with serum LH and with testosterone concentrations. Other authors have attempted to correlate predictors for the diagnostic criteria of women with PCOS. For example Fox and colleagues found that a combination of the free androgen index (FAI) with serum LH concentration was the most accurate for making the diagnosis of PCOS in women with oligomenorrhea.[5] However, this group also found that the progestogen challenge test, as an assay of estrogenization, was as good a predictor and did not require the measurement of sex hormone binding globulin (SHBG) – an expensive and less commonly used test. In another series of women with oligomenorrhea, independent correlations with ovarian morphology were identified with LH concentrations and androgen levels.[6] Furthermore, markers of insulin resistance correlated with ovarian volume and stromal echogenicity, which in turn have been correlated with androgen production.[6-8]

Population-based studies

Estimates of the prevalence of PCOS are greatly affected by the nature of the population which is being assessed. Populations of women who are selected on the basis of the presence of a symptom associated with the syndrome (e.g. hirsutism, acne, and menstrual cycle disturbances) would be expected to demonstrate a prevalence of PCOS greater than that which exists in the general population.

In a study of 173 women presenting with anovulation or hirsutism, Adams et al found the prevalence of polycystic ovaries (using ultrasound criteria for diagnosis) to be 26% in women with amenorrhea, 87% in women with oligomenorrhea and 92% in women with hirsutism and regular cycles.[9] In another study of 389 women presenting with menstrual cycle disturbances, Gadir et al found the prevalence of polycystic ovaries to be 65%.[10] Whereas in a third study of 350 women presenting with hirsutism and/or androgenic alopecia, O'Driscoll et al identified polycystic ovaries in 60% of 282 women whose

ovaries were successfully visualized by ultrasound.[11] In a fourth study examining 119 women with acne, but no menstrual disorders, obesity, or hirsutism, Peserico et al found the prevalence to be 45% in this group.[12] This reflects that polycystic ovaries, and by definition PCOS, are very common in these specifically defined groups of women. However the prevalence of PCOS in the general population has not been definitively determined. A cross-sectional study by Knochenhauer et al examined the prevalence of PCOS in a population of American women and determined a prevalence rate of 4%.[13] However this study applied the US definition of PCOS and did not include polycystic ovarian morphology on ultrasound as part of the defining criteria.

Several studies have been performed to attempt to determine the prevalence of polycystic ovaries as detected by ultrasound alone in the general population, and have found remarkably similar prevalence rates in the order of 17–22%. The study designs and results are summarized in Table 3.3. All of the studies used transabdominal ultrasound for the diagnosis of polycystic ovaries except for Cresswell et al, who converted to a transvaginal scan if the transabdominal picture was unclear.[19]

The study populations recruited by Polson et al, Tayob et al, and by Botsis et al, were all subject to a degree of selection bias due to the fact that they recruited women from hospital-associated populations (although Polson's study admittedly recruited hospital workers and not patients) and not from the general population.[14,15,18] The low response rates achieved in the community-based studies by Clayton et al and Farquhar et al might reduce confidence in the validity of their estimates of prevalence,[16,17] but reassuringly Cresswell et al, who achieved a much higher response rate in their sample, determined a very similar prevalence.[19] In the study by Cresswell et al, women were first interviewed at home by a trained fieldworker before being invited to attend for a scan.[19] The establishment of this personal rapport may have contributed to the higher response rate achieved in this cross-sectional study than in the studies by Clayton et al and Farquhar et al, which required participants to attend for a scan outright.[16,17] However, in the absence of a large, cross-sectional population-based study, the prevalence rates detected above provide the best estimates of the occurrence of

Table 3.3 The prevalence of polycystic ovaries in the general population

Authors	Polson et al (1988)[14]	Tayob et al (1990)[15]	Clayton et al (1992)[16]	Farquhar et al (1994)[17]	Botsis et al (1995)[18]	Cresswell et al (1997)[19]
Study population	Volunteers recruited from clinical and secretarial staff at St Mary's Hospital, London	Volunteers using a low dose combined oral contraceptive pill, recruited from routine clinics at the Margaret Pyke Centre and the Royal Free Hospital, London	Volunteers born between 1952 and 1969, recruited from a list of a group practice in Harrow, London, by random postal invitation	Volunteers recruited from two electoral rolls in Auckland, NZ, by random postal invitation	Volunteers recruited from women presenting to an outpatient clinic for routine pap smear	Volunteers born between 1952 and 1953 recruited from records of the Jessop Hospital, Sheffield, by invitation and personal interview
	n = 257	n = 120	n = 190	n = 183	n = 1078	n = 235
Response rate	Unknown	Unknown	18%	16%	Unknown	68%
Age range (years)	18–36	18–30 mean = 24	18–36	18–45 mean = 33	17–40	40–42
Prevalence (%)	22	22	22	21	17	21
95% CI (%)	17–27	14–30	16–28	14–27	14–19	16–26

CI = Confidence interval

polycystic ovaries in the 'normal' population. The pooled prevalence is 19%, indicating that polycystic ovaries (as defined by their ultrasound appearance) are extremely common.

The study by Tayob et al was primarily designed to identify women who were at risk of breakthrough ovulation while taking the combined oral contraceptive pill.[15] Although the ovaries were assessed by transabdominal ultrasound, blood samples were not collected, and clinical symptoms of PCOS were not recorded. In the other studies, clinical and biochemical features associated with PCOS were compared between women with and without polycystic ovaries. In all of the studies, hirsutism was identified more commonly in women with polycystic ovaries. Menstrual cycle abnormalities were also found to be more common in the polycystic ovary groups, except in the study by Clayton et al which detected no significant difference in menstrual patterns when comparing women with polycystic ovaries *versus* those with normal ovaries.[16] In the study by Polson et al, a surprisingly low frequency of irregular menstrual cycles was detected in those women with normal ovaries.[14]

The explanation for this is not clear as the definition of 'irregular cycles' is similar to that used in other studies, but may be related to the way in which menstrual histories were recorded from the participants. Botsis et al noted a greater tendency towards obesity in their group of women with polycystic ovaries, but significant differences in obesity were not identified in the other reports.[18] All of these studies determined higher mean ovarian volumes in women with polycystic ovaries when compared with women with normal ovaries. The frequency of symptoms and signs identified in women with and without polycystic ovaries is summarized in Table 3.4.

The inconsistencies between these studies may be due in part to differences in the definitions used for each symptom or sign that was recorded. However, the method of recruitment may also be relevant as the community-based studies of Clayton et al, Farquhar et al, and Cresswell et al show frequencies of menstrual cycle disturbances and of hirsutism that are much lower than those recorded in the larger studies of women with PCOS recruited from reproductive/endocrine clinics (see Table 3.1).[16,17,19] The study by Botsis et

Table 3.4 Frequency of clinical symptoms and signs in women with and without polycystic ovaries

	Percentage frequency									
	Polson et al (1988)[14]		Clayton et al (1992)[16]		Farquhar et al (1994)[17]		Botsis et al (1995)[18]		Cresswell et al (1997)[19]	
	PCO n = 33[a]	Normal n = 116[a]	PCO n = 43	Normal n = 165	PCO n = 39	Normal n = 144	PCO n = 183	Normal n = 823	PCO n = 49	Normal n = 186
Menstrual cycle disturbance	76	1	29[a]	27	46[b]	20	80	–	41	27
Hirsutism	–	–	14	2	23	4	40	10	14	2
Obesity	–	–	33	29	23	19	41	10	35	48
Infertility[c] primary/ secondary	–	–	12	10	26	11	–	–	16	15

– Denotes feature not recorded.
PCO: Polycystic ovaries.
[a]Value includes only non-oral contraceptive pill users with PCO.
[b]Percentage calculated for non-oral contraceptive pill users with PCO where n = 34.
[c]Includes only women who have tested their fertility.

al (and by Polson et al, which records clinical information about menstrual irregularities only),[14,18] records frequencies that resemble more closely those previously determined in the hospital-based studies, suggesting that their population was subject to greater selection bias.

Comparison of hormone levels between women with and without polycystic ovaries was further complicated by the high proportion of women using the oral contraceptive pill (OCP) in these populations. This necessitated division of the 'normal' and 'polycystic ovary' groups of women into further subgroups dependent upon their oral contraceptive status. The differences in hormone levels that were detected were by no means consistent across the studies. Polson et al did not detect any significant difference in the mean level of serum LH or testosterone concentrations between women with and without polycystic ovaries, but did identify a difference in the numbers of LH and testosterone observations that were above the normal range in the women with polycystic ovaries.[14] Clayton et al detected significantly higher LH levels in women with polycystic ovaries, compared with those with normal ovaries in their group of non-OCP users, but found no significant differences between the

groups for any of the other hormones measured.[16] Farquhar et al were only able to identify higher levels of free testosterone in their non-OCP group with polycystic ovaries.[17] Botsis et al, who subdivided their group of women with polycystic ovaries into those with and without menstrual irregularities, determined significantly higher LH/follicle stimulating hormone (FSH) ratios and testosterone levels in those women with polycystic ovaries who had menstrual symptoms when compared with controls.[18] Cresswell et al reported significantly higher mean plasma concentrations of LH and testosterone in their group of women with polycystic ovaries, and a higher ratio of LH to FSH.[19]

Despite the problems of small sample populations and inconsistent methodology, these studies indicate a high prevalence (19%) of polycystic ovaries in the 'normal' population. They have also shown that many of these women have symptoms and signs that may be attributable to PCOS, but reinforce the observation that in some women with polycystic ovaries, no clinical or biochemical abnormalities are detected. The question of whether polycystic ovaries alone are pathological or a normal variant of ovarian morphology is still debated. While the spectrum of 'normality' might include the presence of polycystic ovaries in the absence of signs or symptoms of PCOS, there is evidence that women with polycystic morphology alone show typical responses to stresses such as gonadotrophin stimulation during in vitro fertilization (IVF) treatment or to weight gain as stimulated by sodium valproate therapy.[20,21] The difficulty in answering this question lies in the fact that to date there are no large-scale, longitudinal prospective studies of women with polycystic ovaries, and that the pathophysiology of polycystic ovaries has not been fully determined.

We studied 224 normal female volunteers between the ages of 18 and 25 years and identified polycystic ovaries using ultrasound in 33% of participants.[22] Fifty per cent of the participants were using some form of hormonal contraception, but the prevalence of polycystic ovaries in users and non-users of hormonal contraception was identical. Polycystic ovaries in the non-users of hormonal contraception were associated with irregular menstrual cycles and significantly higher serum testosterone concentrations when compared with women with normal ovaries, however only a small proportion of women with polycystic ovaries (15%) had 'elevated' serum testosterone concentrations outside the normal range. Interestingly there were no significant differences in acne, hirsutism, BMI or body fat percentage between women with polycystic and normal ovaries, and hyperinsulinism and reduced insulin sensitivity were not associated with polycystic ovaries in this group. Also, no significant differences were identified for beta-cell function between the groups, unlike other studies which have shown pancreatic beta-cell dysfunction in women with PCOS when compared with controls.[23]

In our study, the prevalence of PCOS was as low as 8% using the North American National Institute of Health (NIH) 'consensus' definition for PCOS*, or as high as 26% if the broader European criteria were applied. However, features included in the European criteria (menstrual irregularity, acne, hirsutism, BMI >25 kg/m^2, raised serum testosterone, or raised LH) were found to occur frequently in women without polycystic ovaries, and 75% of women with normal ovaries had one or more of these attributes. Subgroup analyses of women according to the presence of normal ovaries, polycystic ovaries alone, or polycystic ovaries and features of PCOS, revealed greater mean BMI in women with PCOS, but also indicated lower fasting insulin concentrations and greater insulin sensitivity in polycystic ovary and PCOS groups when compared with women with normal ovaries, which is in contrast to studies of older women.[24,25] These interesting findings were difficult to interpret in the light of current understanding of PCOS, but forced us to consider the possibility that this young, mainly non-overweight population, might reflect women early in the natural history of the development of PCOS, and that abnormalities of insulin metabolism might evolve following weight gain in later life.

In our study we were also able to determine genotype frequencies for the insulin gene minisatellite (*INS VNTR*) which has been linked to anovulatory PCOS (see also Chapter 5).[29] Genotype frequency distributions were found to be similar in women with polycystic ovaries and those with normal ovaries. However, subdivision of those women with polycystic ovaries according to the 'severity' of PCOS revealed increasing frequency of the III/III genotype with increasing severity of the PCOS phenotype.[22] This could suggest that the *INS VNTR* locus may determine clinical severity of PCOS in women with polycystic ovaries; however, larger studies would be necessary to determine this conclusively.

---

*The defining features of PCOS in the UK and much of Europe have been the presence of menstrual disturbance and/or hyperandrogenism in association with an ultrasound picture of polycystic ovaries,[26] while the 1990 National Institute of Health Conference on PCOS recommended that diagnostic criteria should include evidence of hyperandrogenism and ovulatory dysfunction, in the absence of non-classic adrenal hyperplasia, and that evidence of polycystic ovarian morphology was not essential.[27] At a recent joint ESHRE/ASRM (European Society of Human Reproduction and Endocrinology/American Society for Reproductive Medicine) consensus meeting, a refined definition of the PCOS was agreed: namely the presence of two out of the following three criteria: oligo- and/or anovulation; hyperandrogenism (clinical and/or biochemical); polycystic ovaries, with the exclusion of other etiologies (see Chapter 2).[28]

National and racial differences in expression of polycystic ovary syndrome

Michelmore et al demonstrated that 80% of those with polycystic ovaries (PCO) (which was 26% of those from the community) had features of PCOS based on the UK/European definition of PCOS, in their post menarchal years (i.e. ages 18–24).[30] However, using the much more stringent US criteria which do not utilize ovarian morphology, the prevalence rate for PCOS ranged from 4.5–11.2% from an unselected group of white Europeans and blacks in a population-based study in Alabama,[13] 9% in Greece,[31] and 6.5% in Spain.[32]

The highest reported prevalence of PCO has been 52% amongst South Asian immigrants in Britain, of whom 49.1% had menstrual irregularity.[33] They demonstrated that South Asian women with PCO have a comparable degree of insulin resistance to age-matched South Asian women with established type 2 diabetes mellitus and normal ovaries. Nonetheless, there has been a paucity of data about the prevalence of PCOS among women of South Asian origin, both among migrant and native groups. Type 2 diabetes and insulin resistance have a high prevalence among indigenous populations in South Asia, with a rising prevalence among women. Insulin resistance and hyperinsulinemia are common antecedents of type 2 diabetes, with a high prevalence in South Asians. Type 2 diabetes also has a familial basis, inherited as a complex genetic trait that interacts with environmental factors, chiefly nutrition, commencing from fetal life. We are currently exploring the hypothesis that ethnic variations in the overt features of PCOS (i.e. symptoms of hyperandrogenism, menstrual irregularity, and obesity) in women of South Asian descent are linked to the higher prevalence and degree of insulin resistance in South Asians. We have already found that South Asians with anovular PCOS have greater insulin resistance and more severe symptoms of the syndrome than anovular Caucasians with PCOS.[34] Furthermore, we have found that women from South Asia, living in the UK appear to express symptoms at an earlier age than their Caucasian British counterparts.

Generally, ethnic differences in the prevalence of PCOS have not been well explored. Dunaif and coworkers reported an increased rate of PCOS among Caribbean Hispanic women.[35] However, Knochenhauer et al, in a sample of 195 black women and 174 white women in the US, found that the prevalence of PCOS among black women was comparable to that of whites (3.4% versus 4.7%).[13] There may also be ethnic variation in overt features of PCOS when the prevalence of biochemical manifestations is similar across the races.[36] A study carried out comparing women with PCOS from the USA, Japan and Italy reported less obesity in Japanese women, yet comparable rates of androgen excess and insulin resistance.[37] The question remains as to whether differences in expression of the syndrome are due to dietary and lifestyle factors or genetic variations in hormone actions, such as polymorphisms in gonadotrophin subunits or receptor function (affecting the expression of androgens, gonadotrophins or insulin). The genetics of PCOS is discussed in detail in Chapter 5 and there are a number of candidate genes that have been proposed. It may be that some families or racial groups have genetic differences that affect the expression or presentation of PCOS – and we and others are working to try and identify such variations.

Conclusions

PCOS is one of the most common endocrine disorders and may present, at one end of the spectrum, with the single finding of polycystic ovarian morphology as detected by pelvic ultrasound. At the other end of the spectrum symptoms such as obesity, hyperandrogenism, menstrual cycle disturbance and infertility may occur either singly or in combination. Women with PCOS are characterized by the presence of insulin resistance, central obesity, and dyslipidemia, which appears to place them at a higher risk of developing diabetes as well as cardiovascular disease. There are a number of environmental factors that may influence the expression of the syndrome – in particular a tendency to insulin-resistant states induced by overeating and under-exercising. A plausible hypothesis for the survival of PCOS in the population is that of the 'thrifty phenotype/genotype' whereby in times of famine, individuals who have a tendency to obesity

---

Key points

- A number of correlations have been made of biochemical changes with clinical features of PCOS: high serum testosterone concentrations correlate with clinical hyperandrogenism and infertility; high LH concentrations are associated with infertility and menstrual cycle disturbances; and insulin resistance correlates with ovarian volume and androgen concentrations.
- The degree of insulin resistance correlates with intermenstrual interval.
- PCOS accounts for 95% of cases of hyperandrogenism, 95% of cases of acne in adult women, 90% of women with oligomenorrhea and 30–50% of women with amenorrhea.
- Polycystic ovaries are seen on ultrasound in between 22% and 33% of Caucasian women, of whom approximately three-quarters have clinical manifestations of the syndrome.
- There are significant racial differences in clinical presentation, most noticeably with respect to hirsutism.
- There are racial differences in the rate of insulin resistance, for example this has led to approximately 50% of women from South Asia who live in the UK having PCOS.

---

preserve the population by maintaining fertility, while those of normal body weight fall below the threshold body weight for fertility. This might explain the greater prevalence of PCOS among South Asians in the UK, where there is relatively greater nutrition and thus the right environment to express PCOS.

PCOS is probably the same the world over, although there may be factors that affect expression and presentation – whether because of racial differences in the color and distribution of hair (e.g. Japanese vs Mediterranean women) or variations in hormone production and receptor activity. Fundamentally the underlying condition is likely to be the same.

References

1. Balen AH, Conway GS, Kaltsas G, Techatrasak K et al. Polycystic ovary syndrome: the spectrum of the disorder in 1741 patients. Hum Reprod 1995; 10:2107–2111.
2. Franks S. Polycystic ovary syndrome: a changing perspective. Clin Endocrinol (Oxf) 1989; 31:87–120.
3. Goldzieher JW. Polycystic ovarian disease. Fertil Steril 1981; 35:371–394.
4. Conway GS, Honour JW, Jacobs HS. Heterogeneity of the polycystic ovary syndrome: clinical, endocrine and ultrasound features in 556 patients. Clin Endocrinol (Oxf) 1989; 30:459–470.
5 Fox R, Corrigan E, Thomas PA, Hull MG. The diagnosis of polycystic ovaries in women with oligo-amenorrhoea: predictive power of endocrine tests. Clin Endocrinol (Oxf) 1991; 34:127–131.
6. Pache TD, de Jong FH, Hop WC, Fauser BCJM. Association between ovarian changes assessed by transvaginal sonogrophy and clinical and endocrine signs of the polycystic ovary syndrome. Fertil Steril 1993; 59:544–549.
7. Dewailly D, Robert Y, Helin I, Ardaens Y et al. Ovarian stromal hypertrophy in hyperandrogenic women. Clin Endocrinol (Oxf) 1994; 41:557–562.
8. Kyei-Mensah A, Maconochie N, Zaidi J, Pittrof R et al. Transvaginal three-dimensional ultrasound: reproducibility of ovarian and endometrial volume measurements. Fertil Steril 1996; 5:718–722.
9. Adams J, Polson DW, Franks S. Prevalence of polycystic ovaries in women with anovulation and idiopathic hirsutism. Br Med J Clin Res Ed 1986; 293:355–359.
10. Gadir AA, Khatim MS, Mowafi RS, Alnaser HM et al. Implications of ultrasonically diagnosed polycystic ovaries. I. Correlations with basal hormonal profiles. Hum Reprod 1992; 7:453–457.
11. O'Driscoll JB, Mamtora H, Higginson J, Pollock A et al. A prospective study of the prevalence of clear-cut endocrine disorders and polycystic ovaries in 350 patients presenting with hirsutism or androgenic alopecia. Clin Endocrinol (Oxf) 1994; 41:231–236.
12. Peserico A, Angeloni G, Bertoli P et al. Prevalence of polycystic ovaries in women with acne. Arch Dermatol Res 1989; 281:502–503.
13. Knochenhauer ES, Key TJ, Kahsar-Miller M, Waggoner W et al. Prevalence of the polycystic ovary syndrome in unselected Black and White

Women of the Southeastern United States: A prospective study. J Clin Endocrinol Metab 1998; 83:3078–3082.

14. Polson DW, Adams J, Wadsworth J, Franks S. Polycystic ovaries – a common finding in normal women. Lancet 1988; 1:870–872.

15. Tayob Y, Robinson G, Adams J et al. Ultrasound appearance of the ovaries during the pill-free interval. Br J Fam Plann 1990; 16:94–96.

16. Clayton RN, Ogden V, Hodgkinson J et al. How common are polycystic ovaries in normal women and what is their significance for the fertility of the population? [see comments]. Clin Endocrinol (Oxf) 1992; 37:127–134.

17. Farquhar CM, Birdsall M, Manning P, Mitchell JM. Transabdominal versus transvaginal ultrasound in the diagnosis of polycystic ovaries in a population of randomly selected women. Ultrasound Obstet Gynecol 1994; 4:54–59.

18. Botsis D, Kassanos D, Pyrgiotis E, Zourlas PA. Sonographic incidence of polycystic ovaries in a gynecological population. Ultrasound Obstet Gynecol 1995; 6:182–185.

19. Cresswell JL, Barker DJ, Osmond C, Egger P et al. Fetal growth, length of gestation, and polycystic ovaries in adult life. Lancet 1997; 350:1131–1135.

20. MacDougall MJ, Tan SL, Balen A, Jacobs HS. A controlled study comparing patients with and without polycystic ovaries undergoing in-vitro fertilization. Hum Reprod 1993; 8:233–236.

21. Isojarvi IT, Laatikainen T, Pakarinen AJ, Juntunen KTS, Myllyla VV. Polycystic ovaries and hyperandrogenism in women taking valproate for epilepsy. N Engl J Med 1993; 329:1383–1388.

22. Michelmore KF, Ong K, Mason S, Bennett S et al. Clinical features in women with polycystic ovaries: relationships to insulin sensitivity, insulin gene VNTR and birth weight. Clin Endocrinol (Oxf) 2001; 55:439–446.

23. Dunaif A, Finegood DT. Beta-cell dysfunction independent of obesity and glucose intolerance in the polycystic ovary syndrome. J Clin Endocrinol Metab 1996; 81:942–947.

24. Dunaif A. Insulin resistance and the polycystic ovary syndrome: mechanism and implications for pathogenesis. Endocrinol Rev 1997; 18:774–800.

25. Conway GS, Clark PM, Wong D. Hyperinsulinaemia in the polycystic ovary syndrome confirmed with a specific immunoradiometric assay for insulin. Clin Endocrinol (Oxf) 1993; 38:219–222.

26. Balen AH. The pathogenesis of polycystic ovary syndrome: the enigma unravels. Lancet 1999; 354:966–967.

27. Zawadzki JA, Dunaif A. Diagnostic criteria for polycystic ovary syndrome: towards a rational approach. In: Dunaif A, Givens JR, Haseltine FP, Merriam GR, eds. Polycystic ovary syndrome. Boston: Blackwell Scientific, 1992:377–384.

28. The Rotterdam ESHRE/ASRM-sponsored PCOS consensus workshop group: Fauser B, Tarlatzis B, Chang J, Azziz R et al. Revised 2003 consensus on diagnostic criteria and long-term health risks related to polycystic ovary syndrome (PCOS). Hum Reprod 2004; 19:41–47.

29. Waterworth DM, Bennett ST, Gharani N, McCarthy MI et al. Linkage and association of insulin gene VNTR regulatory polymorphism with polycystic ovary syndrome. Lancet 1997; 349:986–990.

30. Michelmore KF, Balen AH, Dunger DB, Vessey MP. Polycystic ovaries and associated clinical and biochemical features in young women. Clin Endocrinol (Oxf) 1999; 51:779–786.

31. Diamanti-Kandarakis E, Kouli CR, Bergiele AT, Filandra FA et al. A survey of the polycystic ovary syndrome in the Greek island of Lesbos: hormonal and metabolic profile. J Clin Endocrinol Metab 1999; 84:4006–4011.

32. Asunción M, Calvo RM, San Millán JL, Sancho J et al. A prospective study of the prevalence of the polycystic ovary syndrome in unselected Caucasian women in Spain. J Clin Endocrinol Metab 2000; 85:2434–2438.

33. Rodin DA, Bano G, Bland JM, Taylor K, Nussey SS. Polycystic ovaries and associated metabolic abnormalities in Indian subcontinent Asian women. Clin Endocrinol (Oxf) 1998; 49:91–99.

34. Wijeyaratne CN, Balen AH, Barth J, Belchetz PE. Clinical manifestations and insulin resistance (IR) in polycystic ovary syndrome (PCOS) among South Asians and Caucasians: is there a difference? Clin Endocrinol (Oxf) 2002; 57:343–350.

35. Dunaif A, Sorbara L, Delson R, Green G. Ethnicity and polycystic ovary syndrome are associated with independent and additive decreases in insulin action in Caribbean Hispanic women. Diabetes 1993; 42:1462–1468.

36. Solomon CG. The epidemiology of polycystic ovary syndrome- prevalence and associated disease risks. Endocrinol Metab Clin North Am 1999; 28:247–263.

37. Carmina E, Koyama T, Chang L, Stanczyk FZ, Lobo RA. Does ethnicity influence the prevalence of adrenal hyperandrogenism and insulin resistance in polycystic ovary syndrome? Am J Obstet Gynecol 1992; 167:1807–1812.

38. Franks S, Gharani N, McCarthy M. Candidate genes in polycystic ovary syndrome. Hum Reprod Update 2001; 7:405–410.

Chapter 4

The pathophysiology of polycystic ovary syndrome

Introduction

Polycystic ovary syndrome (PCOS) is a heterogeneous collection of signs and symptoms that gathered together form a spectrum of a disorder with a mild presentation in some, while in others a severe disturbance of reproductive, endocrine and metabolic function is seen. The pathophysiology of PCOS appears to be multifactorial and polygenic. Because the phenotype of women with polycystic ovaries (PCO) and the polycystic ovary syndrome may be very variable, it is then difficult to elucidate the genotype (see Chapter 5).[1] It is also likely that different combinations of genetic variants may result in differential expression of the separate components of the syndrome.[2]

The highest reported prevalence of PCO has been 52% amongst South Asian immigrants in Britain, of whom 49.1% had menstrual irregularity.[3] Rodin et al demonstrated that South Asian women with PCO had a comparable degree of insulin resistance to controls with established type 2 diabetes mellitus.[3] Type 2 diabetes and insulin resistance have a high prevalence among indigenous populations in South Asia, with a rising prevalence among women. Insulin resistance and hyperinsulinemia are common antecedents of type 2 diabetes, with a high prevalence in South Asians. Type 2 diabetes also has a familial basis, inherited as a complex genetic trait that interacts with environmental factors, chiefly nutrition, commencing from fetal life. We have already found that South Asians with anovular PCOS have greater insulin resistance and more severe symptoms of the syndrome than anovular Caucasians with PCOS.[4] Furthermore, we have found that women from South Asia, living in the UK appear to express symptoms at an earlier age than their Caucasian British counterparts.[4]

In understanding the pathophysiology of PCOS, one has to consider both the nature of the dysfunction within the ovary and the external influences that prevail to modify ovarian behavior.

Ovarian biochemistry and hyperandrogenism

Clinical phenotyping of PCOS involves determining the presence of clinical and/or biochemical androgen excess (hyperandrogenism), while excluding related disorders. The primary clinical sign of androgen excess is the presence of hirsutism. The assessment of hirsutism is relatively subjective, and few physicians in clinical practice actually use standardized scoring methods. There are also significant racial differences with hirsutism being significantly less prevalent in hyperandrogenic women of Eastern Asian origin and more so in those from Southern Asia.[4,5] The sole presence of acne is also felt to be a relatively good indicator of hyperandrogenism, although studies are somewhat conflicting regarding the exact prevalence of androgen excess in these patients.[6] The sole presence of androgenic alopecia as an indicator of hyperandrogenism has been less well studied. However, it appears to be a relatively poor marker of androgen excess, unless present in the oligo-ovulatory patient.[7]

While some studies have found that most patients with PCOS have evidence of hyperandrogenemia,[8] others have not.[1,9–11] In a study of over 1700 women with PCOS, we found that a third had an elevated serum total testosterone concentration and that the 95 percentile for total testosterone was 4.8 nmol/l.[1] We therefore use this value in practice as the cut-off for screening for

CHOLESTEROL

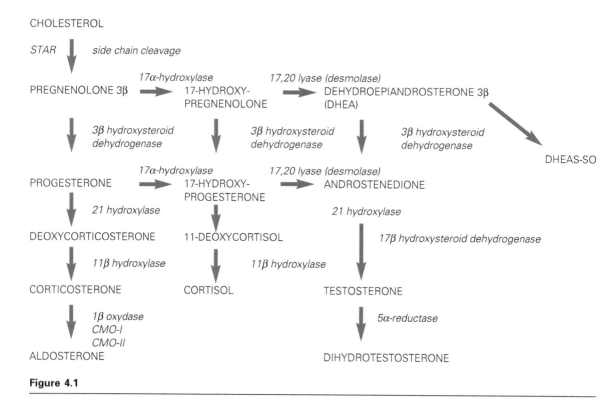

Figure 4.1

The steroidogenic pathway.

other causes of androgen excess. If the value is greater than 4.8 nmol/l it is only then necessary to assess the androgen profile in greater detail in order to exclude other causes such as androgen-secreting tumors of the ovary or adrenals (in which case the clinical history of hyperandrogenism is usually of more acute onset), late onset congenital adrenal hyperplasia (CAH) or Cushing's syndrome.

The measurement of free testosterone (T) or the free T (free androgen) index (FAI), are thought to be sensitive methods of assessing for hyperandrogenemia,[12,13] and methods for the assessment of free T include equilibrium dialysis,[14,15] calculation of free T from the measurement of sex hormone binding globulin (SHBG) and total T, or ammonium sulfate precipitation.[16]

Women with the 'classical' syndrome have the highest levels of androgens, although even women with polycystic ovaries and mild or no symptoms have mean serum concentrations of testosterone that are higher than in those with normal ovaries.[17] The bulk of evidence points to the ovary being the source of excess androgens, which appears to result from an abnormal regulation (dysregulation) of steroidogenesis.[18]

The ovary and adrenal cortex share the bulk of the steroid biosynthesis pathways, by making equal contributions to the circulating concentrations of androstenedione and testosterone, in a normal pre-menopausal woman. Both glands secrete androstenedione in significantly greater quantities than testosterone, while 50% of circulating testosterone is derived from the peripheral metabolism of androstenedione.[19] Androgen production in the ovary is by the theca interna layer of the ovarian follicle, while the zona fasciculata of the adrenal cortex synthesizes adrenal androgens. The enzymes utilized in the formation of androstenedione from the initial substrate, cholesterol, are similar in both glands, under the endocrine control of luteinizing hormone (LH) in the ovary and adrenocorticotrophic hormone (ACTH), in the adrenal glands.[20,21]

The initial step in the biosynthesis of all steroid hormones is the conversion of cholesterol to pregnenolone, by a two-stage process involving cholesterol side chain cleavage enzyme and the acute steroidogenic regulatory protein. Pregnenolone is then converted to dehydroepiandrosterone (DHEA) by a two-step process along the Δ^5-steroid pathway, the conversion being catalyzed by cytochrome P450c17α. Progesterone undergoes a parallel transformation to androstenedione in the Δ^4-steroid pathway. In humans the cytochrome P450c17 gene product seems to play a minor role in terms of 17,20-lyase activity in the Δ^4-pathway. In the adrenal gland, 17-hydroxyprogesterone is either converted to cortisol or sex hormones, depending on whether it undergoes 21-hydroxylation to cortisol, or 17,20-lysis to be converted to 17-ketosteroids. The action of 17β-hydroxydehydrogenase on the 17-ketosteroids is essential for their conversion to testosterone, dihydrotestosterone, and estradiol (Figure 4.1).

Androgen secretion in normal women undergoes about two-fold episodic, diurnal, and cyclic variation. The rate-limiting step in steroidogenesis is the formation of pregnenolone from cholesterol, which is regulated by trophic hormones. The rate-limiting step in androgen formation is the gene expression of P450c17, which is absolutely dependent on trophic hormones, LH in the ovary and ACTH in the adrenal cortex. The steroidogenic response to the trophic hormones is modulated by an array of small peptides, which include insulin and insulin-like growth factors (IGFs).

A certain amount of intra-ovarian androgens are essential for normal follicular growth, and for the synthesis of estradiol. Nonetheless, when the synthesis of androgens is not co-ordinated with the needs of a developing follicle, and is in excess, poor follicle maturation and increased folliclular atresia results. In the normal ovary, LH acts on thecal-interstitial-stromal cells, while follicle stimulating hormone (FSH) acts on granulosa cells. According to the 'two-gonadotropin, two-cell theory' of estrogen biosynthesis, the thecal compartment secretes androgens in response to LH, and the androstenedione thus formed is converted in the granulosa cell to estrogens, by the action of aromatase, which in turn is under the influence of FSH (Figure 4.2). When a dominant follicle emerges, the estrogen content dominates

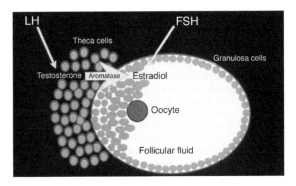

Figure 4.2

Two gonadotropin, two-cell mechanism of estrogen biosynthesis.

over androgens and is not driven by long-loop negative feedback effects. The intra-ovarian modulation of androgen synthesis by LH plays a critical regulatory role. As LH stimulation increases, a homologous desensitization sets in. Overstimulation with LH, in a time- and dose-dependent manner, causes downregulation of LH receptors, reduces cholesterol side-chain cleavage activity, 17,20 lyase activity, and finally activity of 17-hydroxylase. Thus the ratio of 17-hydroxyprogesterone to androgen increases.[22]

Autocrine, paracrine and hormonal factors modulate the co-ordination of thecal and granulosa cell function, in terms of androgen synthesis. Androgens and estrogens are negative modulators of LH effects, while IGFs play a positive modulator role. Insulin also augments LH-stimulated androgen production, either via its own receptors or via IGF-1 receptors. Inhibin promotes androgen synthesis, while androgens in turn stimulate inhibin production. Activin opposes the effects of inhibin. Furthermore, prostaglandins and angiotensin also play a promoter role, while corticotrophin releasing hormone, transforming growth factor-β, epidermal growth factor, tumor necrosis factor, and cytokines play an inhibitory role in androgen biosynthesis.

Granulosa cell development, and thereby the increase of aromatase activity, also determines androgen production. A healthy follicle which is 8 mm or more in diameter, converts androstenedione to estradiol efficiently. Conversely atretic and/or cystic follicles have a high androstenedione to estradiol ratio. The action of FSH on granulosa cells determines the growth of healthy follicles that are greater than 2–5 mm in diameter, partly mediated by the IGF system and insulin in physiological concentrations, all of which stimulate the production of estradiol. IGF-binding proteins inhibit FSH bioactivity and are markedly expressed in atretic follicles. Transforming growth factor and epidermal growth factor inhibit aromatase, while activin promotes granulosa cell estrogen production while inhibiting thecal androgen secretion.

Nearly half of the circulating testosterone in normal adult women is derived from the peripheral conversion of androstenedione, and the remainder is derived from the ovary and adrenal cortex. The important tissues in which this conversion takes place are the lung, liver, adipose tissue and skin. Adipose tissue also forms estrone from androstenedione, which explains the mild estrogen excess of obesity. Plasma dihydrotestosterone is produced virtually entirely by 5α-reductase activity in the periphery, with plasma androstenedione being its major precursor.[23]

Ovarian function in PCOS

The presence of enlarged polycystic ovaries suggests that the ovary is the primary site of endocrine abnormality, particularly the hyperandrogenism. In 1990, Rosenfield et al suggested that derangement of P450c17α activity played a central role in excess ovarian androgen production.[18] This was subsequently confirmed by other workers who assessed the response of the pituitary and ovary to a single dose of the gonadotropin releasing hormone agonist (GnRHa), nafarelin, in hyperandrogenemic women with PCOS in whom adrenal androgen production had been suppressed by administering dexamethasone.[22] The observations were that GnRHa yielded a significant elevation of androstenedione and 17-hydroxyprogesterone. Franks et al, extended this study to anovulatory and ovulating hyperandrogenemic women, and reported a small but significant increase in androstenedione levels in both groups in response to GnRHa, and a similar response in 17-hydroxyprogesterone levels, which were signifi-

cantly higher in the anovulatory women.[17] They also demonstrated that there was no significant rise in these two hormones in response to an ACTH injection, which excluded a significant role of adrenal androgen production. These data indicate that hyperandrogenemia, in both ovulatory and anovulatory women with PCOS, is predominantly of ovarian origin. This also confirmed that the primary cause of excess androgen production by the polycystic ovary was not due to hypersecretion of LH alone and it was reasonable to conclude that the intrinsic defect was due to an ovarian theca-interstitial cell dysfunction, or other stimulatory influences such as insulin, IGF-I, etc.

Further research confirmed that women with classic PCOS when injected with a single dose of GnRHa, had a surge of FSH and LH of preovulatory magnitude, a hyper-responsive secretion of 17-hydroxyprogesterone, and to a lesser extent, of androstenedione, testosterone, estrone and estradiol.[22] This is highly suggestive of a generalized dysregulation of ovarian androgen secretion, and currently P450c17 is the favored route for this dysfunction.

Both in vivo and in vitro data confirm that the theca cells of PCOS patients have a generalized overactive steroidogenesis. PCOS patients have a tendency to an excess of estradiol at all stages of follicular maturation. This is partly due to availability of excess androgen substrate for aromatase activity, as well as an excessive response of follicle development and estradiol secretion to FSH.[24] Granulosa cells from PCO in vitro have also been reported to lose FSH responsiveness, and produce low amounts of progesterone.[25]

The distinct ovarian morphology is pathognomonic for the syndrome (see Chapter 2), its major marker being hyperandrogenemia arising from the theca cells. Follicular development is disturbed, with antral follicles arrested at a diameter of 2–9 mm. It is thought that the abnormal endocrine environment adversely affects follicular maturation, although it is uncertain whether there is in addition an intrinsic abnormality within the follicle of polycystic ovaries. The whole process of follicle development from primordial to pre-ovulatory takes about six months, with only the final two weeks being gonadotropin dependent. Pre-antral follicle development is dependent on local growth factors which determine growth and survival of those follicles that escape death by atresia. A recent study of follicle densities from normal and polycystic ovaries found that normal ovaries contained 11.4 small preantral follicles/m^3 (4–34); ovulatory polycystic ovaries had a density of 27.4 follicles/m^3 (9–81); and anovulatory polycystic ovaries had a density of 73.0 follicles/m^3 (31–94). This significant difference was also demonstrated for primary follicles.[26] Anovulatory polycystic ovaries had the highest overall density of follicles, although there was no significant difference between those from anovulatory and ovulatory polycystic ovaries or between ovulatory polycystic ovaries and normal ovaries. Primordial follicle density was similar in all three groups, although the follicles from polycystic ovaries were less likely to be healthy. Thus there appears to be a significantly higher density of small pre-antral follicles particularly in anovulatory polycystic ovaries. This is thought to be due to a higher rate of recruitment from the resting follicle pool in polycystic ovaries, rather than a reduced rate of atresia (which if anything may be slightly increased). The observation that women with polycystic ovary syndrome do not have an early menopause suggests that there may be a higher starting follicle pool, although this is yet to be proven.

LH excess is considered to be the cause of the ovarian hyperandrogenism of PCOS, in view of the stimulatory effect of LH on theca cells. Nevertheless, some women with PCOS have normal LH levels while being hyperandrogenic, while yet others who had downregulation of LH secretion with long-term GnRHa displayed hyper-responsiveness of 17-hydroxyprogesterone to human chorionic gonadotrophin (hCG) injection (i.e. challenge with LH). These findings argue against a sole role of LH in the androgen excess of PCOS. They favor the theory that theca cells of PCOS women hyper-respond to gonadotropins and produce excess androgens due to an escape of their normal downregulation to gonadotropins, thereby linking this dysregulation to excess of insulin and IGF-I. Prelevic and colleagues supported this theory by demonstrating that suppression of insulin secretion by a somatostatin analogue lowers serum LH and androgens in PCOS women.[27] Indeed insulin acts as a 'co-gonadotropin' and also amplifies the effects of testosterone by suppressing SHBG.

Inhibin is an FSH-inducible factor, which is capable of interfering with the downregulation of steroidogenesis. Plasma inhibin and androstenedione concentrations correlate, and women with PCOS have elevated serum inhibin-B.[28] This helps to explain the relatively low serum concentrations of FSH compared with LH in anovulatory women with PCOS. Since inhibin stimulates androgen production, and androgens in turn stimulate inhibin secretion, there is a potential for the development of a vicious cycle within the ovary that would inhibit follicle development. Alternatively, a defect in the IGF system could cause an alteration of the set point for the response of the granulosa cell to FSH. Mason and coworkers suggested that LH acts on granulosa cells in the presence of insulin, thereby leading to premature luteinization, maturational arrest and excess androgen production.[25]

In summary, as a consequence of dysregulation of androgen synthesis within the ovary, women with PCOS have ovarian hyper-responsiveness to gonadotropins: that of thecal cells to LH explaining the excess androgens, and that of granulosa cells to FSH leading to increased estrogens.

The hypothalamic–pituitary–ovarian axis

Serum LH concentrations are significantly elevated in PCOS women as compared with controls.[29,30] This is due to an increased amplitude and frequency of LH pulses.[31] Elevated LH concentrations (above the 95th percentile of normal) can be observed in approximately 40–60% of PCOS women.[1,11,32] An elevated serum LH concentration has been associated with a reduced chance of conception and an increased risk of miscarriage.[33] LH levels are influenced by the temporal relation to ovulation, which transiently normalizes LH due to the suppressive effect of progesterone, and by body weight, which is higher in lean women with PCOS. While an elevation in serum LH concentration is pathognomonic of PCOS (in the absence of the mid-cycle preovulatory LH surge or the menopause transition), a measured elevation of LH is not required to make the diagnosis. No longer either is an elevated LH to FSH ratio required or useful.[34]

The pituitary gonadotroph is central to reproductive function – its production and secretion of FSH and LH is directly stimulated by

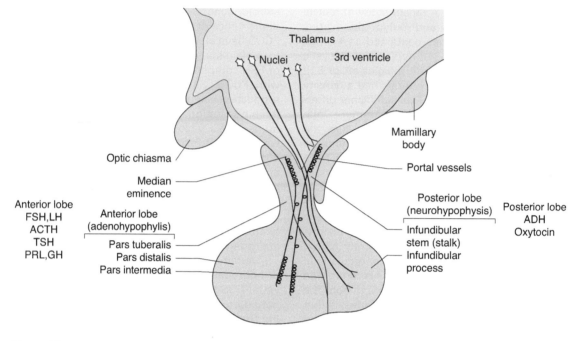

Figure 4.3

The hypothalamus and pituitary. TSH: thyroid stimulating hormone; PRL: prolactin; GH: growth hormone; ADH: antidiuretic hormone.

hypothalamic GnRH and is also influenced by integrated feedback mechanisms. FSH provides the initial stimulus for follicular development and also promotes granulosa cell conversion of androgens to estrogens by stimulating the aromatase enzymes. LH, classically known for its role in the luteal phase by promoting progesterone secretion, also has a vital role in the follicular phase, inducing thecal androgen production (the substrate for estrogen synthesis) and initiating oocyte maturation at midcycle.

A single hypothalamic decapeptide, GnRH, stimulates the release of both LH and FSH from the gonadotroph.[35] Pulsatile GnRH stimulation is required to maintain gonadotropin secretion, whereas the continuous exposure of the pituitary to GnRH results in desensitization and a suppression of gonadotropin secretion.[36] Changes in the pulsatility of GnRH are thought to alter the ratio of secretion of the two pituitary gonadotropins throughout the menstrual cycle. When GnRH pulsatility is slow, FSH secretion predominates,

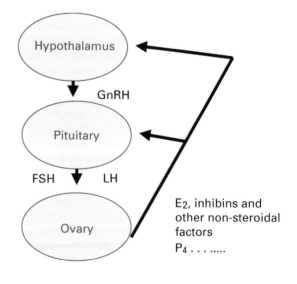

Figure 4.4

The hypothalamic–pituitary–ovarian axis.

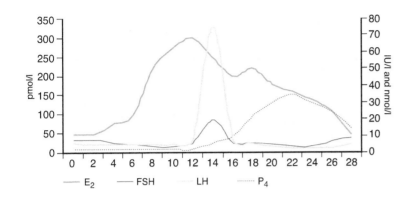

Figure 4.5

The normal menstrual cycle.
E_2: estradiol
FSH: follicle stimulating hormone
LH: luteinizing hormone
P_4: progesterone

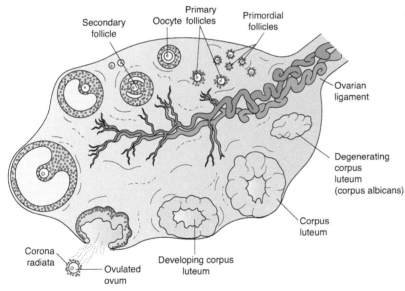

Figure 4.6

Structure of an ovary

and when rapid LH secretion predominates.[37] The action of GnRH is modulated at the level of the pituitary, thereby resulting in differential production and secretion of the two gonadotropins. GnRH both causes release of LH and FSH and has a self-potentiating effect on the gonadotroph.[38] The primary release of gonadotropins, and their secondary synthesis and storage have been termed the first and second pools of gonadotropins respectively. Pituitary responsive-ness to GnRH is increased by the self-priming action of GnRH, which is defined as the protein synthesis-dependent increase in GnRH-stimulated gonadotropin secretion, caused by previous exposure of the pituitary gland to GnRH.[39]

The sensitivity of the pituitary to GnRH varies during the menstrual cycle in synchrony with changes in circulating estradiol (E_2) concentrations.[40] In the early follicular phase, when E_2 levels are low, pituitary sensitivity and gonadotropin

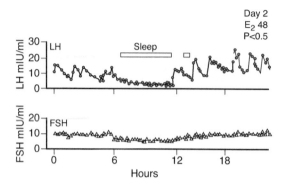

Figure 4.7

Normal female gonadotropin physiology. Early follicular phase (days −13 to −9). Sampling every 10 minutes. Pulse frequency 90 minutes. Absence during sleep.[131]

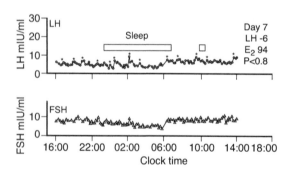

Figure 4.8

Mid-follicular phase (days −8 to −5). Pulse frequency 60 minutes. Reduced amplitude. No suppression during sleep.[137]

content are at a minimum; as E_2 levels rise, consequent upon follicular development, both sensitivity and content increase – particularly the latter, as E_2 has a stimulating effect on pituitary synthesis and storage and promotes the self-priming effect of GnRH on the pituitary.[40] At the time of the midcycle surge, sensitivity to GnRH is maximal, with the resultant release of large amounts of gonadotropins. Estradiol also potentiates GnRH

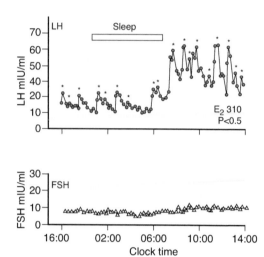

Figure 4.9

Late follicular phase (days −4 to 0). Shown on day of surge. Pulse frequency ≤60 minutes. Increased amplitude.[137]

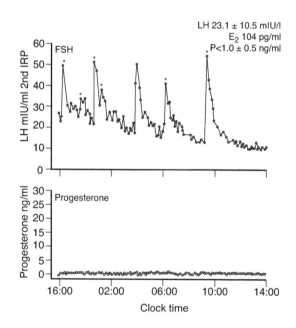

Figure 4.10

Early luteal phase (days +1 to +4). Pulse frequency 100 minutes. Bimodal LH; tonic progesterone secretion.[137]

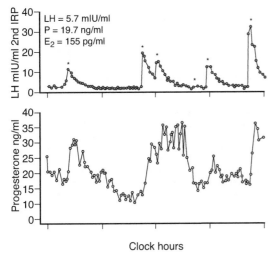

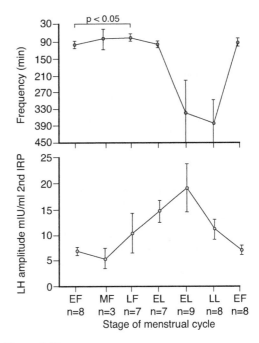

Figure 4.11

Mid-luteal phase (days +5 to +9). Pulse frequency 240 minutes pulsatile progesterone secretion.[137]

Figure 4.13

LH pulse frequency and amplitude through the menstrual cycle.[137]

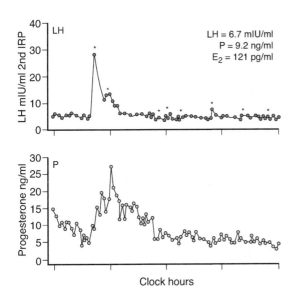

Figure 4.12

Late luteal phase (days +10 to +14). Pulse frequency increasing. Low amplitude – lowest before menses. Return of sleep-associated suspension.[137]

responsiveness, increasing the number of GnRH receptors by directly stimulating the protein synthesis required for receptor formation.

The arcuate nucleus of the hypothalamus acts as a transducer for neuronal into endocrine signals, although the cellular nature of the GnRH 'pulse generator' is still unknown. Here the GnRH-secreting neurons act in a pulsatile manner, with varying frequencies throughout the normal ovulatory cycle, resulting in variable frequencies and amplitudes of gonadotropin release. The control of the rhythmicity of the GnRH pulse generator is not fully understood. Although there does not appear to be feedback from within the pituitary itself.[41] Gonadal steroids and other factors modulate GnRH action at the pituitary level, and possibly also at the level of the hypothalamus.

Some of the factors that influence GnRH activity include β-endorphin and opiate peptides, angiotensin II, serotonin, neuropeptide-Y, neurotensin, somatostatin, corticotropin releasing factor, dopamine, melatonin, norepinephrine (noradenaline), oxytocin and substance P. The interrelationship of these factors is unclear. Endogenous opioid tone is important in the regulation of LH and prolactin secretion. Opioids, such as β-endorphin, inhibit GnRH release from the human mediobasal hypothalamus. It has been postulated that withdrawal of endogenous opioid tone in the presence of sufficient quantities of estradiol may contribute to the initiation of the LH surge. When opioid tone decreases, a chain of neurosecretory events is initiated, which, in the rat, activates neuropeptide-Y neurons which in turn, either alone or together with adrenergic transmitters, stimulate secretion of GnRH. The effects of opioids appear to be dependent upon the steroid hormone environment, in particular estrogen, whose effect is augmented by progesterone:[42] thus the administration of an opioid antagonist, such as naloxone, during the early follicular phase has little effect on gonadotropin levels, while greater effects are observed midcycle and the greatest effects are seen in the luteal phase.[42]

Circulating steroid levels also influence GnRH metabolism by altering the activity of proteolytic enzymes in the pituitary and peripheral circulation. For example, estradiol has been shown to inhibit degradation of GnRH in rat and monkey pituitaries, and may thus enhance GnRH activity under conditions of high serum estradiol concentrations.[43] Perhaps steroids also play such a role in women with PCOS.

Tonic hypersecretion of LH in women with PCOS has been suggested as being caused by, at least in part, a combination of diminished opioid and dopaminergic tone.[44,45] There is also evidence that adrenergic activity is altered in women who hypersecrete LH.[46,47] Women with PCOS were found to be very sensitive to exogenous dopamine and it was proposed that these women had a deficiency in endogenous dopaminergic inhibition of GnRH secretion.[44] In normal women, both dopamine receptor antagonists such as metoclopramide, and opiate receptor antagonists such as naloxone, elicit a rise in serum LH concentrations.[45] Conversely, administration of synthetic β-endorphin elicits a fall in serum LH concentration. In women with PCOS, the administration of metoclopramide, naloxone and β-endorphin did not alter LH secretory activity. It was therefore proposed that an underlying hypothalamic defect

might lead to hypersecretion of LH, through a reduction in endogenous dopaminergic and opioid control of GnRH secretion.[45]

Barnes and Lobo in 1985 performed naloxone infusion experiments in women with PCOS and weight-matched controls, and found that LH responses were similar. Pretreatment with L-dopa-carbidopa for one week resulted in an absence of naloxone-stimulated LH increase in normal women, but an exaggerated response of the rise in LH after naloxone in women with PCOS.[48] It was suggested that central opioid tone is not decreased in PCOS and that dopaminergic tone and/or the interaction between the dopamine and opioid system might be altered in PCOS. Further studies failed to demonstrate major alterations in brain dopaminergic activity in women with PCOS,[49] although it is difficult to study the physiology of brain dopamine. Berga and Yen administered both progestogens and opioid antagonists to women with PCOS, and found that there was an apparent link between an impairment of opioid and progesterone secretion in the genesis of hypersecretion of LH.[50] Yoshino et al. studied women with PCOS and found abnormalities not only in dopamine metabolites but also in adrenergic metabolites.[47] It was also demonstrated that four weeks' treatment with naltrexone reduced pituitary sensitivity to GnRH in PCOS patients,[51] and so the question of the precise role of endogenous opioids in the control of LH secretion is unresolved.

The interactions of factors at the level of the hypothalamus are therefore complex, and the factors that predominate in influencing LH secretion are unknown. Schoemaker reviewed the subject of neuroendocrine control in PCOS and found a number of contrasting and sometimes contradictory theories.[52] He concluded that central disturbances in PCOS (that is at the level of the hypothalamus and pituitary) are secondary to 'one or more peripheral factors, which may be ovarian in origin'.

An area of some further controversy is whether there is an increase in GnRH pulse frequency in women who hypersecrete LH. This is important for, if steroids are the main ovarian product to influence LH secretion, they are able to cross the blood–brain barrier and so might be expected to affect GnRH pulsatility also. If, however, the primary defect is through perturbed secretion of an ovarian peptide, it would not be predicted to cross the blood–brain barrier to affect GnRH pulse frequency. While there is no disputing the increase in pulse amplitude, some studies have also described an increase in pulse frequency of LH.[31,53,54] Many groups, however, have failed to detect an increase in pulse frequency.[55–60] Some studies have also demonstrated an alteration of the circadian rhythm of LH secretion, with a persistance of high-amplitude LH pulses during the night.[58] The differing conclusions may result from different study populations; for this reason, differences in pulse frequency that have been detected may be too small to represent a central role for a primary disturbance of the hypothalamus in the hypersecretion of LH. Murdoch and coworkers, who extensively investigated the variability of LH measurements in women with PCOS, found good reproducibility with repeated studies over a one-year period.[60] They also assessed LH pulsatility by time-series analysis, which takes into consideration the complicated patterns of LH secretion that occur as superimposed pulses of differing frequency. No difference in pulse frequency was detected between nine patients with PCOS and 12 normal women.[60]

It has been found that some women with HH also have polycystic ovaries detected by pelvic ultrasound, and when these women were treated with pulsatile GnRH to induce ovulation they had significantly higher serum LH concentrations than women with HH and normal ovaries.[61] Furthermore, the elevation in LH concentration was observed before serum estradiol concentrations rose. Thus hypersecretion of LH occurred in these women when the hypothalamus was replaced by an artificial GnRH pulse generator (i.e. the GnRH pump), with a fixed GnRH pulse interval of 90 minutes (equivalent to the pulse interval in the early follicular phase). These results suggest that the cause of hypersecretion of LH involves a perturbation of ovarian–pituitary feedback, rather than a primary disturbance of hypothalamic pulse regulation.

The data collected in women with PCOS undergoing laparoscopic ovarian diathermy are also consistent with the hypothesis that it is altered ovarian–pituitary feedback that causes hypersecretion of LH. In these patients, LH pulse amplitude decreased but no change in the (normal) pulse frequency was detected after the procedure.[62] Rossmanith et al found an attenuation of GnRH-stimulated LH secretion after laparoscopic ovarian diathermy, a result consistent with abnormalities in the production of an ovarian factor(s) that regulates LH secretion, rather than with the theory that the disorder starts at the level of either the hypothalamus or pituitary.[63]

Glycosylation of luteinizing hormone

LH exists in multiple forms in both the pituitary gland and the peripheral circulation, primarily because of the considerable variations in the oligosaccharide side chains which may result in numerous LH 'glycoforms'.[64] The alpha- and beta-subunits of LH each have two N-linked glycosylation sites, and oligosaccharides form about 30% of the molecule. Individual glycoforms cannot be isolated and even the recently available recombinant gonadotrophins are likely to have a variety of glycoforms. The glycosylation isoforms that are more basic have a shorter half-life and a lower in vivo activity than the acidic isoforms, although, conversely, the basic isoforms have a higher biopotency, with higher receptor binding, steroidogenic and intracellular cAMP-stimulating ability in vitro. These differences are not recognized by either immunoassays (as antibodies do not recognize oligosaccharides) or in vitro bioassays, which are not dependent on in vivo clearance mechanisms. Lectins bind to oligosaccharides and might have a future role to play in two-site lectin/antibody assays.

LH is probably modified in the circulation, for example by proteolytic cleavage of part of the beta-chain ('nicking').[65] Human chorionic gonadotropin (hCG) differs from LH by having a single additional C-terminal peptide. There is evidence that hCG itself is secreted by the normal pituitary and may circulate at concentrations of about 1% of that of LH.[64]

Exposure of the pituitary to different serum concentrations of steroids may affect glycosylation and hence bioactivity of LH, which in turn may influence ovarian steroid production. While animal studies have shown that gonadal steroids may act directly at the pituitary to control the biopotency of stored and secreted gonadotropins, it is uncertain whether LH bioactivity is affected by the chronic alterations in steroid hormone secretion that are seen in women with the polycystic ovary syndrome. Some studies have shown that bioactive serum concentrations of LH are elevated in these patients [66–70]. Lobo et al[66] suggested that the level of bioactive LH may be a more useful marker than the immunoactive LH concentration or the LH:FSH ratio, although the degree of bioactivity did not correlate with dopaminergic activity or serum estradiol concentrations.[67] Fauser et al[68] found that bioactive LH levels correlated better with symptoms of PCOS (oligo-/amenorrhea) than did serum LH concentrations as measured by immunoradiometric assay (IRMA).[29] It has been suggested that women with PCOS may secrete LH isoforms with a high biological activity.[66] Further evidence for this was obtained by Ding and Huhtaniemi[69] who performed isoelectric focusing on serum from women with normal and elevated concentrations of LH. They found that those with high serum LH concentrations had the majority of LH isoforms distributed with an alkaline isoelectric point and this correlated with a high biological activity.

Circulating serum concentrations of estradiol, estrone, androstenedione, testosterone or dehydroepiandrosterone sulfate (DHEAS) were not found to correlate with either the bioactive or immunoreactive LH levels.[69] Experiments in non-human primates have demonstrated that the administration of different doses of GnRH results in pituitary secretion of LH isoforms of varying bioactivity.[70] The pituitaries of women with PCOS might be sensitized to GnRH such that higher-activity LH isoforms are secreted than in women with normal ovaries. It might be that a nonsteroidal messenger from the ovary affects this phenomenon.

A genetic variant of LH (vLH) has been described with two missense point mutations in the LHβ gene (Trp^{8}Arg and Ile^{15}Thr), initially reported from Finland but now recognized as a common polymorphism with worldwide distribution and a mean population carrier frequency of 18.5% (28.9% in Finland, 16.8% in the UK, 14.1% in the US and 11.2% in the Netherlands).[71] The biological activity of vLH is greater than wild-type LH in vitro, while its half-life in the circulation is shorter and the overall effect on in vivo bioactivity is unclear. The vLH carrier frequency appears similar in obese and non-obese controls but lower in obese subjects with PCOS. The authors suggest that obese women with

vLH might be protected from developing symptomatic PCOS while those with wild-type LH may be more liable to develop the syndrome. Interestingly, of the four countries studied, this relationship was true for all but those from the UK who exhibited a higher frequency of vLH in obese PCOS individuals than obese controls.

Insulin stimulates pituitary gonadotropin secretion, at least in vitro.[72] It has therefore been proposed that the hyperinsulinemia that is seen in many women with PCOS might have a causal relationship with hypersecretion of LH. Antilla et al studied obese and non-obese women with PCOS and found that the non-obese women had elevated serum concentrations of bioactive LH and the obese women tended to have normal serum concentrations of bioactive LH.[72] These differences could not be attributed to serum androgen concentrations. It was noted that bioactive, but not immunoactive, LH levels related to the serum insulin concentration, and Antilla proposed that the degree of hyperinsulinemia in obese, insulin-resistant subjects had a direct effect on the glycosylation of LH.[72]

Women with PCOS often hypersecrete LH and this may result in increased theca cell androgen secretion. A study of 556 women with polycystic ovaries demonstrated that the patients with the highest serum LH concentrations did not have the highest serum testosterone concentrations.[74] Indeed, it has been shown that lean women with PCOS and normal fasting serum insulin concentrations have higher serum LH concentrations than lean or obese women with polycystic ovaries, and elevated fasting insulin levels.[75] Furthermore, it was found that lean and obese women with polycystic ovaries and elevated fasting insulin levels had higher serum testosterone concentrations than women with normal insulin levels, suggesting a stronger relationship between androgen secretion and circulating insulin levels than with LH.

Steroidal feedback on LH secretion

In their studies on the functional capacity of the human gonadotroph, with respect to its sensitivity to GnRH and its reserve storage of gonadotropins, Lasley et al examined the effects of estradiol and progesterone administration on GnRH-stimulated gonadotropin secretion in normal women in the follicular phase of their cycle.[76] They found that estradiol increased pituitary gonadotropin secretion and this was augmented by the addition of progesterone – the effects being similar on FSH and LH secretion. The physiological significance of the amplification effect of progesterone on the estrogen-primed pituitary is uncertain. Many studies have shown that various doses of exogenous estrogen are able to induce an LH surge in monkeys and women.[77,78] Both estradiol and progesterone also inhibit pituitary gonadotrophin secretion, and the differential effects may be dose- and time-dependent.[79] The main effect of progesterone has been proposed as being at the level of the hypothalamus,[77] although the finding of progesterone receptors on monkey gonadotrophs suggests a direct effect at the level of the pituitary also.[78] It is unlikely that progesterone plays a role in hypersecretion of LH as it is secreted in negligible quantities during the follicular phase of women with both normal and high serum concentrations of LH.[80]

In a study of women with PCOS, Baird and coworkers found that serum LH concentrations were lower after an ovulatory cycle than after a period of anovulation.[55] They also found that anovulatory women responded to exogenous GnRH by secreting larger pulses of LH than ovulatory women with PCOS, who did not differ in their response from women with normal ovaries. From these observations it was suggested that hypersecretion of LH was secondary to the increased secretion of ovarian steroids during periods of anovulation – in particular androgens which were then metabolized to estrone in the peripheral fat. Ovulatory women with polycystic ovaries, however, have also been shown to have higher serum concentrations of LH than ovulatory women with normal ovaries.[80,81] Women with polycystic ovaries treated with gonadotropins to induce ovulation have also been shown to have an elevated serum concentration of LH at a time when they might be expected to have suppressed LH levels due to the ovarian secretion of LH-inhibitory factor(s).[82,83] These data support the notion that women with PCOS have a perturbation of ovarian–pituitary feedback control of LH secretion – even in the presence of exogenous gonadotrophins.

The precise role of estrone in gonadotropin secretion is not known. Plasma concentrations of estrone are elevated in some women with PCOS,

and it has been postulated that estrone may play a role in the hypersecretion of LH that is seen in these women.[53,84] The administration of exogenous estrone to women with normal or polycystic ovaries over periods of 5–15 days did not, however, increase serum LH levels or the sensitivity of the pituitary to exogenously administered GnRH.[85]

Estrogens have also been shown to be inhibitory to GnRH-mediated gonadotropin secretion, usually in a biphasic pattern, with a subsequent stimulatory effect that may be secondary to a direct effect on the number of available GnRH receptors.[86–88] It appears that in pituitary cell cultures a four-hour exposure to estradiol decreases the rat pituitary response to GnRH, while a longer exposure of 24–48 hours is required before the response to GnRH is augmented. The cellular mechanisms that result in this inhibitory effect are still to be elucidated. The concentration of estradiol is critical, as high concentrations decrease the response, creating a bell-shaped dose–response curve.[88] When estradiol was administered to both anovulatory and ovulatory hyperandrogenemic women with PCOS, there was no difference in the suppression of serum LH concentrations, which were also no different from those in normal controls.[89]

Androgens have been shown to inhibit gonadotropin secretion by decreasing the number of GnRH receptors in a pituicyte culture,[90] and post-receptor events also appear to be affected by androgens. Studies in female-to-male transsexuals demonstrated that large doses of testosterone failed to block an estradiol-induced LH surge.[91] It therefore appears that androgens do not play a significant role in the genesis of the LH surge, or, for that matter, in normal secretion of LH. The polycystic ovary often over-secretes androgens, which are metabolized to estrogens. Exogenously administered androgens do not result in an elevation of either LH pulse amplitude or frequency, whether administered acutely or long term. Indeed supraphysiological levels of testosterone suppress LH secretion.[92]

Non-steroidal feedback on luteinizing hormone secretion

Since the isolation and characterization of inhibin it has become apparent that not only are there several members of the inhibin family of glyco-protein hormones, but there are also other non-steroidal gonadal signals that influence gonadotropin secretion and help to fine-tune reproductive function. It has been established that ovarian inhibin exerts negative feedback on pituitary gonadotropin production, preferentially affecting FSH.[93] More recently a feedback pathway that influences pituitary LH secretion has been proposed, following in vivo and in vitro evidence that has suggested the presence of a putative inhibitory peptide which has been named gonadotropin surge-inhibiting or -attenu-ating factor (GnSIF/GnSAF).[94,95] The proposed actions of GnSIF and GnSAF are similar, although this will only be confirmed if and when they are purified.

Before the recognition of the complex endocrine and paracrine mechanisms that control ovulation, the hypothesized mechanism for the pre-ovulatory gonadotropin surge was, perhaps, improbably simple (Figure 4.5). The classical theory was that when a critical level of estradiol was secreted by the ovary, this steroid hormone switched from a negative to a positive feedback effect both on hypothalamic pulsatility of GnRH and pituitary secretion of the gonadotropins. In recent years, the use of superovulation regimens for assisted conception procedures has provided further insight into the mechanism of ovulation itself: for, in spite of supraphysiological levels of estradiol in the early follicular phase of stimulated cycles, the pre-ovulatory LH surge does not commence earlier in the cycle and when it does occur it is usually significantly attenuated. This phenomenon has led to the realization that there may be an additional factor(s) produced by the developing ovarian follicle(s) that suppresses pituitary secretion of LH.

An area of controversy is whether there is an increase in GnRH pulse frequency in women who hypersecrete LH. This is important for, if steroids are the main ovarian product to influence LH secre-tion, they are able to cross the blood–brain barrier and so might be expected to affect GnRH pulsatility also. If, however, the primary defect is through perturbed secretion of an ovarian peptide, it would not be predicted to cross the blood–brain barrier to affect GnRH pulse frequency.

We have described the observation that women with HH and polycystic ovaries, when treated with pulsatile GnRH had significantly higher serum LH concentrations than women with HH and normal ovaries.[61] Furthermore, the elevation in LH concentration was observed before serum estra-diol concentrations rose. Thus hypersecretion of LH occurred in these women when the hypothala-mus was replaced by an artificial GnRH pulse generator. These results suggest that the cause of hypersecretion of LH involves a perturbation of ovarian–pituitary feedback, and are also consis-tent with the notion that there may be a non-steroidal factor(s) that disturbs ovarian–pituitary feedback control of LH secretion.[61]

The data collected in women with PCOS under-going laparoscopic ovarian diathermy are also consistent with the hypothesis that it is altered ovarian–pituitary feedback that causes hyper-secretion of LH. In these patients, LH pulse ampli-tude decreased but no change in the (normal) pulse frequency was detected after the proce-dure.[62,63]

We performed a prospective study to compare unilateral with bilateral ovarian diathermy in order to observe which ovary responded by ovulating.[96] Three of the four patients who received unilateral diathermy ovulated, all from the contralateral ovary in the first cycle and then alternately from each ovary. There were no signif-icant differences between the baseline hormone measurements of the responders and those of the non-responders. When the pre- and post-treat-ment values were compared, there were no differ-ences in the serum FSH and testosterone concentrations in either the responders or the non-responders. In the responders, however, there was a significant fall of the serum LH concentration after LOD ($p = 0.045$, 95% confi-dence interval (CI) 0.2–13.4), while in the non-responders there was no difference in the LH concentrations before and after treatment.

The mechanism of ovulation induction by LOD is uncertain. It appears, however, that minimal damage to an unresponsive ovary either restores an ovulatory cycle or increases the sensitivity of the ovary to exogenous stimulation. Furthermore, the finding of an attenuated response of LH secre-tion to stimulation with GnRH suggests an affect on ovarian–pituitary feedback and hence pituitary sensitivity to GnRH. Our study goes one step further by demonstrating that unilateral dia-thermy leads to bilateral ovarian activity, showing conclusively for the first time, that ovarian diathermy achieves its effect by correcting a perturbation of ovarian–pituitary feedback. Our own hypothesis is that the response of the ovary to injury leads to a local cascade of growth factors and those such as IGF-I, which interact with FSH, result in stimulation of follicular growth and then ovarian–pituitary feedback leads to a fall in serum LH concentrations.[96]

Ovarian peptide hormones have important effects on pituitary gonadotropin secretion. Inhibin and its related peptides act primarily on FSH secretion. Inhibin has been shown to have effects, at different concentrations and in differing conditions, on both basal secretion of FSH and GnRH-stimulated FSH and LH.[97] The proposed existence of GnSAF is an attractive, although unproven hypothesis for the differential regulation of LH secretion. GnSAF is an inhibitory factor, different from inhibin, that is produced by ovarian follicles and which suppresses GnRH-stimulated LH, and possibly also FSH, secretion. The hypothesis is that GnSAF antagonizes the priming of the pituitary gland by GnRH, and raises its threshold to the action of GnRH, preventing a premature LH surge. The surge may then occur when elevated serum estradiol concentrations increase the sensitivity of the pituitary to GnRH, so overriding the inhibitory factor.[98]

There has been debate as to whether the putative GnSAF could in fact be inhibin. Culler gave FSH to rats and found that the pre-ovulatory gonadotrophin surge of FSH and LH was inhibited; this effect was reversed by the administration of an anti-inhibin antibody, which suggested that inhibin was responsible for these observations.[99] However, using Culler's anti-inhibin antibody we demonstrated that GnSAF bioactivity in human follicular fluid is retained after treatment with anti-inhibin.[100] It would seem reasonable to postulate that inhibin and other non-steroidal hormones have effects at different stages of the cycle and at different serum concentrations in the 'fine-tuning' of pituitary secretion of the gonadotropins.

Abnormalities of inhibin secretion have long been implicated in the pathogenesis of PCOS, with the notion that hypersecretion of inhibin-B by the ovary suppresses pituitary secretion of FSH, to cause the relative imbalance in gonadotropin concentrations observed in these patients.[101] A series of experiments has demonstrated significantly elevated serum levels of inhibin-B in women with PCOS, which has been postulated as being responsible both for the reversed FSH:LH ratio and the increased sensitivity of the polycystic ovary to exogenous FSH.[102]

Gonadotropin biosynthesis and secretion are influenced by hypothalamic, paracrine, and endocrine factors and there is considerable overlap between all three. The influence of non-steroidal factors on pituitary and hypothalamic function is still being elucidated. Further work is required to examine both the pathophysiology of hypersecretion of LH and its effects at the level of the oocyte.

Hyperinsulinemia

The association between insulin resistance, compensatory hyperinsulinemia and hyperandrogenism has provided insight into the pathogenesis of PCOS.[103] The cellular and molecular mechanisms of insulin resistance in PCOS have been extensively investigated and it is evident that the major defect is a decrease in insulin sensitivity secondary to a post-binding abnormality in insulin receptor-mediated signal transduction, with a less substantial, but significant, decrease in insulin responsiveness.[104] It appears that decreased insulin sensitivity in PCOS is potentially an intrinsic defect in genetically susceptible women, since it is independent of obesity, metabolic abnormalities, body fat topography and sex hormone levels. There may be genetic abnormalities in the regulation of insulin receptor phosphorylation, resulting in increased insulin-independent serine phosphorylation, and decreased insulin-dependent tyrosine phosphorylation.[104,105]

Although the insulin resistance may occur irrespective of BMI, the common association of PCOS with obesity has a synergistic deleterious impact on glucose homeostasis and can worsen both hyperandrogenism and anovulation. An assessment of BMI alone is not thought to provide a reliable prediction of cardiovascular risk. It has been reported that the association between BMI and coronary heart disease almost disappeared after correction for dyslipidemia, hyperglycemia and hypertension.[106] Some women have profound metabolic abnormalities in the presence of a normal BMI and others have few risk factors with an elevated BMI.[107,108] It has been suggested that rather than BMI itself, it is the distribution of fat that is important, with android obesity being more

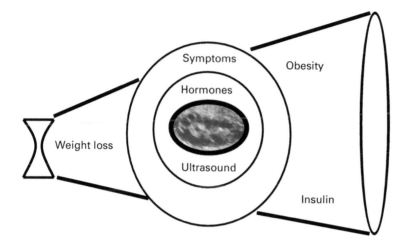

Figure 4.14

Amplification of signs and symptoms of polycystic ovary syndrome with increasing obesity and insulin resistance.

of a risk factor than gynecoid obesity.[107] Hence the value of measuring waist:hip ratio, or waist circumference, which detects abdominal visceral fat rather than subcutaneous fat. It is the visceral fat which is metabolically active and which, when increased, results in increased rates of insulin resistance, type 2 diabetes, dyslipidemia, hypertension and left ventricular enlargement (Figure 4.15).[107] Exercise has a significant effect on reducing visceral fat and reducing cardiovascular risk.

Lord and colleagues have found a closer link between waist circumference and visceral fat mass, as assessed by computed tomography (CT) scan, than with waist:hip ratio or BMI (Figure 7.2).[107] Waist circumference should ideally be less than 79 cm, while a measurement that is greater than 87 cm carries a significant risk.

Insulin acts through multiple sites to increase endogenous androgen levels. Increased peripheral insulin resistance results in a higher serum insulin concentration. Excess insulin binds to the IGF-1 receptors which enhances the theca cells' androgen production in response to LH stimulation.[109] Hyperinsulinemia also decreases the synthesis of SHBG by the liver. Therefore, there is an increase in serum free-testosterone (T) concentration, and consequent peripheral androgen action. In addition, hyperinsulinemia inhibits the hepatic secretion of insulin-like growth factor binding protein-1 (IGFBP-1) leading to increased bio-availability of IGF-1 and 2,[110,111] the important regulators of ovarian follicular maturation and steroidogenesis.[112] Together with more IGF-2

'Compensated' insulin resistance
with normal glucose tolerance
↓
Impaired glucose tolerance (IGT)
Pancreatic β-cell dysfunction
↓
Type 2 diabetes

Figure 4.15

Progression through to impaired glucose tolerance and type 2 diabetes mellitus.

secretion from the theca cells, IGF-1 and 2 further augment ovarian androgen production by acting on IGF-1 receptors.[113,114]

Insulin may also increase endogenous androgen concentrations by increased cytochrome P450c17α enzyme activity, which is important for ovarian and adrenal steroid hormone biosynthesis. Insulin-induced overactivity of P450c17α and an exaggerated serum 17-hydroxyprogesterone (17-OHP) response to stimulation by GnRHa have also been demonstrated.[18,115,116] Intra-ovarian androgen excess is responsible for anovulation by acting directly on the ovary promoting the process of follicular atresia.[79,117] This latter process is characterized by apoptosis of granulosa cells. As a consequence there is an increasingly larger stromal compartment, which retains LH responsiveness and continues to secrete androgens.

Insulin resistance is defined as a reduced glucose response to a given amount of insulin and may occur secondary to resistance at the insulin receptor, decreased hepatic clearance of insulin and/or increased pancreatic sensitivity. Both obese and non-obese women with PCOS are more insulin-resistant and hyperinsulinemic than age- and weight-matched women with normal ovaries.[118,119] Thus there appear to be factors in women with PCOS that promote insulin resistance and that are independent of obesity.[120] Pancreatic beta-cell dysfunction has been described in women with PCOS, whereby there is increased basal secretion of insulin yet an inadequate post-prandial response.[121] This defect remains even after weight loss, despite an improvement in glucose tolerance.[122]

Insulin acts through its receptor to initiate a cascade of post-receptor events within the target cell. Phosphorylation causes insulin receptor substrates (IRS1–4) to promote glucose uptake via the transmembrane glucose transporter (GLUT4), and also intracellular protein synthesis. Tyrosine phosphorylation increases the tyrosine kinase activity of the insulin receptor, while serine phosphorylation inhibits it, and it appears that at least 50% of women with PCOS have excessive serine phosphorylation and inhibition of normal signaling.[120] This affects only glucose homeostasis and not the other pleiotropic actions of insulin, so that cell growth and protein synthesis may continue.[121] Serine phosphorylation also increases activity of P450c17 in both the ovary and adrenal, thus promoting androgen synthesis,[122] and so this may be a mechanism for both insulin resistance and hyperandrogenism in some women with PCOS (see Figures 5.5 and 5.6).

The evolution of polycystic ovary syndrome through adolescence

PCOS appears to have its origins during adolescence and is thought to be associated with increased weight gain during puberty.[123] However, the polycystic ovary gene(s) has not yet been identified and the effect of environmental influences such as weight changes and circulating hormone concentrations, and the age at which these occur

are still being unravelled. Detecting polycystic ovaries in girls relies upon transabdominal scanning, which in a study by Fox et al in adults failed to detect 30% of polycystic ovaries, compared with a 100% detection rate with a transvaginal scan.[124] Bridges et al performed 428 ovarian scans in girls aged between three and 18 years, and found polycystic ovaries in 101 girls (24% of the total).[125] The rate of detection of polycystic ovaries was 6% in six-year-old girls, rising to 18% in those aged 10 years and 26% in those aged 15 years. The implication of this study is that polycystic ovaries are present before puberty and are more easy to detect in older girls as the ovaries increase in size.

Prior to puberty, there appear to be two periods of increased ovarian growth. The first is at adrenarche in response to increased concentrations of circulating androgens, and the second is just before and during puberty due to rising gonadotropin levels, the actions of growth hormone and IGF-1 and insulin on the ovary. Sampaolo et al reported a study of 49 obese girls at different stages of puberty, comparing their pelvic ultrasound features and endocrine profiles with 35 age- and pubertal stage-matched controls.[126] They found that obesity was associated with a significant increase in uterine and ovarian volume. They also found obese post-menarchal girls with polycystic ovaries had larger uterine and ovarian volumes than obese post-menarchal girls with normal ovaries. Sampaolo concluded that obesity leads to hyperinsulinism, which causes both hyperandrogenemia and raised IGF-1 levels, which augments the ovarian response to gonadotropins.[126] This implies that obesity may be important in the pathogenesis of polycystic ovaries, but further study is required to evaluate this. It is known that obesity is not a prerequisite for PCOS. Indeed, in a series of 1741 women with polycystic ovaries in a study by Balen et al, only 38.4% of patients were overweight (BMI >25 kg/m²).[127]

As well as association of tall stature and obesity with PCOS, a high prevalence has also been noted in a number of conditions associated with hyperinsulinemia. PCOS is common in subjects with genetic defects of the insulin receptor, and congenital lypodystrophy. It has also been observed in children with glycogen storage disease treated with high doses of oral glucose, and in adolescents with type 1 diabetes where there are inappropriately high levels of circulating insulin. Thus during childhood, as in adult life, high circulating levels of insulin from whatever cause may be a trigger for the subsequent development of polycystic ovaries.

Adrenarche and PCOS

In the study reported by Bridges et al adrenarche was associated with an increased prevalence of PCOS on ultrasound.[125] Adrenarche has always been considered to be a benign condition, but recent work from several groups has suggested that, along with premature pubarche, it may in some populations be associated with insulin resistance. In a series of elegant studies, Ibanez et al have shown that girls presenting with premature adrenarche and pubarche may be more insulin resistant than controls and are at high risk of developing ovarian hyperandrogenism after menarche.[128] This association was particularly strong in girls who are born small for gestational age. However, this low birth weight, premature pubarche, insulin resistance, ovarian hyperandrogenism sequence is not necessarily associated with ovarian morphological features of polycystic ovaries; instead small ovaries have been reported.

The association between PCOS and insulin resistance, together with links with type 2 diabetes and gestational diabetes (GDM), have led to the suggestion that PCOS could be related to a 'thrifty ovary'; this would enhance fertility during periods of poor nutrition and only lead to infertility and associated problems with improved nutrition. Similarly, insulin resistance per se may be a survival mechanism whereby growth is maintained during poor nutrition, and risks for GDM and type 2 diabetes only become apparent with increased weight gain. The INS VNTR class III/III genotype, as well as links with PCOS, GDM and type 2 diabetes, may also represent a putative 'thrifty genotype' by conferring larger size at birth, and thus potentially increased perinatal survival in the face of maternal/fetal nutritional deprivation (see also Chapter 5).

Higher birthweight has been associated with adult risk of polycystic ovaries in historical,[129] and more contemporary, cohorts.[130] These data indicate that the risk for PCOS may originate in early prenatal development and could be influenced by both uterine environment and/or fetal genotype. The larger size at birth associated with INS VNTR III/III genotype may reflect intrinsic

insulin resistance in the fetus. In other infants, larger size at birth could reflect fetal hyperinsulinemia secondary to increased placental transfer of glucose, as observed in infants of diabetic mothers. Exposure to high levels of insulin, by either mechanism, could predispose to the development of polycystic ovaries.

Paradoxically, insulin resistance, ovarian hyperandrogenism and ovarian dysfunction have also been associated with low birthweight. These links with low birthweight and postnatal catch-up growth are seen not only in girls presenting with premature pubarche (PP) but also in non-selected low birthweight infants,[128,131] and correspond to well-replicated low birthweight associations with type 2 diabetes risk.[132] Our recent data indicate that this phenotype in PP girls is independently associated with both low birthweight and the INS VNTR genotype class I allele, which although associated with lower birthweight, confers increased postnatal insulin secretion and greater weight gain. However, this low birthweight, postnatal catch-up growth, hyperinsulinemia and ovarian hyperandrogenism sequence is not associated with polycystic ovarian changes, but rather with small ovaries and reduced volume percentage of primordial follicles.

These apparently paradoxical pathways to the classical PCOS symptomatology of anovulation and ovarian hyperandrogenism (the one being associated with higher birthweight, class III INS VNTR genotype and polycystic ovaries on ultrasound, and the other with a lower birthweight, class I INS VNTR genotype and no polycystic ovarian changes) may accurately reflect the dichotomy in the definitions of PCOS.

There may well be important genetic and ethnic differences between populations that determine the severity and characteristics of the PCOS phenotype. Insulin resistance is thought to be particularly severe in Hispanic PCOS women compared with non-Hispanic women matched for age, weight and body composition. Within the UK, the Indian and Pakistani populations appear to have a high background risk for insulin resistance and a high prevalence of PCOS.[133]

Puberty and PCOS

The prevalence of polycystic ovaries increases dramatically at puberty. Normal pubertal development is associated with an increase in insulin resistance which is most marked in peripheral glucose uptake rather than hepatic glucose production. There is compensatory hyperinsulinemia which has an active rather than a passive role in pubertal growth and development. The high insulin levels lead to a gradual fall in SHBG and IGFBP-1 production by the liver. The exposure of the ovary to high levels of insulin may be important in ovarian development, directly or indirectly through falls in IGFBP-1 and a rise in IGF-1. Insulin resistance at puberty is thought to be driven by increases in growth hormone secretion and both growth hormone and IGF-1 may be important for ovarian development.

Nobels and Dewailly suggested that PCOS was a result of the effects of the progressively rising levels of insulin and IGF-1 on the ovary during puberty.[134] They speculated that polycystic ovarian changes may persist in some girls due to an abnormal continuance of hyperinsulinemia after puberty. However, this is only likely to be the case in those programed or genetically predisposed to insulin resistance.

Excessive weight gain during puberty will lead to an exacerbation of any underlying insulin resistance and compensatory hyperinsulinemia. The trends towards an ever increasing prevalence of obesity during childhood and adolescence could increase the rate of expression of PCOS during puberty. The recent rise in the prevalence of type 2 diabetes presenting earlier during childhood in several ethnic minority groups in the US and other parts of the world may also be accompanied by an increasing prevalence of PCOS.

The diagnosis of PCOS in children and adolescents

There is an increasing awareness of the increased prevalence of PCOS in children with genetic forms of insulin resistance and in those with conditions such as glycogen storage disease and type 1 diabetes, where hyperinsulinemia may be the result of therapy. However, the increasing background prevalence of obesity in western society should also increase our awareness of the possiblity of PCOS developing in genetically susceptible individuals in the UK. PCOS is likely to parallel the increasing prevalence of insulin resis-

tance and type 2 diabetes which is currently being observed in the Asian population. Other ethnic groups known to be at increased risk of insulin resistance may also be at risk of PCOS. The low birthweight, premature pubarche, ovarian hyperandrogenism sequence has, thus far, only been described in a few populations, but more active investigation and follow up of patients presenting with adrenarche or pubarche is indicated. Presentation of PCOS during adolescence is likely to be similar to that seen in adults with either menstrual disturbance or evidence of hyperandrogenism, acne and hirsutism. Acanthosis nigricans may be an important marker of insulin resistance. Cryptogenic congenital adrenal hyperplasia (CAH) needs to be carefully excluded, and evidence of polycystic ovaries ought to be sought on transabdominal ultrasound.

Although obesity and PCOS are clearly linked, the mechanism underlying the relationship is uncertain. Obesity is associated with hyperinsulinemia and this could, by driving down levels of SHBG, lead to higher free androgen levels and an increase in symptomatology. The association between obesity and raised free androgen levels is, however, even stronger in women with increased central obesity, a phenotype known to be associated with insulin resistance.

Leptin is a 167-amino acid peptide that is secreted by fat cells in response to insulin and glucocorticoids. Leptin is transported by a protein which appears to be the extracellular domain of the leptin receptor itself.[135] Leptin receptors are found in the choroid plexus, on the hypothalamus and ovary and at many other sites. Leptin decreases the intake of food and stimulates thermogenesis, it also appears to inhibit the hypothalamic peptide neuropeptide-Y, which is an inhibitor of GnRH pulsatility. Leptin appears to serve as the signal from the body fat to the brain about the adequacy of fat stores for reproduction. Thus menstruation will only occur if fat stores are adequate. Obesity, on the other hand, is associated with high circulating concentrations of leptin and this in turn might be a mechanism for hypersecretion of LH in women with PCOS. To date most studies have been in the leptin-deficient and consequently obese *Ob/Ob* mouse. Starvation of the *Ob/Ob* mouse leads to weight loss, yet fertility is only restored after the administration of leptin.[136] Leptin administration to overweight, infertile women may not be as straightforward as

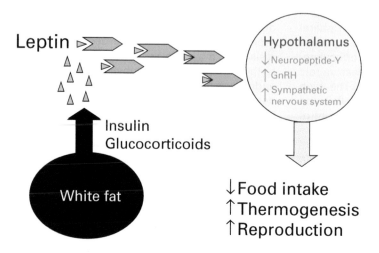

Leptin

Insulin
Glucocorticoids

White fat

Hypothalamus
↓ Neuropeptide-Y
↑ GnRH
↑ Sympathetic
nervous system

↓ Food intake
↑ Thermogenesis
↑ Reproduction

Figure 4.16

The leptin pathway.

it might initially seem, because of the complex nature of leptin transport into the brain. Nonetheless, the role of leptin in human reproduction is an area of ongoing research (Figure 4.16). Recently, there has been interest in whether abnormalities of leptin secretion could predispose to weight gain in women with PCOS. Evidence for 'leptin resistance', i.e. leptin levels that are greater than might be predicted by BMI, have been noted in PCOS and in general populations of women who are overweight. 'Leptin resistance' is common in other insulin-resistant states and its role, if any, in the pathophysiology of PCOS is yet to be determined (see also p. 89).

Conclusions

In summary, PCOS is a heterogeneous condition. Ovarian dysfunction leads to the main signs and symptoms and the ovary is influenced by external factors in particular the gonadotrophins, insulin and other growth factors, which are dependent upon both genetic and environmental influences. The diagnosis relies upon the presence of at least two of the features of menstrual disturbance, hyperandrogenism and/or the presence of polycystic ovaries. In 2003, international consensus definitions were agreed both for the morphological characteristics of the polycystic ovary and the diagnostic criteria for the syndrome. There are likely to be several potential routes by which an individual may develop PCOS, due to a combination of genetic and environmental factors. At the heart of the pathophysiology for many is insulin

Key points

- In understanding the pathophysiology of PCOS, one has to consider both the nature of the dysfunction within the ovary and the external influences that modify ovarian behavior.
- Both in vivo and in vitro data confirm that the theca cells of PCOS patients have a generalized overactive steroidogenesis.
- LH and insulin stimulate theca cell androgen production and insulin also amplifies the effects of testosterone by suppressing SHBG.
- Serum LH concentrations are significantly elevated in PCOS due to an increased amplitude and frequency of LH pulses.
- Hyperinsulinemia is a key component to the pathogenesis of PCOS but is not ubiquitous.

resistance and hyperinsulinemia, and even if this is not the initiating cause in some it is certainly an amplifier of hyperandrogenism in those that gain weight (Figure 4.14). PCOS is a familial condition and appears to have its origins during adolescence when it is thought to be associated with increased weight gain during puberty. In the management of young women with menstrual disturbances or mild signs of hyperandrogenism there is an increasing awareness among physicians about the possibility of PCOS. This awareness should be enhanced if there is a family history.

References

1. Balen AH, Conway GS, Kaltsas G, Techatraisak K et al. Polycystic ovary syndrome: The spectrum of the disorder in 1741 patients. Hum Reprod 1995; 10:2705–2712.

2. Balen AH, Michelmore K. What is polycystic ovary syndrome? Are national views important? Hum Reprod 2002; 17:2219–2227.

3. Rodin DA, Bano G, Bland JM, Taylor K, Nussey SS. Polycystic ovaries and associated metabolic abnormalities in Indian subcontinent Asian women. Clin Endocrinol (Oxf) 1998; 49:91–99.

4. Wijeyaratne CN, Balen AH, Barth J, Belchetz PE. Clinical manifestations and insulin resistance (IR) in polycystic ovary syndrome (PCOS) among South Asians and Caucasians: is there a difference? Clin Endocrinol (Oxf) 2002; 57:343–350.

5. Carmina E, Koyama T, Chang L, Stanczyk FZ, Lobo RA. Does ethnicity influence the prevalence of adrenal hyperandrogenism in insulin resistance in the polycystic ovary syndrome? Am J Obstet Gynecol 1992; 167:1807–1112.

6. Slayden SM, Moran C, Sams WM, Jr, Boots LR, Azziz R. Hyperandrogenemia in patients presenting with acne. Fertil Steril 2001; 75:889–892.

7. Futterweit W, Dunaif A, Yeh C, Kingsley P. The prevalence of hyperandrogenism in 109 consecutive female patients with diffuse alopecia. J Am Acad Dermatol 1988; 19:831–836.

8. Legro RS, Driscoll D, Strauss JF 3rd, Fox J, Dunaif A. Evidence for a genetic basis for hyperandrogenemia in polycystic ovary syndrome. Proc Natl Acad Sci USA 1998; 95:14956–14960.

9. Knochenhauer ES, Key TJ, Kahsar-Miller M, Waggoner W et al. Prevalence of the polycystic ovary syndrome in unselected black and white women in the Southeastern United States: A prospective study. J Clin Endocrinol Metab 1988; 83:3078–3082.

10. Pugeat M, Nicolas MH, Craves JC, Alvarado-Dubost C et al. Androgens in polycystic ovarian syndrome. Ann NY, Acad Sci 1993; 687:124–135.

11. Laven JS, Imani B, Eijkemans MJ, Fauser BC. New approaches to PCOS and other forms of anovulation. Obstet Gynecol Surv 2002; 57:755–767.

12. Cibula D, Hill M, Starka L. The best correlation of the new index of hyperandrogenism with the grade of increased hair. Eur J Endocrinol 2000; 143: 405–408.

13. Imani B, Eijkemans MJ, de Jong FH, Payne NN et al. Free androgen index and leptin are the most prominent endocrine predictors of ovarian response during clomiphene citrate induction of ovulation in normogonadotropic oligoamenorrheic infertility. J Clin Endocrinol Metab 2000; 85:676–682.

14. Rosner W. Errors in the measurement of plasma free testosterone. J Clin Endocrinol Metab 1997; 82:2014–2015.

15. Vermeulen A, Verdonck L, Kaufman JM. A critical evaluation of simple methods for the estimation of free testosterone in serum. J Clin Endocrinol Metab 1999; 84:3666–3672.

16. Tremblay RR, Dube JY. Plasma concentration of free and non-TeBG bound testosterone in women on oral contraceptives. Contraception 1974; 10:599–605.

17. Franks S, White D, Gilling-Smith C, Carey A et al. Hypersecretion of androgens by polycystic ovaries: the role of genetic factors in the regulation of cytochrome P450c17a. Balliere's Clin Endocrinol Metab 1996; 10:193–203.

18. Rosenfield RL, Barnes RB, Cara JF, Lucky AW. Dysregulation of cytochrome P450c17a as the cause of polycystic ovarian syndrome. Fertil Steril 1990; 53:785–791.

19. Ehrmann DA, Barnes RB, Rosenfield RL. Polycystic ovary syndrome as a form of functional ovarian hypernadrogenism due to dysregulation of androgen secretion. Endocrinol Rev 1995; 16:322–353.

20. Kirschner MA, Bardin CW. Androgen production and metabolism in normal and virilized women Metabolism 1972; 21:667–688.

21. Rivarola M, Singleton R, Migoen C. Splanchnic extraction and interconversion of testosterone and androstenedione in man. J Clin Invest 1967; 46:2095–2099.

22. White DW, Leigh A, Wilson C et al. Gonadotrophin and gonadal steriod response to a single dose of a long-acting agonist of gonadotrophin-releasing hormone in ovulatory and anovulatory women with polycystic ovary syndrome. Clin Endocrinol (Oxf) 1995; 42:475–481.

23. Barnes RB, Rosenfield RL, Burstein S, Ehrmann D. Pituitary-ovarian response to nafarelin testing in the polycystic ovary syndrome. N Engl J Med 1989; 320:559–65

24. Erickson GF, Magoffin DA, Garza VG, Cheung AP, Chang RJ. Granulosa cells of polycystic ovaries: are they normal or abnormal? Hum Reprod 1992; 7:293–9.

25. Mason HD, Willis DS, Beard RW et al. Estradiol production by granulosa cells of normal and polycystic ovaries (PCO): relationship to menstrual cycle history and to concentrations of gonadotrophins and sex steroids in follicular fluid. J Clin Endocrinol Metab 1994; 79:1355.

26. Webber LJ, Stubbs S, Stark J, Trew GH, Franks S. Formation and early development of follicles in the polycystic ovary. Lancet 2003; 362:1017–1021.

27. Prelevic G, Wurzburger M, Balint-Peri C, Nesic JS. Inhibitory effect of sandostatin on secretion of luteinizing hormone and ovarian steroids in polycystic ovary syndrome. Lancet 1990; 336:900–3.

28. Anderson R, Groome N, Baird D. Inhibin A and inhibin B in women with polycystic ovarian syndrome during treatment with FSH to induce mono-ovulation. Clin Endocrinol (Oxf) 1998; 48:577–84.

29. Fauser BCJM, Pache TD, Lamberts WJ, Hop WCJ et al. Serum bioactive and immunoreactive luteinising hormone and follicle stimulating hormone levels in women with cycle abnormalities, with or without polycystic ovary disease. J Clin Endocrinol Metab 1991; 73:811–817.

30. Taylor AE, McCourt B, Martin K, Anderson EJ et al. Determinants of abnormal gonadotropin secretion in clinically defined women with PCOS J Clin Endocrinol Metab 1997; 82:2248–2256.

31. Waldstreicher J, Santoro NF, Hall HJE, Filicori M, Crowley WF. Hyperfunction of the hypothalamic-pituitary axis in women with polycystic ovarian disease: Indirect evidence of partial gonadotroph desensitization. J Clin Endocrinol Metab 1998; 66:165–172.

32. van Santbrink EJ, Hop WC, Fauser BC. Classification of normogonadotropin infertility: Polycystic ovaries diagnosed by ultrasound versus endocrine characteristics of PCOS. Fertil Steril 1997; 67:452–458.

33. Balen AH, Tan SL, Jacobs HS. Hypersecretion of luteinising hormone – a significant cause of subfertility and miscarriage. Br J Obstet Gynaecol 1993; 100:1082–1089.

34. The Rotterdam ESHRE/ASRM-sponsored PCOS consensus workshop group: Fauser B, Tarlatzis B, Chang J, Azziz R et al. Revised 2003 consensus on diagnostic criteria and long-term health risks related to polycystic ovary syndrome (PCOS). Hum Reprod 2004; 19:41–47.

35. Schally AV, Arimura A, Kastin AJ, Matsuo H et al. Gonadotropin-releasing hormone: one polypeptide regulates secretion of luteinizing and follicle stimulating hormones. Science 1971; 173:1036–1037.

36. Belchetz PE, Plant TM, Nakai Y, Keogh EG, Knobil E. Hypophyseal responses to continuous intermittent delivery of hypothalamic GnRH. Science 1978; 202:631–633.

37. Dalkin AC, Haisenleder DJ, Ortolano GA, Ellis TR, Marshall JC. The frequency of GnRH stimulation differentially regulates gonadotropin subunit mRNA expression. Endocrinol 1989; 125:917–924.

38. Pickering AJMC, Fink G. Priming effect of luteinising hormone-releasing factor: in-vitro and in-vivo evidence consistent with its dependence upon protein and RNA synthesis. J Endocrinol Metab 1976; 69:373–379.

39. Aiyer MS, Chiappa SA, Fink G. A priming effect of luteinizing releasing factor on the pituitary gland in the female rat. J Endocrinol 1974; 62:573–588.

40. Wang CF, Lasley BL, Lein A, Yen SSC. The functional changes of the pituitary gonadotrophs during the menstrual cycle. J Clin Endocrinol Metab 1976; 42:718–728.

41. Knobil E. Electrophysiological approaches to the hypothalamic GnRH pulse generator. In: Yen SSC, Vale WW, eds. Neuroendocrine regulation of reproduction. Norwell, USA: Serono Symposia, 1990:3–8.

42. Rosmanith WG, Wirth U, Sterzik K, Yen SS. The effects of prolonged opioidergic blockade on LH pulsatile secretion during the menstrual cycle. J Endocrinol Invest 1989; 12:245–252.

43. Danforth DR, Elkind-Hirsch K, Hodgen G. In-vivo and in-vitro modulation of GnRH metabolism by estradiol and progesterone. Endocrinology 1990; 127:319–324.

44. Quigley M, Rakoff J, Yen SSC. Increased luteinising hormone sensitivity to dopamine inhibition in the polycystic ovary syndrome. J Clin Endocrinol Metab 1981; 52:231.

45. Cumming DC, Reid RL, Quigley ME, Rebar RW, Yen SS. Evidence for decreased endogenous dopamine and opioid inhibitory influences on LH secretion in polycystic ovary syndrome. Clin Endocrinol (Oxf) 1984; 20:643–648.

46. Shoupe D, Lobo RA. Evidence for altered catecholamine metabolism in polycystic ovary syndrome. Am J Obstet Gynecol 1984; 150:566–570.

47. Yoshino K, Takahashi K, Shirai T, Nishigaki A et al. Changes in plasma catecholamines and pulsatile patterns of gonadotropins in subjects with a normal ovulatory cycle and with polycystic ovary syndrome. Int J Fertil 1990; 35:34–39.

48. Barnes R, Lobo R. Central opioid activity in the polycystic ovary syndrome with and without dopaminergic modulation. J Clin Endocrinol Metab 1985; 61:779.

49. Barnes RB, Mileikowsky GN, Cha KY, Spencer CA et al. Effects of dopamine and metoclopramide in

polycystic ovary syndrome. J Clin Endocrinol Metab 1986; 63:506–509.

50. Berga SL, Yen SSC. Opioidergic regulation of LH pulsatility in women with polycystic ovary syndrome. Clin Endocrinol (Oxf) 1989; 30:177–184.

51. Lanzone A, Apa R, Fulghesu AM, Cutillo G et al. Long-term naltrexone treatment normalizes the pituitary response to gonadotrophin-releasing hormone in polycystic ovarian syndrome. Fertil Steril 1993; 59:734–737.

52. Schoemaker J. Neuroendocrine control in polycystic ovary-like syndrome. Gynecol Endocrinol 1991; 5:277–288.

53. Rebar R, Judd HL, Yen SCC, Rakoff J et al. Characterization of the inappropriate gonadotropin secretion in polycystic ovary syndrome. J Clin Invest 1976; 57:1320–1329.

54. Burger CW, Korsen T, Van Kessel H, Van Dop PA et al. Pulsatile luteinizing hormone patterns in the follicular phase of the menstrual cycle, polycystic ovarian disease (PCOD) and non PCOD secondary amenorrhoea. J Clin Endocrinol Metab 1985; 61:1126–1132.

55. Baird DT, Corker CS, Davison DW, Hunter WM et al. Pituitary ovarian relationships in polycystic ovary syndrome. J Clin Endocrinol Metab 1977; 45:798–809.

56. Kazer RR, Kessel B, Yen SS. Circulating luteinizing hormone pulse frequency in women with polycystic ovary syndrome. J Clin Endocrinol Metab 1987; 65:233–236.

57. Sagle M, Kiddy D, Mason HD, Dobriansky D et al. Evidence for normal hypothalamic regulation of LH in ovulatory women with the polycystic ovary syndrome. In: Rolland R, Heineman MJ et al. eds. Neuroendocrinology of reproduction, Amsterdam: Excerpta Medica, 1987.

58. Venturoli S, Porcu E, Fabbri R, Magrini O et al. Episodic pulsatile secretion of FSH LH, prolactin, oestradiol, oestrone and LH circadian variations in polycystic ovary syndrome. Clin Endocrinol (Oxf) 1988; 28:93–107.

59. Couzinet B, Thomas G, Thalabard JC, Brailly S, Schaison G. Effects of a pure antiandrogen on gonadotropin secretion in normal women and in polycystic ovarian disease. Fertil Steril 1989; 52:42–47.

60. Murdoch AP, Diggle PJ, White MC, Kendall-Taylor P, Dunlop W. LH in polycystic ovary syndrome: reproducibility and pulsatile secretion. J Endocrinol 1989; 121:185–191.

61. Schachter M, Balen AH, Patel A, Jacobs HS. Hypogonadotrophic patients with ultrasonographically diagnosed polycystic ovaries have aberrant gonadotropin secretion when treated with pulsatile gonadotrophin releasing hormone – a new insight into the pathophysiology of polycystic

ovary syndrome. Gynecol Endocrinol 1996; 10:327–335.

62. Gadir AA, Mowafi RS, Alnaser HMI, Alnaser HMI et al. Ovarian electrocautery versus hMG and pure FSH therapy in the treatment of patients with polycystic ovarian disease. Clin Endocrinol (Oxf) 1990; 33:585–592.

63. Rossmanith WG, Keckstein J, Spatzier K, Lauritzen C. The impact of ovarian laser surgery on the gonadotrophin secretion in women with PCOD. Clin Endocrinol (Oxf) 1991; 34:223–230.

64. Jeffcoate SL. Analytical and clinical significance of peptide hormone heterogeneity with particular reference to growth hormone and luteinising hormone in serum. Clin Endocrinol (Oxf) 1993; 38:113–121.

65. Iles RK, Lee CL, Howes I, Davies S et al. Immunoreactive ß-core-like material in normal postmenopausal urine: human chorionic gonadotrophin or LH origin? Evidence for the existence of LH core. J Endocrinol 1992; 133:459–466.

66. Lobo RA, Kletzky OA, Campeau J, di Zerega G. Elevated bioactive luteinising hormone in women with polycystic ovary syndrome. Fertil Steril 1983; 39:674–679.

67. Lobo RA, Shoupe D, Chang SP, Campeau J. The control of bioactive luteinising hormone secretion in women with polycystic ovary syndrome. Am J Obstet Gynecol 1984; 148:423–428.

68. Fauser BCJM, Pache TD, Hop WCJ, de Jong FH, Dahl KD. The significance of a single serum LH measurement in women with cycle disturbances: discrepancies between immunoreactive and bioactive hormone estimates. Clin Endocrinol (Oxf) 1992; 37:445–452.

69. Ding Y-Q, Huhtaniemi I. Preponderance of basic isoforms of serum LH is associated with the high bio/immuno ratio of LH in healthy women and in women with polycystic ovarian disease. Hum Reprod 1991; 6:346–350.

70. Matteri RL, Djiershke DJ, Bridson WE, Rhutasel NS, Robinson JA. Regulation of the biopotency of primate LH by GnRH in-vitro and in-vivo. Biol Reprod 1990; 43:1045–1049.

71. Tapanainen JS, Koivunen Riitta, Fauser BCJM, Taylor AE et al. A new contributing factor to polycystic ovary syndrome: The genetic variant of luteinizing hormone. J Clin Endocrinol Metab 1999; 84:711–1715.

72. Antilla L, Ding Y-Q, Ruutiainen K, Erkkola R et al. Clinical features and circulating gonadotropin, insulin and androgen interactions in women with polycystic ovarian disease. Fertil Steril 1991; 55:1057–1061.

73. Adashi EY, Hsueh AJW, Yen SSC. Insulin enhancement of luteinising hormone and follicle stimulat-

ing hormone release by cultured pituitary cells. Endocrinol 1981; 108:1441–1449.

74. Conway GS, Honour JW, Jacobs HS. Heterogeneity of the polycystic ovary syndrome: clinical, endocrine and ultrasound features in 556 patients. Clin Endocrinol (Oxf) 1989; 30:459–470.

75. Conway GS, Clark PMS, Wong D. Hyperinsulinaemia in the polycystic ovary syndrome confirmed with a specific immunoradiometric assay for insulin. Clin Endocrinol (Oxf) 1993; 38:219–222.

76. Lasley BL, Wang CF, Yen SSC. The effects of estrogen and progesterone on the functional capacity of the gonadotrophs. J Clin Endocrinol Metab 1975; 41:820–826.

77. Karsch FJ. Central actions of ovarian steroids in the feedback regulation of pulsatile secretion of luteinising hormone. Ann Rev Physiol 1987; 49:365–382.

78. Sprangers SA, Brenner RM, Bethea CL. Estrogen and progesterone receptor immunocytochemistry in lactotropes versus gonadotropes of monkey pituitary cell cultures. Endocrinology 1989; 124:1462–1470.

79. Hsueh ADW, Billig H, Tsafiri A. Ovarian follicle atresia: A hormonally controlled apoptotic process. Endocrinol Rev 1994; 15:707–724.

80. Abdulwahid NA, Adams J, Van der Spuy ZM, Jacobs HS. Gonadotrophin control of follicular development Clin Endocrinol (Oxf) 1985; 23:613–626.

81. Eden JA. The polycystic ovary syndrome. Aust NZ J Obstet Gynaecol 1989; 29:403–416.

82. McFaul PB, Traub AI, Thompson W. Premature luteinization and ovulation induction using human menopausal gonadotrophin or pure follicle stimulating hormone in patients with polycystic ovary syndrome. Acta Eur Fertil 1989; 20:157–161.

83. Mizunuma H, Andoh K, Yamada K, Takagi T et al. Prediction and prevention of ovarian hyperstimulation by monitoring endogenous luteinising hormone release during purified follicle stimulating hormone therapy. Fertil Steril 1992; 58:46–50.

84. DeVane GM, Czekala NM, Judd HL, Yen SSC. Circulating gonadotropins, estragens and androgens in polycystic ovarian disease. Am J Obstet Gynecol 1974; 38:476–481.

85. Chang RJ, Mandfdel FP, Lu JK, Judd HL. Enhanced disparity of gonadotropin secretion by estrone in women with polycystic ovarian disease. J Clin Endocrinol Metab 1982; 54:490–494.

86. Frawley LS, Neill JD. Biphasic effects of estrogen on GnRH-induced LH release in monolayer cultures of rat and monkey pituitary cells. Endocrinol 1984; 114:659–663.

87. Menon M, Peegel H, Katta V. Estradiol potentiation of gonadotrophin-releasing hormone responsiveness in the anterior pituitary is mediated by an increase in gonadotrophin-releasing hormone

receptors. Am J Obstet Gynaecol 1985; 151:534–540.

88. Emons G, Hoffmann HG, Brack C, Ortmann O et al. Modulation of GnRH receptor concentration in cultured female pituitary cells by estradiol treatment. J Steroid Biochem 1988; 31:751–756.

89. Pemberton P, White DM, Franks S. The feedback effect of oestradiol on secretion of LH in ovulatory and anovulatory women with polycystic ovary syndrome. J Endocrinol Supp 1992; 135:P97.

90. Giguere V, Lefebvre F-A, Labrie F. Androgens decrease LHRH binding sites in rat anterior pituitary cells in culture. Endocrinology 1981; 108:350–352.

91. Spinder T, Spijkstra JJ, van den Tweel JG, Burger CW et al. The effects of long term testosterone administration on pulsatile luteinizing hormone secretion and on ovarian histology in eugonadal female to male transsexual subjects. J Clin Endocrinol Metab 1989; 69:151–157.

92. Goh HH, Ratnam SS. The gonadotrophin surge in humans: Its mechanism and role in ovulatory function – a review. Ann Acad Med 1990; 19:524–529.

93. Burger HG, Igarashi M. Inhibin – definition and nomenclature. J Clin Endocrinol Metab 1988; 66:885–886.

94. Sopelak VM, Hodgen GD. Blockade of the estrogen-induced LH surge in monkeys: a nonsteroidal, antigenic factor in porcine follicular fluid. Fertil Steril 1984; 41:108–113.

95. Messinis IE, Templeton A. Pituitary response to exogenous LHRH in superovulated women. J Reprod Fert 1989; 87:633–639.

96. Balen AH, Jacobs HS. A prospective study comparing unilateral and bilateral laparoscopic ovarian diathermy in women with the polycystic ovary syndrome. Fertil Steril 1994; 62:921–925.

97. Burger HG. Inhibin: review. Reprod Med Rev 1992; 1:1–20.

98. Balen AH, Rose M. The control of luteinising hormone secretion in the polycystic ovary syndrome (review). Contem Rev Obstet Gynaecol 1994; 6:201–207.

99. Culler MD. In-vivo evidence that inhibin is a gonadotrophin surge-inhibiting factor. Endocrinol 1992; 131:1556–1558.

100. Balen AH, Er J, Rafferty B, Rose M. (1995b) Evidence that gonadotrophin surge attenuating factor is not inhibin. J Reprod Fertil 1995; 104:285–289.

101. Lockwood GM, Muttukrishna S, Groome NP, Matthews DR, Ledger WL. Mid-follicular phase pulses of inhibin B are absent in polycystic ovary syndrome and are initiated by successful laparoscopic ovarian diathermy: a possible mechanism for the emergence of the dominant follicle. J Clin Endocrinol Metab 1998; 83:1730–1735.

102. Lockwood GM. The role of inhibin in PCOS, Hum Fertil 2000; 3:86–92.

103. Balen AH. The pathogenesis of polycystic ovary syndrome: the enigma unravels. Lancet 1999; 354:966–967.

104. Dunaif A. Insulin resistance and the polycystic ovary syndrome: mechanisms and implication for pathogenesis. Endocrine Rev 1997; 18:774–800.

105. Franks S, Gharani N, McCarthy M. Candidate genes in polycystic ovary syndrome. Hum Reprod Update 2001; 7:405–410.

106. Ashton WD, Nanchahal K, Wood DA. Body mass index and metabolic risk factors for coronary heart disease in women. Eur Heart J 2001; 22:46–55.

107. Lord J, Wilkin T. Polycystic ovary syndrome and fat distribution: the central issue? Hum Fertil 2002; 5:67–71.

108. Despres JP, Lemieux I, Prud'homme D. Treatment of obesity: need to focus on high risk, abdominally obese patients. Br Med J 2001; 322:716–720.

109. Bergh C, Carlsson B, Olsson JH, Selleskog U, Hillensjo T. Regulation of androgen production in cultured human thecal cells by insulin-like growth factor I and insulin. Fertil Steril 1993; 59:323–331.

110. Leroith D, Werner H, Beitner-Johnson D, Roberts CT, Jr. Molecular and cellular aspects of the insulin-like growth factor I receptor. Endocrinol Rev 1995; 16:143–163.

111. De Leo V, la Marca A, Orvieto R, Morgante G. Effect of metformin on insulin-like growth factor (IGF) I and IGF-binding protein I in polycystic ovary syndrome. J Clin Endocrinol Metab 2000; 85:1598–1600.

112. Adashi E. Intraovarian regulation: the proposed role of insulin-like growth factors. Ann NY Acad Sci 1993; 687:10–12.

113. Erickson GF, Magoffin D, Cragun J, Chang R. The effects of insulin and insulin-like growth factors-I and II on estradiol production by granulosa cells of polycystic ovaries. J Clin Endocrinol Metab 1990; 70:894–901.

114. Voutilainen R, Franks S, Mason HD, Martikainen H. Expression of insulin-like growth factor (IGF), IGF-binding protein, and IGF receptor messenger ribonucleic acids in normal and polycystic ovaries. J Clinical Endocrinol Metab 1996; 81:1003.

115. Nestler JE, Jacobowicz DJ. Decreases in ovarian cytochrome p450c17µ activity and serum free testosterone after reduction of insulin secretion in polycystic ovary syndrome. New England Journal of Medicine. 1996; 335:617–623.

116. la Marca A, Egbe TO, Morgante G, Paglia T et al. Metformin treatment reduces ovarian cytochrome P450c17a response to human chorionic gonadotrophin in women with insulin resistance-related polycystic ovary syndrome. Hum Reprod 2000; 15:21–23.

117. Uilenbroek JTJ, Wonlersen PJA, van der Schoot P. Atresia in preovulatory follicles: Gonadotropin binding in steroidogenic activity. Biol Reprod 1980; 23:219–229.

118. Dunaif A, Segal KR, Futterweit W, Dobrjansky A. Profound peripheral insulin resistance, independent of obesity in polycystic ovary syndrome. Diabetes 1989; 38:1165–1174.

119. Dunaif A, Segal KR, Shelley DR, Green G et al. Evidence for distinctive and intrinsic defects in insulin action in polycystic ovary syndrome. Diabetes 1992; 41:1257–1266.

120. Tsilchorozidou T, Overton C, Conway GS. The pathophysiology of polycystic ovary syndrome. Clin Endocrinol (Oxf) 2004; 60:1–17.

121. Ehrmann DA, Sturis J, Byrne MM, Karrison T et al. Insulin seceretory defects in polycystic ovary syndrome. Relationship to insulin sensitivity and family history of non-insulin dependent diabetes mellitus. J Clin Invest 1995; 96:520–527.

122. Zhang LH, Rodriguez H, Ohno S, Miller WL. Serine phosphorylation of human P450c17 increases 17,20-lyase actvitiy: implications for adrenarche and the polycystic ovary syndrome. Proc Nat Acad Sci USA 1995; 92:10619–10623.

123. Balen AH, Dunger D. Pubertal maturation of the internal genitalia (Commentary). Ultrasound Obstet Gynaecol 1995; 6:164–165.

124. Fox R, Corrigan E, Thomas PA, Hull MGR. The diagnosis of polycystic ovaries in women with oligo-amenorrhoea: predictive power of endocrine tests. Clin Endocrinol (Oxf) 1991; 34:127–131.

125. Bridges NA, Cooke A, Healy MJR, Hindmarsh PC, Brook CGD. Standards for ovarian volume in childhood and puberty. Fertil Steril 1993; 60:456–460.

126. Sampaolo P, Livien C, Montanari L, Paganelli A et al. Precocious signs of polycystic ovaries in obese girls. Ultrasound Obstet Gynaecol 1994; 4:1–6.

127. Balen AH, Conway GS, Kaltsas G, Techatraisak K et al. Polycystic ovary syndrome: The spectrum of the disorder in 1741 patients. Hum Reprod 1995; 10: 2705–2712.

128. Ibanez L, Potau N, Enriquez G, de Zegher F. Reduced uterine and ovarian size in adolescent girls born small for gestational age. Pediatr Res 2000; 47:575–577.

129. Cresswell JL, Barker DJ, Osmond C, Egger P et al. Fetal growth, length of gestation, and polycystic ovaries in adult life. Lancet 1997; 350:1131–1135.

130. Michelmore KF, Balen AH, Dunger DB, Vessey MP. Polycystic ovaries and associated clinical and biochemical features in young women. Clin Endcrinol 1999; 51:779–786.

131. Ibanez L, Potau N, Francois I, de Zegher F. Precocious pubarche, hyperinsulinism, and ovarian hyperandrogenism in girls: relation to reduced fetal

growth. Clin Endocrinol Metab. 1998; 83:3558–3562.

132. Hales CN, Barker DJ, Clark PM et al. Fetal and infant growth and impaired glucose tolerance at age 64. Br Med J 1991; 303:1019–1022.

133. Balen AH, Michelmore K. Polycystic ovary syndrome: are national views important? Hum Reprod 2002; 17:2219–2227.

134. Nobels, Dewailly D. Puberty and polycystic ovary syndrome: the insulin/insulin-like growth factor 1 hypothesis. Fertil Steril 1992; 58:655–666.

135. Tartaglia LA, Dembski M, Weng X et al. Identification and expression cloning of a leptin receptor, Ob-R. Cell 1995; 83:1–20.

136. Chehab FF, Mounzih K, Lu R, Lim ME. Early onset of reproductive function in normal female mice treated with leptin. Science 1997; 275:88–90.

137. Crowley WF, Flicori M, Spratt DI, Santorro NF. The physiology of gonadotropin releasing hormone (GnRH) secretion in men and women. Recent Progress in Hormone Research 1985; 41:473–531.

Chapter 5

The genetics of polycystic ovary syndrome

Introduction

Polycystic ovary syndrome (PCOS) is a heterogeneous collection of signs and symptoms that gathered together form a spectrum of a disorder with a mild presentation in some, while in others there is a severe disturbance of reproductive, endocrine and metabolic function. The pathophysiology of the PCOS appears to be multifactorial and polygenic. The definition of the syndrome has been much debated (see Chapter 2) yet this is pivotal to any discussion about genetic origins. Furthermore, there is considerable heterogeneity of symptoms and signs amongst women with PCOS.[1] PCOS is familial and various aspects of the syndrome may be differentially inherited. Polycystic ovaries can exist without clinical signs of the syndrome, which may then become expressed over time. There are a number of interlinking factors that affect expression of PCOS. A gain in weight, for example, is associated with a worsening of symptoms.

Genetic studies have identified a link between PCOS and disordered insulin metabolism, and indicate that the syndrome may be the presentation of a complex genetic trait disorder.[2] The features of obesity, hyperinsulinemia, and hyperandrogenemia, which are commonly seen in PCOS, are also known to be factors that confer an increased risk of cardiovascular disease and non-insulin dependent diabetes mellitus (NIDDM).[3] Evidence of women with PCOS having long-term health risks caused by increased cardiovascular risk has prompted debate on the need for screening women for polycystic ovaries. Since the phenotype of women with polycystic ovaries and the polycystic ovary syndrome can vary,[1] it is difficult to elucidate the genotype. It is also likely that different combinations of genetic variants may result in differential expression of the separate components of the syndrome.

Genetic origins of PCOS

Genetics: from phenotype to genotype

A familial basis for PCOS has long been noted, and the differential inheritance of the individual components of the syndrome has been proposed.[4] Detailed analysis of families with many members affected by PCOS would help elucidate the genetic basis. Nevertheless, family studies reported so far have been hampered by the inconsistency in assigning a phenotype for PCOS. Assigning a phenotype to first-degree relatives of women with PCOS is the first step in performing genetic analysis. The next step is to identify specific markers in the genome that segregate with the syndrome. The final step is to locate the disease genes that determine the phenotype, which lie in the proximity of the genetic marker.[5]

Most of the criteria used for diagnosing PCOS are continuous traits, such as degree of hirsutism, level of circulating androgens, extent of menstrual irregularity, and ovarian volume and morphology. To perform genetic analyses, these continuous variables have to be transformed into nominal variables. Such definitions must also be based on comparison with normal controls that are matched for racial origin, age, sex and weight. Even then some of these criteria, despite being nominal variables, are more likely to represent continuous variables, and have an arbitrary cut-off for assigning abnormal status. A classic example of this is the diagnosis by ovarian ultrasound, based on the number of follicles, rather than by ovarian volume. Is the number of follicles constant in an individual? If she has 13 follicles one month and has by definition 'polycystic' ovaries but the following month has only 11, does she no longer have PCOS? Inevitably such continuous variables will have some overlap between affected populations and normal controls.

Genetics: family studies

In view of the features of PCOS being expressed during the reproductive years, the focus of research on the segregation of PCOS in sisters is sensible. Family studies revealed that sisters of women with PCOS had a substantial risk of being affected by a variety of traits of PCOS. On average, the occurrence of hirsutism and oligomenorrhea among sisters has been around 50% in most studies thus suggesting a dominant mode of Mendelian inheritance. However, these studies have been hampered by the use of varying criteria to assign affected status, and the ascertainment bias in the selection of multiply affected families. Common problems affecting the assigning of affected status to first-degree female relatives were the use of questionnaires alone, the determination of affected status of post-menopausal women and the lack of detailed endocrine profile of family members.[5] All studies have had an element of ascertainment bias, in that families with multiply affected females have been selected, and those with few affected women disregarded.

Cooper and Clayton performed the first large study of familial PCOS, where all of the probands were identified as having Stein–Leventhal syndrome by wedge resection biopsy of the ovary.[6] First-degree female relatives were compared with controls, which revealed oligomenorrhea was more common in mothers and sisters of the proband. The inheritance was suggested to be autosomal dominant with decreased penetrance. Givens et al studied multiple kindred showing affected members in many generations.[6] They did not specify ethnicity and

had no control arm, but studied male family members and proposed an X-linked mode of inheritance. This group was the first to report the severe metabolic sequelae of PCOS such as cardiovascular risks and diabetes mellitus. Ferriman and Purdie reported a higher prevalence of hirsutism, oligomenorrhea and infertility among first-degree relatives of the proband, when compared with controls.[7] The data were questionnaire based with no detailed endocrine assessment, and a modified dominant mode of inheritance was concluded. Lunde et al identified affected status by wedge resection of ovaries, menstrual irregularity, hirsutism, infertility and obesity.[8] The familial segregation, was similar to that reported by Ferriman and Purdie,[7] suggesting an autosomal dominant mode of inheritance. Hague and coworkers used high-resolution ultrasonography to identify polycystic ovaries in 50 women with menstrual irregularity, hyperandrogenism and obesity, and studied their female first-degree relatives by ovarian ultrasound.[9] The segregation ratios for ultrasound features were in excess of an autosomal dominant mode of inheritance, with 67% of mothers and 87% of sisters of the probands being affected.

Carey and coworkers characterized in detail the affected proband and their families, and suggested a single gene mutation with an autosomal dominant mode of transmission as the cause of PCOS.[10] The proband and female family members were identified by utilizing currently accepted ultrasound criteria for the diagnosis of polycystic ovaries, medical history, measurement of physical indices, serum androgens, 17-hydroxy-progesterone, gonadotropins, and prolactin, and an assessment of insulin resistance in those who were obese based oral glucose tolerance tests. Norman et al also utilized intensive phenotyping criteria and demonstrated the occurrence of ultrasound-diagnosed polycystic ovaries among sisters to be 73%, hyperandrogenemia 87%, and hyperinsulinemia 66%.[11] However, the sample size was small and likely to have been affected by ascertainment bias. They also reported a high prevalence of hyperinsulinemia and hypertriglyceridemia in family members when compared with controls. However, they studied a much smaller number of families, and utilized low sex hormone binding globulin (SHBG) as a diagnostic criterion, which in turn is a feature of hyperinsulinemia – albeit a 'surrogate marker'.

Legro and coworkers carried out more intensive phenotyping of PCOS families: 115 sisters of 80 probands with PCOS (defined as oligomenorrhea and hyperandrogenemia), from unrelated families, were examined.[12] The control group was 70 healthy women who were age- and weight-matched; 22% of the sisters had PCOS, and an additional 24% had hyperandrogenemia and regular menstrual cycles – a total of 46% affected versus 14% in the controls, demonstrating a relative risk of 3.3 for hyperandrogenemia occurring in sisters of affected women.[12] This increased risk in sisters confirms that PCOS is likely to have a genetic origin. Legro argues that his study provides insight to the heterogeneity of PCOS by demonstrating that several phenotypes of PCOS occur within one family, and that the heterogeneity has a genetic basis, suggesting a variable expression of a monogenic trait or an oligogenic (i.e. small number of causative genes) trait.[12] The familial aggregation of hyperandrogenemia, with or without menstrual disturbance led Legro to suggest hyperandrogenemia as the key feature to be used to assign affected status in linkage studies. This was further supported by the same group in a study of 307 sisters of a cohort of 336 women with PCOS, showing a strong association of the markers of insulin resistance with hyperandrogenemia rather than with menstrual irregularity.[13] Yildiz et al, who studied assessed glucose tolerance and insulin resistance in 102 first-degree relatives (including fathers and brothers) of 52 women with PCOS, reported a high risk of diabetes mellitus and insulin resistance with mothers and sisters also having higher androgen levels than controls.[14]

A study of the mothers and sisters of 93 patients with PCOS (defined by a history of oligomenorrhea, clinical or biochemical hyperandrogenism, and the exclusion of other disorders) found that of the 78 mothers and 50 sisters, respectively 24% and 32% had PCOS.[15] When only pre-menopausal women not taking any hormone therapy were included, the rates of PCOS were 35% and 40% respectively. This compared with the expected rate in the general population of 4% using their diagnostic criteria – a 5–6-fold increase in incidence among first-degree relatives.[16] The association with hyperandrogenemia in the absence of a menstrual disturbance, however, was not demonstrated – once more identifying the problems with diagnosis and potential population differences.

Thus studies of first-degree relatives show differences that may be explained either by the use of different diagnostic criteria or more general racial/population effects. An interesting recent study also explored the family history of various diseases in 41 women with PCOS and 66 controls.[17] The proportion of women with a positive family history of breast cancer was greater in those with PCOS (20% vs 5% in controls, $p < 0.05$), as was a positive family history of myocardial infarction (35% vs 15%, $p < 0.05$).

Male phenotype

Although several phenotypes have been proposed, there is a notable absence of an equivalent male phenotype to that of PCOS in a woman of reproductive age.[18] Identifying the male phenotype is of importance for performing genetic analysis of kindred and for assisting in genetic counseling.[5] Cooper and Clayton identified increased 'pilosity' as the male phenotype.[6] Givens reported oligospermia and abnormal gonadotropin secretion as problems in male family members.[19] Stronger paternal transmission was reported and an X-linked dominant inheritance was suggested. Ferriman and Purdie were the first to report an increased prevalence of baldness among male relatives of a large cohort of women with PCOS.[7] Lunde et al reported that the first-degree male relatives of the affected women were more likely to have early baldness or excessive hairiness when compared with controls.[8] Premature male pattern baldness was accepted as the male phenotype by Carey et al, with the segregation being consistent with an autosomal dominant inheritance.[10] Norman et al confirmed male pattern baldness as a common phenomenon in first-degree male relatives, and included hyperinsulinemia and hypertriglyceridemia in the male phenotype.[20] Govind et al, examined first-degree male and female relatives of 29 probands with PCOS (defined by ultrasound scan and symptoms) and found that 52% of mothers, 66% of sisters, 21% of fathers and 22% of brothers could be assigned affected status.[21] The history of premature male pattern balding was higher than expected for non-affected families, and the sisters with polycystic ovaries were less likely to have endocrine abnormalities.[21] These data strongly suggested an autosomal dominant mode of inheritance with nearly complete penetrance. Not all investigators have found increased balding in first-degree male relatives. Legro et al studied 119 brothers of 87 unrelated women with PCOS, and 68 weight- and ethnicity-comparable unrelated control men were examined and had fasting blood samples obtained.[13] The odds of balding did not differ in the brothers of PCOS women compared with control men. Brothers of women with PCOS had significantly elevated dehydroepiandrosterone sulfate (DHEAS) levels and further there was a significant positive linear relationship between DHEAS levels in PCOS probands and their brothers. These findings supported hyperandrogenemia as a potential male phenotype and familial trait in PCOS families.[13]

Twin studies in PCOS

Twin studies are often employed to help establish the genetic origins of disease yet there are few in the field of PCOS. In 1995, Jahanfar et al reported the largest twin study in PCOS, which did not support a strong genetic component.[22] They studied 34 pairs of monozygotic and dizygotic twins from 500 female pairs invited from a twin registry. The incidence of polycystic ovaries was high at 50%, but showed a strong degree of discordance. However, there was greater concordance among affected twins with respect to biochemical parameters, including fasting insulin levels and androgens. These investigators proposed that PCOS has a complex inheritance pattern, perhaps polygenic, with environmental factors playing a significant role.

Methods for performing genetic studies in PCOS

Epidemiological studies for the genetic mapping of highly polymorphic genetic markers may be carried out as twin studies, studying the relative risk for a relative of an affected person to carry the gene, or segregation analysis by fitting an inheritance pattern of a trait in pedigrees.

The methods available are:

- *linkage analysis* by proposing a model to explain the inheritance pattern of phenotype and genotype in a pedigree
- *allele sharing methods* such as study of affected sibling pairs, and identity by descent (this method tracks the inheritance of putative disease-associated alleles from the parent to the affected sibling)
- *association studies*, which use case-control studies, based on a comparison of unrelated affected and unaffected individuals from a population.[23]

Association studies are most meaningful when applied to a functionally significant variation of genes having a clear biological relation to the trait. An allele is considered to be significantly associated with the trait if it is found more often in the affected group than the unaffected group.[5] Nevertheless, association studies can be hampered by statistical error. Most commonly a small sample size is used to test multiple alleles, and a false-positive association arises by chance. Hence, it is suggested that any positive association with allele(s) be followed up by a detailed study of the allele status of parents, in order to determine the pattern of inheritance by using the transmission disequilibrium test.[24]

Franks and coworkers recruited 23 multiply affected families with well-characterized PCOS.[25] Their extensive pedigrees demonstrated the heterogeneity of the symptoms of PCOS between the probands and their sisters, the problems of assigning definite affected status to more than one generation in view of unreliable data from post-menopausal women, and the difficulties in assigning affected status for men. They acknowledge that PCOS should be treated as a quantitative trait disorder, which could possibly explain the variable phenotype based on a small number of causative genes as the basis of the disease. A candidate gene approach would be of greater validity than performing linkage studies using a single-gene autosomal dominant model. Franks et al used a linkage analysis program that makes no assumption of the mode of inheritance, along with association studies, for candidate genes coding for steroidogenic enzymes in the androgen biosynthetic pathway, and those involved with the secretion and action of insulin.[25]

Genetics: steroidogenesis and polycystic ovary syndrome

As hyperandrogenism is a key feature of PCOS it is logical to explore the critical steps in steroidogenesis and potential enzyme dysfunction. A number of studies have therefore looked at key stages in the steroidogenic pathway. The main conclusion is a possible abnormality with the cholesterol side chain cleavage gene (CYP11a).

Cholesterol side chain cleavage gene (CYP11a)

The cholesterol side chain cleavage enzyme CYP11a converts cholesterol to pregnenolone, and is an important rate-limiting step in steroidogenesis (Figure 4.1). Franks and coworkers showed that polycystic ovary theca cells produce an excess of both androgens and progesterone.[26,27] This prompted them to examine CYP11a (encoding P450 side chain cleavage (p450scc)) as a possible candidate gene for abnormal steroidogenesis. Gharani et al reported in 1997, that CYP11a is a major genetic susceptibility locus for PCOS. They examined the segregation of CYP11a in 20 families and performed association studies in consecutively recruited women of European descent with classical PCOS, and matched controls. They demonstrated that variation in the CYP11a gene was associated with both PCOS and elevated serum testosterone concentrations. They allowed for genetic heterogeneity and estimated that approximately 60% of their 20 families had linkage with the cholesterol side chain cleavage enzyme. Thus CYP11a was suggested as a major susceptibility locus for the hyperandrogenism of PCOS.[25]

Urbanek et al in 1999 reported the results of 150 families with multiply affected PCOS women, of whom 148 were of white European descent, and who were studied extensively for 37 candidate genes linked to PCOS.[28] They studied their identity by descent, as well as the extent of association between specific alleles at the candidate gene markers and PCOS, by using transmission disequilibrium. They confirmed the evidence for a significant linkage of the CYP11a gene with PCOS. However, after very stringent correction made to these results for multiple testing, they concluded that the association was not significant.

17-hydroxylase/17,20 lyase gene (CYP17)

Carey et al reported in 1994 of a possible association between a variant allele of CYP17 (the gene encoding P450c17α) and PCOS.[29] Their findings were based on a relatively small population of 71 affected subjects and 33 controls. These authors and others have subsequently been unable to demonstrate the same association with a larger numbers of subjects, suggesting a type I error.[30,31] None of these studies found any relationship between the variant CYP17 and serum androgen levels.[25]

The aromatase gene (CYP19)

Gharani et al also studied, both by case-control and linkage analysis, alleles of the CYP19 gene, which encodes P450 aromatase, and found no association with PCOS.

Genetics: insulin resistance and polycystic ovary syndrome

The risk of developing PCOS is partly genetic and disturbances in insulin metabolism play a key role. Linkage was reported with common allelic variation (Class I and Class III allele) at the variable number of tandem repeat (VNTR) locus in the promotor region of the insulin gene (INS).[32] The III/III genotype and class III allele were linked to PCOS, but only in women who were anovulatory and hyperinsulinemic. The INS VNTR III/III genotype has also been associated with large size at birth,[33] and with an increased risk for type 2 diabetes.[34] These data would favor the theory that genetic variations that regulate fetal growth could influence perinatal survival and predispose to the development of adult disease.[33]

A review of research into the molecular basis of insulin resistance in PCOS suggests a genetic basis for PCOS with reports of some kindreds being linked to premature baldness as the male phenotype.[10] In these families, linkage to the VNTR locus upstream of the insulin gene has been

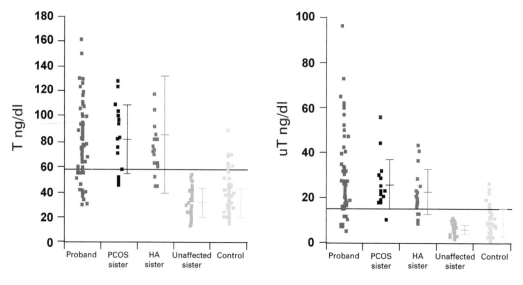

Figure 5.1

Elevated testosterone (total T) and bioavailable (uT) levels in affected sisters. Probands used to identify the family are on the left of the graph. PCOS sisters have elevated androgens and chronic anovulation. HA is hyperandrogenemia alone in the sisters who have regular menses. Unaffected sisters have normal androgens and menses. Adapted from Legro et al, 1998.[81]

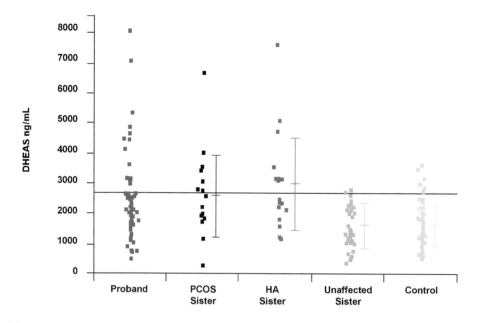

Figure 5.2

DHEAS adrenal androgen levels are also elevated in affected sisters. Probands used to identify the family are on the left of the graph. PCOS sisters have elevated androgens and chronic anovulation. HA is hyperandrogenemia alone in the sisters who have regular menses. Unaffected sisters have normal androgens and menses. Adapted from Legro et al, 1998.[81]

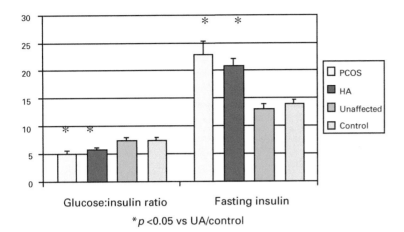

Figure 5.3

Hyperandrogenemia, with or without chronic anovulation identifies insulin resistance in PCOS sisters. Probands used to identify the family are on the left of the graph. PCOS sisters have elevated androgens and chronic anovulation. HA is hyperandrogenemia alone in the sisters who have regular menses. Unaffected sisters have normal androgens and menses. Adapted from Legro et al, 2002.[13]

demonstrated.[32] In view of the strong association of PCOS with insulin resistance, and the insulin receptor or a related regulatory element being very likely to have central control in its expression, the insulin receptor (*INSR*) gene has also long been thought to be a candidate gene of PCOS.

Legro et al suggest that familial aggregation of PCOS supports a genetic origin.[34] In view of the finding that not all hyperandrogenemic women in PCOS families have chronic anovulation and insulin resistance, they suggest the variable penetrance of a single genetic trait or that an additional gene(s) confer insulin resistance.

Family and twin studies also suggest that insulin resistance is a genetic trait in PCOS kindreds (Figures 5.1–5.4).[12,13,81] Thus, substantial evidence suggests that abnormalities in steroidogenesis and insulin action are genetic defects in PCOS.

The insulin receptor

Insulin acts through its receptor to initiate a cascade of intracellular events that both promote glucose uptake into the cell and also activate

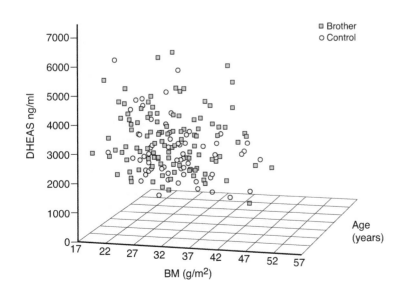

Figure 5.4

Elevated DHEAS levels in brothers of PCOS probands displayed by BMI and with age- and weight-matched control males. Adapted from Legro et al, 2002.[13]

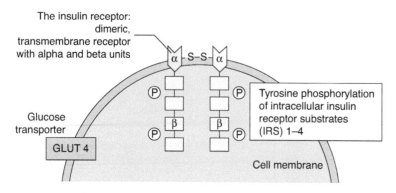

The insulin receptor: dimeric, transmembrane receptor with alpha and beta units

Glucose transporter

GLUT 4

Tyrosine phosphorylation of intracellular insulin receptor substrates (IRS) 1–4

Cell membrane

Activation of:
1. phosphotidyl inositol kinase (PIK) to permit glucose uptake via GLUT4
2. Cascade of cell growth and differentiation

Figure 5.5

Insulin acts through its receptor to cause tyrosine phosphorylation of insulin-receptor substrates, which then initiate both glucose uptake and trophic actions within the cell.

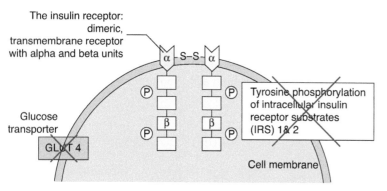

The insulin receptor: dimeric, transmembrane receptor with alpha and beta units

Glucose transporter

GLUT 4

Tyrosine phosphorylation of intracellular insulin receptor substrates (IRS) 1 & 2

Cell membrane

Activation of:
1. phosphotidyl inositol kinase (PIK) to permit glucose uptake via GLUT4
2. Cascade of cell growth and differentiation

Figure 5.6

In PCOS serine phosphorylation rather than tyrosine phosphorylation reduces glucose uptake whilst the trophic effects remain.

protein synthesis and steroidogenesis (Figure 5.5). The receptor is phosphorylated – usually undergoing tyrosine phosphorylation, although in insulin-resistant states it undergoes serine phosphorylation, which impedes the normal action of insulin (Figure 5.6). Insulin-receptor substrates are activated, and a cascade of intracellular messengers are then mobilized. Various steps in this pathway have been explored to ascertain potential dysfunction in individuals with insulin resistance and PCOS.

Extensive studies failed to detect any abnormalities in the tyrosine kinase domain of the insulin receptor gene in a cohort of hyperinsulinemic PCOS women.[35] Talbot et al performed scanning of the entire coding region of the insulin receptor gene (*INSR*) on DNA samples from 24 well-characterized women with PCOS.[36] Common polymorphisms were detected in the intron 5′ and exon 3, but no missense or nonsense mutations (i.e. those that would be expected to result in marked impairment of receptor function) were found.[36,37]

Tucci et al performed association studies in a total of 85 Caucasian PCOS patients and 87 age-matched Caucasian controls.[38] They demonstrated a strong association between PCOS and marker D19S884 located 1 cM telomeric to the *INSR* gene, while they found no association with the INSR microsatellite located inside the *INSR* gene. They proposed three possibilities to explain their finding, namely:

- the susceptibility gene on 19p13 (the closer marker) may be a regulatory element of the *INSR* gene located close to D19S884 (the distant marker)
- the closer marker has a higher mutation rate than that of the distant marker
- the more distant marker shows greater linkage disequilibrium with PCOS than the closer marker.

The marker D19S884 has been subsequently associated with PCOS, in a family-based association study using the transmission disequilibrium test (TDT).[28] Hence it is possible that this gene mediates its effects by influencing *INSR* gene expression in the ovary. Since insulin stimulates androgen secretion by ovarian stroma, it is likely that changes in the *INSR* or its signaling pathway in the ovary could explain some of the genetic susceptibility to PCOS.

A more recent study from Italy and Spain, however, failed to demonstrate an association between the marker D19S884 at the insulin receptor gene locus and PCOS, suggesting the possibility of racial population differences or environmental factors, such as prevalence of obesity.[39]

In insulin-resistant women with PCOS, there is increased serine phosphorylation, as opposed to tyrosine phosphorylation. This impedes the normal function of the insulin-receptor substrates, which in turn decreases glucose uptake by the cell. Serine phosphorylation of human P450c17 increases androgen biosynthesis.[40] Protein kinase A is a candidate serine kinase that serine phosphorylates the insulin receptor and P450c17 in vitro. If the same factor that serine phosphorylates the insulin receptor, causing insulin resistance, also serine phosphorylates P450c17, causing hyperandrogenism, the association of PCOS and insulin resistance might be explained by a single genetic defect.[41]

It has been hypothesized that polymorphisms in the *INSR* gene that induce mild changes in insulin receptor function may contribute to the development of PCOS, as it is unlikely that a major mutation is present, given the wide variability of insulin resistance in women with PCOS.[42] A case-control study of 99 white women with clinical PCOS and polycystic ovaries compared them with 136 controls. Exon 17 of the *INSR* gene, in the tyrosine kinase domain of the insulin receptor was evaluated. A significant increase in a single nucleotide polymorphism of *INSR* His 1058 C/T was found only in lean women with PCOS (body mass index (BMI) <27 kg/m^2) compared with lean controls.[42] It was unclear why this association was not seen in obese women with PCOS, who have a tendency to be more insulin resistant. The authors postulate that either the sample size was too small or that insulin resistance in lean and obese women with PCOS is caused by different mechanisms.

Other loci involved in the control of intracellular glucose transport have been associated with ovarian hyperandrogenism and insulin resistance. For example:

- the *G972R* variant of the insulin receptor substrate-1 (*IRS-1*) gene, which was found with increased frequency in girls with a history of precocious pubarche[43]
- the *Pro12 Ala* polymorphism of the peroxisome proliferator-activated receptor-γ (*PPARγ*) gene, which was found to be protective against the development of PCOS.[44]

The insulin gene *VNTR*

The insulin gene *VNTR* minisatellite locus lies 5' to the insulin gene on chromosome 11p15.5, and regulates the expression of the insulin gene. Bennett et al implicated the *VNTR* in the susceptibility to type 2 diabetes.[45] This allele was also implicated in hyperinsulinemia related to central obesity in women.[46] At this locus, there is a bimodal distribution of repeats, class I alleles being short (average of 40 repeats) and class III alleles much longer (average 157).

Waterworth et al examined the linkage of PCOS to the 11p15.5 locus in 17 families with several cases of PCOS and male pattern balding.[32] They also looked for an association between the insulin gene *VNTR* (particularly class I and III alleles) and polycystic ovaries in two additional populations of European women presenting to two centers with symptoms of PCOS. They calculated the odds ratio for insulin *VNTR* genotype using the conventional case-control approach and by the use of the family-based controls method (the latter is similar to TDT). They found that the class III allele of the insulin *VNTR* gene was associated with PCOS, and furthermore showed a strong correlation with anovulatory PCOS. Thus, the insulin *VNTR* class III allele correlated with the hyperinsulinemia and insulin resistance of PCOS, as insulin resistance is more prominent in anovulatory women than with equally hyperandrogenemic women with regular menses.[47] Waterworth et al also found that the class III allele was preferentially transmitted from heterozygous fathers to daughters, and not from mother to daughter.[32]

In contrast, Urbanek et al in 1999 did not find any association between the class III allele of the insulin *VNTR* and PCOS.[28] This held for transmission from both parents to daughters with PCOS, and from either fathers or mothers to affected daughters. Neither was an association demonstrated with hyperandrogenism in a study of Spanish women.[48] However, our group found that the class III allele correlated with increasing severity of PCOS phenotype and insulin resistance.[49] The sample was a community-based population of 'normal' volunteers, who belonged to the post-menarchal age group (17–25 years), among whom those with PCOS had a heavier birthweight. A plausible explanation for the latter finding relates to the class III allele of *INS VNTR* being associated with larger size at birth.[33] However, the nature of the association of birthweight with PCO/PCOS is uncertain. Ibanez and coworkers reported a higher incidence of hyperinsulinemic hyperandrogenism in adolescent girls of low birthweight.[50] Fetal insulin resistance may occur in response to intrauterine growth restraint,[51] and may also be associated with the insulin *VNTR* III/III genotype.[34]

Data from the Uppsala group have demonstrated that whereas insulin resistance was largely reversible by weight loss (in the obese PCOS women), an abnormality of first-phase insulin secretion remained despite improved insulin sensitivity, which suggests a fundamental disorder in pancreatic β-cell function.[52]

Genetic aspects of insulin resistance and type 2 diabetes

Insulin resistance and hyperinsulinemia are common abnormalities in individuals at high risk of type 2 diabetes and/or impaired glucose tolerance, as well as their first-degree relatives, which suggests that insulin resistance predicts the development of diabetes.[53] Fasting hyperinsulinemia is a widely accepted surrogate measure of insulin resistance. In a prospective study of Pima Indians with normal glucose tolerance, Weyer and coworkers demonstrated that high fasting insulin concentration was an independent risk factor for diabetes, in addition to insulin resistance and impaired early-phase insulin secretion.[54] They also demonstrated that relative hyperinsulinemia is a highly heritable trait strongly aggregating in families. These data provide one explanation for the high prevalence of diabetes in ethnic groups with marked hyperinsulinemia, such as Native-Americans, Mexican Americans and Pacific Islanders.[55]

An inherited component is strongly involved in the pathogenesis of type 2 diabetes, with lifestyle and environmental factors also contributing. Twin studies have shown high concordance rates for type 2 diabetes in identical twins,[56] although, parenthetically, the only twin study on PCOS proved discordance among identical twins.[22] It is estimated that the lifetime risk of developing type 2 diabetes is between 40 and 60% in first-degree relatives of type 2 diabetic patients.[57] Family studies have also shown that the risk of diabetes in the offspring of affected parents increases two- to four-fold when one or both parents are affected.[58] In addition, some but not all studies in ethnic groups at high risk of diabetes suggest that offspring whose mothers are diabetic are more likely to develop diabetes themselves compared with offspring whose fathers are diabetic. A variety of hypotheses have been advanced to explain this apparent maternal transmission of diabetes.[59,60]

The Framingham Offspring Study, which studied a population predominantly of Caucasian origin, and thus at a low risk for diabetes, showed a simple additive model for parental transmission of diabetes i.e. the offspring of a single diabetic parent had a 3.5-fold higher risk and the offspring of both diabetic parents had a 6-fold higher risk than that of the offspring of non-diabetic parents.[61] These findings were similar to those in Pima Indians, who have a high prevalence of type 2 diabetes, such that the age-adjusted risk ratio of developing diabetes in the offspring of a single diabetic parent was 2.3 and for the offspring of both diabetic parents it was 4.5, when compared with that of the offspring of non-diabetic parents.[62] The similarity of risk ratios in these two study populations suggests that whatever is heritable in diabetes is similar across the races. The Framingham study also demonstrated that the offspring of diabetic mothers were more likely to have milder degrees of glucose homeostasis when compared with the offspring of diabetic fathers.[61]

The intrauterine environment in mothers with diabetes during pregnancy is associated with fetal undernutrition, low birthweight, insulin resistance and adult type 2 diabetes.[63-67] Dabelea et al demonstrated that babies born to diabetic mothers had a significantly higher risk of developing diabetes than the babies born to the same mothers prior to the development of diabetes. They concluded that the intrauterine exposure to diabetes per se confers a risk of obesity and diabetes in the offspring, in excess of the transmitted genetic risk.[68]

Ethnicity, type 2 diabetes and polycystic ovary syndrome

In view of an increased prevalence of PCOS in Caribbean Hispanics, it has been suggested that there may be ethnic variation in overt features and biochemical abnormalities of PCOS.[69] Of the community studies conducted so far to determine the prevalence of polycystic ovaries (PCO), the highest reported prevalence was among South Asian immigrants in Britain (52%).[70] This report demonstrated that South Asian women with PCO have a comparable degree of insulin resistance to age-matched South Asian women with established type 2 diabetes mellitus but without PCO. Nonetheless, there is a paucity of data on the clinical and biochemical features of South Asian women with PCOS. Norman and coworkers demonstrated that Asian Indian women with PCOS had a higher insulin response to a glucose load than their white European counterparts, and suggested the ethnicity of subjects with PCOS

needs consideration when studying its metabolic parameters.[20] Type 2 diabetes has a high prevalence among indigenous populations of South Asia, with central obesity being more strongly associated with diabetes in women than in men.[71-74] The greater prevalence of PCO and type 2 diabetes among South Asian women suggest ethnic differences in the clinical manifestations and metabolic problems of PCOS; this could contribute to a better understanding of the disease mechanism.

An ethnic difference in PCOS has not been well explored. The prevalence of PCO in a population of South Asian women residing in England has been shown to be significantly higher than among white European women, with a significant proportion of the women being symptomatic. Type 2 diabetes and insulin resistance have a high prevalence among indigenous populations in South Asia, with a rising prevalence among women. Insulin resistance and hyperinsulinemia are common antecedents of type 2 diabetes, with a high prevalence in South Asians. Type 2 diabetes also has a familial basis, inherited as a complex genetic trait that interacts with environmental factors, chiefly nutrition, commencing from fetal life.

We performed a case-control cross-sectional observational study of consecutive women with anovular PCOS, 47 South Asians, 40 Caucasians, and their age-matched controls, 11 South Asians and 22 Caucasians.[75] Age-matched unrelated women from the same ethnic backgrounds without PCOS, seeking treatment for male infertility were studied in a similar way to the index subjects. South Asians with PCOS presented at a younger age (26 ± 4 vs 30.1 ± 5 years, $p = 0.005$). BMI and waist:hip ratios were similar in the two affected cohorts. More South Asians had oligomenorrhea commencing at a younger age. Hirsutism (Ferriman Gallwey score, 18 vs 7.5, $p = 0.0001$), acne, acanthosis nigricans, and secondary infertility were significantly more prevalent in South Asians. The fasting glucose was similar (4.52 ± 0.08 vs 4.62 ± 0.09 mmol/l, $p = 0.25$), the fasting insulin was higher (89.4 ± 8.9 vs 48.6 ± 4.8 pmol/l, $p = 0.0001$) and insulin sensitivity (IS) lower (0.335 ± 0.005 vs 0.357 ± 0.002; $p = 0.0001$) among South Asians. Serum SHBG was significantly lower in South Asians (35 ± 3.3 vs 55 ± 9.4 nmol/l, $p = 0.02$), while serum testosterone was similar (2.69 ± 0.11 vs 2.64 ± 0.13 nmol/l, $p = 0.37$). Furthermore there was a significant correlation with an increased rate of the *INS VNTR* III/III genotype in the South Asian women, both with PCOS and normal ovaries.

In an extension to this study, 80 native Sri Lankans (SL) with PCOS and 45 native Sri Lankan controls were compared with the original cohort of 47 British Asians (BA) with PCOS and 11 controls, 40 white Europeans (C) with PCOS and 22 controls were studied.[76] Asian PCOS women were younger than C (27.3 ± 0.7 (SL) and 26 ± 0.4 (BA) vs 30.1 ± 0.5 years (C); $p = 0.008$). BMI of SL PCOS although significantly lower than the other affected groups (26.3 ± 0.95 (SL); 30.59 ± 7.54 (BA); 32.1 ± 5.95 (C) kg/m² ($p = 0.006$) had similar waist:hip ratios (WHR): 0.97 ± 0.01 (SL); 1.04 ± 0.02 (BA); 0.92 ± 0.01 (C), $p = 0.33$). Mean plasma homocysteine (Hcy) was significantly higher in all PCOS groups when compared with their ethnically matched controls ((SL) 10.18 ± 1.9 vs 9.0 ± 3.8, $p = 0.01$; (BA) 7.85 ± 1.9 vs 6.8 ± 2.5, $p < 0.0001$; (C) 8.27 ± 2.3 vs 6.86 ± 1.5, $p = 0.0007$) μmol/l), while SL PCOS had significantly greater Hcy concentrations ($p = 0.0012$) than affected women from other ethnic groups. SL PCOS individuals had significantly greater fasting insulin concentrations: 242.9 ± 38.9 (SL); 89.4 ± 8.9 (BA); 48.6 ± 4.8 (C) pmol/l ($p = 0.0003$) and significantly lower quantitative insulin sensitivity check (QUICKI) (0.308 ± 0.004 (SL); 0.398 ± 0.007 (BA); 0.447 ± 0.014 (C) ($p = 0.0007$)), than BA and C with PCOS. Fasting plasma Hcy correlated positively with fasting insulin concentration $r = 0.49$ ($p < 0.0001$), negatively with insulin sensitivity as assessed by the QUICKI method. $r = -0.52$ ($p < 0.0001$), and did not show a correlation with age and BMI, but had a positive correlation with waist:hip ratio.

Thus PCOS is associated with a significant elevation of fasting plasma homocysteine when compared with ethnically matched controls. Plasma homocysteine concentration in PCOS has a strong correlation with fasting insulin concentrations and insulin resistance, with highest concentrations observed in affected indigenous Sri Lankans. These findings in young Sri Lankan women with PCOS bear major implications for their long-term atherosclerosis risks. Thus South Asians with anovular PCOS seek treatment at a younger age, have more severe symptoms, higher fasting insulin concentrations and lower insulin sensitivity than Caucasians.

We can postulate, based on the Sri Lankan findings, that an ethnic group at a greater risk of insulin resistance and type 2 diabetes, expresses PCOS with greater clinical and metabolic derangements. The effects of environment, in other words urbanization-linked nutrition, may then amplify genetic effects.

Other genes in PCOS

Follistatin gene

Urbanek et al, in their exhaustive analysis of 37 candidate genes and PCOS, reported a significant linkage and association with the follistatin gene, which remained significant even after correction for multiple testing.[28] They argued that since follistatin is an activin-binding protein that neutralizes the biological action of activin, and since activin promotes ovarian follicle development, inhibits thecal cell androgen production, and increases pancreatic β-cell function, an increase in the follistatin level might be expected to lead to an arrest of follicle development, an increase in ovarian androgen production and also inhibition of insulin secretion. Tucci et al in a case-control study of 85 affected Caucasian PCOS women, after correction for multiple testing, failed to demonstrate any association with the follistatin gene.[38] Urbanek et al subsequently reported that despite the finding of 17 allelic variations of the follistatin gene in 19 families with PCOS, 16 of them were too rare to make a major contribution and concluded that any contribution to the etiology of PCOS by the follistatin gene was likely to be very small.[28] They also reported that there was no correlation of messenger RNA levels of follistatin in cultured fibroblasts of women with PCOS. Furthermore, follistatin levels in healthy and atretic ovarian follicles, from normal and PCOS women, have been shown to maintain a similar high steady-state level, indicating it plays no role in PCOS.[51] Liao et al and Calvo have also demonstrated the lack of evidence for a follistatin gene mutation in cohorts of PCOS women of Chinese and Spanish origin.[77,78]

Follicle stimulating hormone β-subunit gene

Based on Urbanek and coworkers' findings,[28] Tong et al searched for mutations in the entire coding region of the follicle stimulating hormone (FSH) β-subunit gene of patients with PCOS.[79,80] The basis of their study of the FSH β-subunit gene was, that PCOS has defects in ovulation that are corrected by exogenous FSH, and that over-expression of follistatin in transgenic mice led to suppression of FSH secretion. They performed case-control association studies in 135 Chinese women with PCOS, and reported only a previously described *Acc1* polymorphism in exon 3 of the gene, especially in the obese hyperandrogenic women with PCOS. This is the only gene tested exclusively in Asian women, and the same group reported similar frequency of the polymorphism in Malay, Chinese and Dravidian Indian women.[80]

Summary

To summarize the genetic basis of PCOS, the steroid synthesis *CYP11a* gene, the insulin gene *VNTR* polymorphism, the follistatin gene and *Acc1* polymorphism of the *β-FSH* gene appear to play a role in the genetic basis of PCOS. The variations in their expression between families and ethnic groups may explain the heterogeneity of the syndrome. These findings remain to be confirmed in larger studies. It is also unlikely that these are the only genes to be involved in the etiology of PCOS. Franks et al postulate that PCOS is an oligogenic disorder, representing a quantitative trait in which a small number of key genes contribute in conjunction with environmental factors (chiefly nutrition), to produce the observed clinical and biochemical heterogeneity.[25] Franks proposes that the underlying problem is the development of the polycystic ovarian morphology, with a primary disorder of folliculogenesis. This predisposes the subject to develop PCOS. However, the genes determining the development of the ovarian morphology remain unknown. Others, ourselves included, favour the notion that it is the environment in which the ovary develops that programmes the expression of PCOS, with hyperinsulinemia either in utero or childhood/adolescence leading to ovarian hyperandrogenism.

References

1. Balen AH, Conway GS, Kaltas G, Techatrasak K et al. Polycystic Ovary Syndrome: the spectrum of the disorder in 1741 patients. Hum Reprod 1995; 10:2107–2111.

2. Franks S, Gharani N, McCarthy M. Candidate genes in polycystic ovary syndrome. Hum Reprod Update 2001; 7:405–410.

3. Rajkhowa M, Talbot JA, Jones PW, Clayton RN. Polymorphism of glycogen synthetase gene in polycystic ovary syndrome. Clin Endocrinol (Oxf) 1996; 44:85–90.

4. Franks S. Medical progress article: polycystic ovary syndrome N Engl J Med 1995; 333:853–861.

5. Legro RS. Polycystic ovary syndrome, phenotype and genotype. Endocrinol Metab Clin North Am 1999; 28:379–396.

6. Cooper DN, Clayton JF. DNA polymorphism and the study of disease associations. Hum Genet 1988; 78:299–312.

7. Ferriman D, Purdie AW. The inheritance of polycystic ovarian disease and a possible relationship to premature balding. Clin Endocrinol (Oxf) 1979; 11:291–300.

8. Lunde O, Magnus P, Sandvik L et al. Familial clustering in the polycystic ovarian disease. Gynaeco Obstet Invest 1989; 28:23–30.

9. Hague WM, Adams J, Reedres ST et al. Familial polycystic ovaries: a genetic disease? Clin Endocrinol (Oxf) 1988; 29:593–605.

10. Carey AH, Chan KL, Short F, White D et al. Evidence for a single gene effect causing polycystic ovaries and male pattern baldness. Clin Endocrinol (Oxf) 1993; 38:653–658.

11. Norman RJ, Masters S, Hague W. Hyperinsulinaemia is common in family members of women with polycystic ovary syndrome. Fertil Steril 1996; 66:942–947.

12. Legro RS, Spielman R, Urbanek M et al. Phenotype and genotype in polycystic ovary syndrome. Recent Prog Horm Res 1998; 53:217–256.

13. Legro RS, Bentley-Lewis R, Driscoll D, Wang SC, Dunaif A. Insulin resistance in the sisters of women with polycystic ovary syndrome: association with hyperandrogenaemia rather than menstrual irregularity. J Clin Endocrinol Metab 2002; 87:2128–2133.

14. Yildiz BO, Yarali H, Oguz H, Bayraktar M. Glucose intolerance, insulin resistance, and hyperandrogenaemia in first degree relatives of women with polycystic ovary syndrome. J Clin Endocrinol Metab 2003; 88:2031–2036.

15. Kahsar-Miller MD, Nixon C, Boots LR, Go RC, Azziz R. Prevalence of polycystic ovary syndrome in first-degree relatives of patients with PCOS. Fertil Steril 2001; 75:53–58.

16. Knochenhauer ES, Key TJ, Kahsar Miller M et al. Prevalence of the polycystic ovary syndrome in unselected black and white women of the Southeastern United Sates: A prospective study. J Clin Endocrinol Metab 1998; 83:3078–3082.

17. Atiomo WU, El-Mahdi E, Hardiman P. Familial associations in women with polycystic ovary syndrome. Fertil Steril 2003; 80:143–145.

18. Xita N, Georgiou I, Tsatsoulis A. The genetic basis of polycystic ovary syndrome. Eur J Endocrinol 2002; 147:717–725.

19. Givens JR. Familial polycystic ovarian disease. Endocrinol Metab Clin North Am 1988; 17:771–781.

20. Norman RA, Bogardus C, Ravussin E. Linkage between obesity and a marker near the tumor necrosis factor a locus in Pima Indians. J Clin Invest 1995; 96:158–162.

21. Govind A, Obhrai MS, Clayton RN. Polycystic ovaries are inherited as an autosomal dominant trait: Analysis of 29 polycystic ovary syndrome and 10 control families. J Clin Endo Met 1999; 84:38–43.

22. Jahanfar S, Eden JA, Warren P et al. A twin study of polycystic ovary syndrome. Fertil Steril 1995; 63:478–486.

23. Lander ES, Schork NJ. Genetic dissection of complex traits. Science 1994; 265:2037–2048.

24. Spielman RS, Ewens WJ. The TDT and other family-based tests for linkage disequilibrium and association [editorial]. Am J Hum Genet 1996; 59:983–989.

25. Franks S, Gharani N, Waterworth D, Batty S et al. The genetic basis of polycystic ovary syndrome. Hum Reprod 1997; 12:2641–2648.

26. Franks S, White D, Gilling-Smith C, Carey A et al. Hypersecretion of androgens by polycystic ovaries: the role of genetic factors in the regulation of cytochrome P450c17a, Balliere's Clin Endocrinol Metab 1996; 10:193–203.

27. Gilling-Smith C, Willis DS, Beard RW, Franks S. Hypersecretion of androstenedione by isolated theca cells from polycystic ovaries. J Clin Endocrinol Metab 1994; 79:1158–1165.

28. Urbanek M, Legro RS, Driscoll DA, Azziz R et al. Thirty seven candidate genes for polycystic ovary syndrome: Strongest evidence for linkage is with follistatin. Proc Natl Acad Sci USA 1999; 96:8573–8578.

29. Carey AH, Waterworth D, Patel K et al. Polycystic ovaries and premature male pattern baldness are associated with one allele of the steroid metabolism gene CYP17. Hum Mol Genet 1994; 3:1873–1876.

30. Gharani N, Waterworth DM, Williamson R et al. 5'polymorphism of the CYP17 gene is not associated with serum testosterone levels in women with polycystic ovaries [letter]. J Clin Endocrinol Metab 1996; 81:4174.

31. Tetchatraisak K, Conway GS, Rumsby G. Frequency of a polumorphism in the regulatory region of 17a hydroxylase-17,20 lyase (CYP17) gene in hyperandrogenic states. Clin Endocrinol (Oxf) 1997; 46:131–134.

32. Waterworth DM, Bennett ST, Gharani N, McCarthy MI et al. Linkage and association of insulin gene VNTR regulatory polymorphism with polycystic ovary syndrome. Lancet 1997; 349:986–990.

33. Dunger DB, Ong KK, Huxtable SJ et al. Association of the INS VNTR with size at birth Nat Genet 1998; 19:98–100.

34. Ong KK, Phillips DI, Fall C et al. The insulin gene VNTR, type 2 diabetes and birth weight. Nat Genet 1999; 21:262–263.

35. Conway GS, Avey C, Rumsby C. The tyrosine kinase domain of the insulin receptor gene is normal in women with hyperinsulinaemia and polycystic ovary syndrome. Hum Reprod 1994; 9:1681–1683.

36. Talbot JA, Bicknell EJ, Rajkhowa M, Krrok A et al. Molecular scanning of the insulin receptor gene in women with polycystic ovarian syndrome J Clin Endocrinol Metab 1996; 81:1979–1983.

37. Sorbara LR, Tang Z, Cama A, Xia J et al. Absence of insulin receptor gene mutations in three insulin resistant women with polycystic ovary syndrome. Metabolism 1994; 43:1568–1574.

38. Tucci S, Futterweit W, Concepcion ES, Greenberg DA et al. Evidence for association of polycystic ovary syndrome in Caucasian women with a marker at the insulin receptor gene locus. J Clin Endocrinol Metab 2001; 86:446–449.

39. Villuendas G, Escobar-Morreale HF, Tosi F, Sancho J et al. Association between the marker D19S884 at the insulin receptor gene locus and polycystic ovary syndrome. Fertil Steril 2003; 79:219–220.

40. Zhang L, Rodriquez H, Ohno S et al. Serine phosphorylation of human P450c17 increases 17,20 lyase activity: Implications for adrenarche and the polycystic ovary syndrome. Proc Natl Acad Sci USA 1995; 92:10619–10623.

41. Dunaif A. Insulin action in the polycystic ovary syndrome. Endocrinol Metab Clin North Am 1999; 28:341–359.

42. Siegel S, Futterweit W, Davies TF, Concepcion ES et al. A C/T single nucleotide polymorphism at the tyrosine kinase domain of the insulin receptor gene is associated with polycystic ovary syndrome. Fertil Steril 2002; 78:1240–1243.

43. Ibanez L, Marcos MV, Potau N, White C et al. Increased frequency of the G972R variant of the insulin receptor substrate-1 (IRS-1) gene amongst girls with a history of precocious pubarche. Fertil Steril 2002; 78:1288–1293.

44. Korhonen S, Heinonen S, Hiltunen M, Helisalmi S et al. Polymorphism in the peroxisome proliferators-activated receptor-γ gene in women with polycystic ovary syndrome. Hum Reprod 2003; 18:540–543.

45. Bennett ST, Lucassen AM, Gough SCL, Powell EE et al. Susceptibility to human type I diabetes and

IDDM2 is determined by tandem repeat variation at the insulin gene minisatellite locus. Nat Genet 1995; 9:284–292.

46. Weaver JU, Kopelman PG, Hitman GA. Cental obesity and hyperinsulinaemia in women are associated with polymorphism in the 5_ flanking region of the human insulin gene Eur J Clin Invest 1992; 22:265–270.

47. Dunaif A, Graf M, Mandeli J, Laumas V, Dobrjansky A. Characterization of groups of hyperandrogenic women with acanthosis nigricans, impaired glucose tolerance and/or hyperinsulinaemia. J Clin Endocrinol Metab 1987; 65:499–507.

48. Calvo RM, Telleria D, Sancho J, San Millan JL et al. Insulin gene variable number of tandem repeats regulatory polymorphism is not associated with hyperandrogenism in Spanish women. Fertil Steril 2002; 77:666–668.

49. Michelmore KF, Ong K, Mason S, Bennett S et al. Clinical features in women with polycystic ovaries: relationships to insulin sensitivity, insulin gene VNTR and birth weight. Clin Endocrinol (Oxf) 2001; 55:439–446.

50. Ibanez L, Potau N, Francois I, de Zegher F. Precocious pubarche, hyperinsulinism, and ovarian hyperandrogenism in girls: relation to reduced fetal growth. J Clin Endocrinol Metab 1998; 83:3558–3562.

51. Simmons RA, Flozak AS, Ogata ES. The effect of insulin and insulin-like growth factor 1 on glucose transport in normal and small for gestational age fetal rats. Endocrinology 1993; 133:1361–1368.

52. Holte J. Disturbances in insulin secretion and sensitivity in women with polycystic ovary syndrome. Bailliere's Clin Endocrinol Metab 1996; 10:221–247.

53. Pratley RE, Weyer C, Borgardus C. Metabolic abnormalities in the development of non-insulin dependent diabetes mellitus. In: Le Roith D, Taylor SI, Olefsky JM, eds. Diabetes Mellitus (2nd edn). Philadelphia: Lippincot-Raven, 2000:549–557.

54. Weyer C, Hanson RL, Tataranni PA et al. A high fasting plasma insulin concentration predicts type 2 diabetes independent of insulin resistance. Evidence for a pathogenic role of relative hyperinsulinaemia. Diabetes 2000; 49:2094–2101.

55. Lillioja S, Mott DM, Sparaul M et al. Insulin resistance, and insulin secretory dysfunction as precursors of non-insulin dependent diabetes mellitus prospective studies of Pima Indians. N Engl J Med 1993; 329:1988–1992.

56. Barnett A, Eff C, Lelsie D et al. Diabetes in identical twins a study of 200 pairs. Diabetologia 1981; 20:87–93.

57. Martin BC, Warram JH, Krolewski AS et al. Role of glucose and insulin resistance in development of type 2 diabetes mellitus: results of a 25 year follow up study. Lancet 1992; 340:925–929.

58. Mitchell BD, Valdez R, Hazuda HP et al. Differences in the prevalence of diabetes and impaired glucose tolerance according to maternal or paternal history of diabetes. Diabetes Care 1993; 16:1262–1267.

59. Kartner AJ, Rowell SC, Ackerson LM et al. Excess maternal transmission of type 2 diabetes: the North Carolina Kaiser Permanente Diabetes Registry. Diabetes Care 1999; 22:938–943.

60. McCarthy M , Cassell P, Tran T et al. Evaluation of the importance of maternal diabetes and of mitochondrial variation in the development of NIDDM. Diabet Med 1996; 13:420–428.

61. Meigs JB, Cupples A, Wilson PWF. Parental transmission of type 2 diabetes: The Framingham Offspring Study. Diabetes 2000; 49:2201–2207.

62. Knowler WC, Pettitt DJ, Savage PJ et al. Diabetes incidence in Pima Indians: contributions of obesity and parental diabetes. Am J Epidemiol 1981; 113:144–156.

63. Hales CN, Barker DJP, Clark PMS et al. Fetal and infant growth and impaired glucose tolerance at age 64. Br Med J 1991; 303:1019–1022.

64. McCance DR, Pettitt DJ, Hanson RL et al. Birthweight and non insulin dependent diabetes: thrifty genotype, or survivng small baby genotype? Br Med J 1994; 308:942–945.

65. Barker DJP, Hales CN, Fall C, Osmond C et al. Type 2 (non insulin-dependent) diabetes mellitus hypertension and hyperlipidaemia (syndrome X): relation to reduced fetal growth. Diabetologia 1993; 36:62–67.

66. Jaquet D, Gaboriau A, Czernihow P, Levy-Marchal C. Insulin resistance early in adulthood in subjects born with intrauetrine growth retardation. J Clin Endocrinol Metab 2000; 85:1401–1406.

67. Dabelea D, Pettitt DJ, Hansen RL et al. Birth weight, type 2 diabetes, and insulin resistance in Pima Indian children and young adults. Diabetes Care 1999; 22:944–950.

68. Dabelea D, Hanson RL, Lindsay RS et al. Intrauterine exposure to diabetes conveys risks for type 2 diabetes and obesity. A study of discordant sibships. Diabetes 2000; 49:2208–2211.

69. Solomons CG. The epidemiology of polycystic ovary syndrome- prevalence and associated disease risks. Endocrinol Metab Clin North Ame 1999; 28:247–263.

70. Rodin DA, Bano G, Bland JM, Taylor K, Nussey SS. Polycystic ovaries and associated metabolic abnormalities in Indian subcontinent Asian women. Clin Endocrinol (Oxf) 1998; 49:91–99.

71. King H, Aubert RE, Herman WH. Global burden of diabetes, 1995–2025: prevalence, numerical estimates, and projections. Diabetes Care 1998; 21:1414–1431.

72. Trevisan R, Vedovato M, Tiengo A. The epidemiology of diabetes mellitus. Nephrol Dial Transplant 1998; 13(suppl 8):2–5.

73. Shera AS, Rafique G, Khawaja IA, Baqai S, King H. Pakistan National Diabetes Survey: prevalence of glucose intolerance and associated factors in Baluchisan province. Diabet Res Clin Pract 1999; 44:49–58.

74. Ramachandran A, Snehalatha C, Latha E, Manoharan M, Vijay V. Impacts of urbanization on the lifestyle and on the prevalence of diabetes in native Asian Indian population. Diabet Res Clin Pract 1999; 44:207–213.

75. Wijeyaratne CN, Balen AH, Barth J, Belchetz PE. Clinical manifestations and insulin resistance (IR) in polycystic ovary syndrome (PCOS) among South Asians and Caucasians: is there a difference? Clin Endocrinol (Oxf) 2002; 57:343–350.

76. Wijeyaratne CN, Pathmakumara A, Warnakulasuriya AM, Gunawardhare AUA et al. Plasma homocysteine in polycystic ovary syndrome: does it correlate with insulin resistance and ethnicity? Clin Endocrinol (Oxf) 2003; 60:560–567.

77. Liao W-X, Roy AC, Ng SC. Preliminary investigation of follistatin gene mutations in women with polycystic ovary syndrome. Mol Hum Reprod 2000; 6:587–590.

78. Calvo RM, Villuendas G, Sancho J, San Millan JL, Escobar-Morreale HF. Role of follistatin gene in women with polycystic ovary syndrome. Fertil Steril 2001; 75:1020–1023.

79. Tong Y, Liao W-X, Roy AC, Ng SC. Association of Acc1 polymorphism in the follicle-stimulating hormone b gene with polycystic ovary syndrome. Fertil Steril 2000; 74:1233–1236.

80. Liao W-X, Tong Y, Roy AC, Ng SC. New Acc1 polymorphism in the follicle stimulating hormone beta subunit gene and its prevalence in three South East Asian populations Hum Heredity 1999; 49:181–182.

81. Legro RS , Driscoll D, Strauss JF, Fox J, Dunaif A. Evidence for a genetic basis for hyperandrogenemia in polycystic ovary syndrome. Proc Natl Acad Sci USA 1998; 95:14956–14960.

Chapter 6
Body image and quality of life with polycystic ovary syndrome

Introduction

Polycystic ovary syndrome (PCOS) is the most common endocrine disturbance affecting women. As has been described elsewhere, there is considerable heterogeneity of symptoms and signs amongst women with PCOS and for an individual these may change over time (see Chapters 2 and 3). Many of the symptoms of PCOS may be associated with psychological disturbances, and any symptom may worsen a pre-existing tendency to psychological dysfunction. While research has been performed on some of the psychological aspects of problems such as obesity, acne and hirsutism – which in women will often include those with PCOS – there is little study of the psychopathology of women defined as having PCOS (by whatever criteria). For example, hirsutism has been shown to cause marked psychological stress,[1] and infertility issues can cause tensions within the family, altered self-perception, and problems at work.[2,3] Despite this, a recent systematic review revealed that limited research had been carried out to assess the impact that the symptoms and associated treatments for PCOS have upon the quality of life of women with the condition.[4]

Symptoms, management and quality of life issues

It is easy to see how PCOS may impact upon a woman's quality of life and psychological wellbeing, yet this area has yet to be fully researched. Most of the literature on PCOS concerns clinical objectives, such as rates of pregnancy with ovulation induction, or changes in acne and hirsutism scores. There is little written on women's assessment of their own state of wellbeing, for example as assessed by 'health-related quality of life' (HRQoL), which is a multi-dimensional concept encompassing physical, psychological and social aspects of a disease process.[5]

A disease-specific questionnaire has been developed for PCOS,[6] although there have been criticisms of its validity and so further work is currently being undertaken to further assess HRQoL.[4] Although HRQoL measurement has an important role in evaluative research, the reliable assessment of quality of life depends upon the psychometric properties of the questionnaire (i.e. the tests underlying the construction and evaluation of the questionnaire), and the statistical methods employed to analyze and interpret the data.[7] It is important therefore that any HRQoL questionnaire to be used is based upon these psychometric properties. At present, one reason for the limited research on the impact of PCOS upon quality of life may be because no validated health outcome measure exists to measure the health status of women with the condition. The disease-specific questionnaire that was developed by Cronin et al, contains 26 items, measuring the following areas of HRQoL: emotions (eight items, e.g. moody as a result of having PCOS?), body hair (five items, e.g. growth of visible hair on chin?), weight (five items, e.g. had trouble dealing with your weight?), infertility problems (four items, e.g. concerned with infertility problems?) and menstrual problems (four items, e.g. irregular menstrual periods?).[6] However, only the content validity of the instrument had been evaluated, thus preventing its use in clinical settings. A study was therefore performed to evaluate the psychometric properties of the PCOS questionnaire (PCOSQ), in particular the reliability, validity and factor structure of the domains when assessing the HRQoL in women with PCOS.[4]

A total of 92 women of reproductive age with PCOS responded to the PCOSQ. Included with the questionnaire was the SF-36,[8] which was used as it was necessary to include another instrument to evaluate the construct validity of the PCOSQ. The PCOSQ has five domains, each relating to a common symptom of PCOS: weight (W), body hair (BH), emotions (EM), infertility (INF) and menstrual problems (MEN). Only those factors that scored >0.5 are recorded in Table 6.1.

Overall weight and infertility produced the worst health in comparison with the body hair domain which had the highest mean score, suggesting that this symptom was causing the least negative impact upon quality of life. The SF-36 questionnaire results indicated that the 'role limitation ± emotional' and 'energy and vitality'

Table 6.1 Analysis of the polycystic ovary syndrome health-related quality of life questionnaire (PCOSQ)[4]

Question		Score
W3.	Concerned about being overweight	0.841
W10.	Had trouble dealing with weight	0.851
W12.	Felt frustration trying to lose weight	0.877
W22.	Felt not sexy because overweight	0.704
W24.	Difficulties staying at ideal weight	0.847
BH1.	Growth of visible hair on chin	0.823
BH9.	Growth of visible hair on upper lip	0.793
BH15.	Growth of visible hair on face	0.873
BH16.	Embarrassment of excess body hair	0.898
BH26.	Growth of visible body hair	0.881
EM2.	Depressed about having PCOS	0.756
EM4.	Easily tired	0.345
EM6.	Moody as a result of having PCOS	0.567
EM17.	Worried about having PCOS	0.765
EM18.	Self-conscious having PCOS	0.744
EM11.	Had low self-esteem having PCOS	0.801
EM14.	Felt frightened of getting cancer	0.497
INF5.	Concerned with infertility problems	0.914
INF13.	Felt afraid of not having children	0.823
INF23.	Felt a lack of control over PCOS	0.652
INF25.	Felt sad because of infertility	0.902
MEN7.	Headaches	0.757
MEN8.	Irregular menstrual periods	0.789
MEN19.	Abdominal bloating	0.722
MEN21.	Menstrual cramps	0.682
EM20.	Late menstrual period	0.797

domains were the areas of poorest health. While generic questionnaires exist to measure HRQoL, such as the SF-36, they do not collect information on all the areas of wellbeing and functioning that may be important to women with PCOS. For example, infertility and hirsutism can place a considerable strain on the emotional wellbeing and personal relationships of women with this disease. However, this information is not collected on the SF-36 generic health measure. The mean scale scores on the PCOSQ reflect the negative impact PCOS can have upon the quality of life of women with the condition.[4] Perhaps not surprisingly, weight and infertility appeared to be the most significant aspects of the illness. Other studies have reported the negative impact infertility can have upon women and their personal relationships.[9,10] The finding that weight caused the most negative impact on quality of life has implications for the management of the condition, especially as it has been estimated that ~50% of women with PCOS suffer from obesity or are overweight.

The women interviewed felt that, on the whole, the questionnaire was addressing the issues relevant to women with PCOS.[4] However, the lack of questions about acne was raised as a serious omission. Acne is recognized as a common symptom of the condition. The finding that 34% of respondents in the study suffered from acne would support this and suggest that the addition of a new acne domain to the PCOSQ would be important if the instrument is to be used in a clinical setting. Another potential limitation to the study is that patients were recruited from a gynecology clinic. Consequently, it could be argued that there was a bias towards PCOS patients with menstrual disturbance and infertility, and not those presenting with other PCOS-related conditions (i.e. weight increase and acne), who are often referred to endocrinology and dermatology clinics.

Obesity

Obesity worsens both symptomatology and the endocrine profile and so obese women (body mass index (BMI) >30 kg/m[2]) should therefore be encouraged to lose weight. Weight loss improves the endocrine profile, reproductive function, and the likelihood of ovulation and a healthy pregnancy. The symptoms of PCOS for many women are a reflection of the 'modern' lifestyle, with a combination of an unhealthy diet and reduced levels of exercise promoting obesity, with secondary insulin resistance, which then increases the symptoms of PCOS in those women with a genetic predisposition.

Weight loss requires significant motivation and a long-term change in lifestyle. Weight loss is usually gradual if it is to be sustained. Women experience significant frustration and require the support of dietitians and clinic nurses in order to encourage adherence to a weight-reducing program. Commercial 'slimming clubs' provide peer support and can also be very valuable. Much has been written about diet and PCOS. The right diet for an individual is one that is practical, sustainable and compatible with her lifestyle. It is sensible to keep carbohydrate content down and to avoid fatty foods. It is often helpful to refer to a dietitian. Anti-obesity drugs may help with weight loss. Metformin may improve insulin resistance and may aid some women with weight loss, combined with a healthy diet and exercise program (see Chapter 7).

Eating disorders

The syndrome develops during adolescent years, at a time when disordered eating patterns are common. Both anorexia nervosa and bulimia have been linked with PCOS. Concerns about body weight may lead to binge eating and a self-perpetuating spiral of despondency and weight gain. Bulimia nervosa is estimated to have a prevalence of between 1 and 2% in adolescent and young adult women,[11-13] and is characterized by recurrent episodes of overeating ('binges'), and extreme behavior designed to control shape and weight.[11] 'Binge-eating disorder', which is not as severe as bulimia nervosa, is much more common with an estimated prevalence of 26% in the general population.[13,14]

The investigation of a potential relationship between PCOS and bulimia nervosa has been prompted by the observation that menstrual irregularity and acne are features that occur commonly in both.[15-18] Several studies have reported an association between the two conditions, but an

etiological link has never been satisfactorily explained.[19-23] Interpretation of existing data is confusing due to limitations of the diagnostic tools used to detect bulimia nervosa, varying criteria applied for diagnosing PCOS, and the influence of selection biases in studies of women recruited from specialist clinics. The possibility that a spurious association may have been identified between the two relatively common conditions of having polycystic ovaries and disordered eating habits must also be considered.

We have explored the reported link between polycystic ovaries, PCOS, and eating disorders using data gathered in our previously reported study of the prevalence of polycystic ovaries in a group of young, post-menarchal women in the normal population.[24] An interviewer-based questionnaire was used for the assessment of behavioral eating patterns. The relationship of abnormal eating behaviors with ultrasound evidence of polycystic ovary morphology and features of PCOS was examined.

Two-hundred and thirty female volunteers aged 18–25 years were recruited by advertisement from Oxford universities and by invitation from general practice surgeries as previously reported.[25] All participants completed the Eating Disorder Examination, 12th edition (EDE).[26] This is an interviewer-based questionnaire which is considered to be the 'gold standard' diagnostic tool for assessment of anorexia nervosa, bulimia nervosa, and their variants.[11] The EDE enables the key aspects of eating disorders: overeating, and the use of extreme measures of weight control, to be assessed and provides frequency ratings for their occurrence over the previous three months. Bulimia nervosa was diagnosed where the individual described recurrent episodes of binge eating, inappropriate compensatory behavior to prevent weight gain (such as self-induced vomiting, misuse of laxatives, diuretics or other medications, fasting, or excessive exercise), and where self-evaluation was unduly influenced by body shape and weight. The diagnosis of 'binge eating disorder' was made where recurrent episodes of binge eating occurred in the absence of inappropriate compensatory behaviors characteristic of bulimia nervosa.

The EDE interview was completed by all 230 participants. Seventy women (30%) described episodes of overeating which could be subdivided into:

- *objective overeating* where a large amount of food was consumed, but where the participant did not feel any loss of control over eating, reported by 56 (24%)
- *objective bulimic episodes* where a large amount of food was consumed and where the participant described a feeling of loss of control over eating, reported by 10 (4%)
- *subjective bulimic episodes* where the participant described a loss of control over eating while consuming amounts that were not objectively large, reported in 14 (6%).

Extreme methods of weight control had been employed by 9 (4%) participants. These included self-induced vomiting in four women, laxative misuse in two women, diuretic misuse in one woman, and intense exercising in six women. None of the 230 participants fulfilled the criteria for anorexia nervosa. Two women (1%) fulfilled the criteria for bulimia nervosa, and five women (2%) fulfilled the criteria for binge-eating disorder. Neither of the women with bulimia nervosa were overweight, defined as a BMI >25 kg/m², but three of the women with binge-eating disorder were overweight.

As frank eating disorders (bulimia nervosa and binge-eating disorder) were identified in only 3% of the total study population, comparisons between women with polycystic and those with normal ovaries were made using the quantitative EDE data. Comparisons were made for three features of disordered eating patterns to determine if polycystic ovarian morphology was associated with (i) binge eating or overeating, (ii) dieting behavior, or (iii) global eating disorder symptoms.

The results for our study group did not confirm any significant associations between polycystic ovaries, or PCOS with bulimia nervosa or binge-eating disorder. Of the 224 women who attended for an ultrasound scan, only one was diagnosed as having frank bulimia nervosa and she was found to have normal ovaries. Binge-eating disorder was diagnosed in three women (4%) in the polycystic ovary group, and in two women (1%) in the normal ovary group but the difference in these proportions was not statistically significant ($p = 0.4$). Analysis of the quantitative EDE data revealed higher mean scores for features of dieting and overall eating disorder symptomatology in women with polycystic ovaries and PCOS,

but these differences were not statistically significant.

The overall prevalence of bulimia nervosa detected in our study is much lower than that described by McCluskey et al who used a self-completed questionnaire (Bulimia Investigation Test, Edinburgh, BITE) to assess the prevalence of bulimia in a group of 375 women presenting to a specialist endocrine clinic.[22] Forty-four per cent of their study population were diagnosed as having PCOS, and bulimia nervosa was diagnosed by a high BITE score in 6% of these women as compared with 1% in their control group. Jahanfar et al using the BITE questionnaire to diagnose subclinical eating disorder and bulimia nervosa, reported that 21% of women with polycystic ovaries (7/34) had abnormal questionnaire scores compared with 2.5% (1/40) of women with normal ovaries.[20] The prevalence of bulimia nervosa in our group closely resembles that of larger population-based studies.[11–13] The discrepancy with the above studies may possibly be explained by the observation that self-reported questionnaires (e.g. BITE), have a lower threshold for diagnosing bulimia and binge eating than the more consistent and reliable interview-based techniques such as the EDE (Table 6.2).[11,26]

Although the prevalence of eating disorders in this population is in keeping with other community-based studies, we must still consider the possibility that a degree of selection bias may have occurred. The study information literature distributed to potential volunteers clearly indicated that participants would be asked to complete a questionnaire about their eating habits. Women with eating disorders are often very secretive about their eating problems and weight control behavior, and in cases of bulimia nervosa, commonly have strong feelings of shame or guilt about their eating habits.[16] Therefore, women with eating disorders may have been reluctant to participate in a study that would require them to expose and discuss their eating behavior. In addition, we must consider the possibility that the prevalence of eating disorders within the study group was in fact higher than detected. Some of the study participants may not have felt comfortable with the interviewer-based EDE setting or questionnaire, and may have therefore provided some inaccurate responses.

Several theories have been advanced to explain the proposed link between polycystic ovaries,

Table 6.2 Items which comprise the four Eating Disorder Examination subscales, with 'normal values' as reported by Fairburn and Cooper, 1992[26]

Restraint
1. Restraint over eating
2. Avoidance of eating
3. Food avoidance
4. Dietary rules
5. Desire for an empty stomach
Normal value = 0.79

Shape concern
1. Desire for a flat stomach
2. Importance of shape
3. Preoccupation with shape or weight
4. Fear of weight gain
5. Discomfort seeing body
6. Avoidance of exposure of body
7. Feelings of fatness
Normal value = 1.14

Eating concern
1. Preoccupation with food, eating, or calories
2. Fear of losing control over eating
3. Concern over eating in social settings
4. Eating in secret
5. Guilt about eating
Normal value = 0.20

Weight concern
1. Importance of weight
2. Reaction to prescribed weighing
3. Preoccupation with shape or weight
4. Dissatisfaction with weight
5. Desire to lose weight
Normal value = 1.00

PCOS, and bulimia nervosa. It has been suggested that emotional distress associated with adverse symptoms of PCOS (menstrual irregularity, obesity, hirsutism, and acne), might act to promote the development of disordered eating habits. This theory is supported by the work of Fairburn et al who performed a large case-control study to investigate risk factors for bulimia nervosa.[27] They identified two broad classes of risk factors for bulimia nervosa; those that are general risk factors for psychiatric disorder (e.g. premorbid psychiatric disorder, behavioral problems, parental psychiatric disorder, disruptive life events), and those that increase the risk of dieting (e.g. critical comments by family about shape or weight, teasing about shape, weight, eating, or appearance, childhood or parental obesity). It seems logical to consider that some symptoms of PCOS (e.g. acne, hirsutism, and weight gain) might contribute towards an increased risk of dieting and a negative self-image, and hence may act as risk factors for the development of bulimia nervosa or subclinical eating disorders. In our population of young women however, where there were no significant differences in acne, hirsutism, or BMI between women with polycystic and women with normal ovaries,[25] we did not detect significant differences in EDE scores for dieting or overall eating disorder symptoms.

It has also been suggested that bulimia nervosa itself creates a hormonal environment that predisposes towards polycystic ovarian changes, as polycystic ovaries have been more commonly identified in bulimic women when compared with controls in some small studies.[19,21] Altered insulin secretion and insulin resistance in bulimic women have been proposed as potential mechanisms,[22,28] but several studies have failed to detect significant differences in fasting insulin and in insulin secretion in bulimic women compared with controls.[19,29–31] The prevalence of frank bulimia nervosa in our study was too low for us confirm or refute the association with polycystic ovaries, however we can note that the frequency of binge eating and overeating was not significantly greater in women with polycystic ovaries or PCOS when compared with women with normal ovaries.

Therefore, using a reliable diagnostic tool for the assessment of eating disorders, it was not found that bulimia nervosa or other binge-eating disorders occur more commonly in women with polycystic ovaries or PCOS.

In addition, women with polycystic ovaries do not demonstrate significantly higher scores for dieting and other features of shape and weight concern when compared with women with normal ovaries. It has been suggested that screening for abnormal eating behavior in women with PCOS should be adopted as routine clinical practice, before dieting is recommended as treatment for symptom control.[32] The suggestion that polycystic ovaries predispose towards development of eating disorders however, is not supported by our study.

Menstrual irregularity

The menstrual cycle is commonly erratic in PCOS, and periods when they occur are often heavy, prolonged and unpredictable. Furthermore, in women with anovulatory cycles, the action of estradiol on the endometrium is unopposed because of the lack of cyclical progesterone secretion. This may result in episodes of irregular uterine bleeding, and in the long term in endometrial hyperplasia and even endometrial cancer.

Menstrual dysfunction brings with it various psychological problems, in particular, mood changes, which are often described as being similar to premenstrual-type symptoms. It is difficult to tease out the specific issues that relate to PCOS although it is likely that 'hormonal imbalance' or the erratic nature of the cycle may lead to altered mood and psychological distress.[33]

Pelvic pain syndrome

Pelvic pain syndrome and pelvic venous congestion have also been linked with PCOS. Again these are common problems and the issue of causality or coincidence has to be proven. Chronic pelvic pain, defined as recurrent pain of at least six months' duration unrelated to periods or sexual intercourse, is said to occur in 24% of women.[34] Pain may both cause and exacerbate depression and a sense of helplessness, and in some cases be a reflection of an underlying psychological morbidity. Pelvic ultrasonography may be helpful in the investigation of patients with pelvic venous congestion in order both to identify the presence of dilated veins and to observe multicystic (as opposed to polycystic) ovaries.[35] In these patients the ovarian volume was found to be greater than in normal controls (6.9 ± 3.4 cm^3 vs 5.1 ± 2.8 cm^3, not significant), with a greater number of follicles (4.6 ± 2.3 vs 2.8 ± 1.6, $p = 0.005$) and similar stromal volume.

These were therefore not typical polycystic ovaries and so the association between PCOS and pelvic venous congestion, contrary to earlier beliefs, has not been proven.

Infertility

PCOS is the most common cause of anovulatory infertility. Obesity impacts negatively on the chance of conception, whether naturally or in response to ovulation induction. Furthermore, obesity is associated with an increased risk of miscarriage. Ovulation can be induced in a number of ways, and careful monitoring is required because of the increased risks of multiple pregnancy and ovarian hyperstimulation syndrome for which women with PCOS are particularly prone (see Chapter 13). Grief explains in some way the infertile patient's sense of loss, but largely negates the often private and self-imposed secrecy experienced by many patients as they struggle with their loss. Patients often report such loss as not being understood or acknowledged by others. As a result, the patient's grief is often expressed in private with their partner, which further adds to the stress and isolation they experience. Indeed, this too can be problematic, as many couples will have defined gender roles in their relationships. Men, for example, may see themselves as 'strong' and having to care for their partner, who is seen as intrinsically 'female', fragile and in need of support. This role is largely socially defined, but places stressors on each of them. The often self-imposed privacy around the patient's grieving then further complicates the grief reaction, and may exacerbate the patient's psychopathology and social functioning. Indeed, evidence does indicate a higher incidence of psychiatric morbidity in infertile couples.[36] It is therefore to be expected that women with PCOS experience significant distress related to infertility,[33] particularly as the subject of ovulation and fertility may be raised early in a patient's care and long before fertility is desired.[38,39] Indeed it is often the mother of an adolescent girl with PCOS who will raise the issue of fertility, when the patient herself simply wants treatment for oligomenorrhea or hirsutism (perhaps because the mother herself has PCOS and experienced difficulty in conceiving).

Hyperandrogenism and hirsutism

It goes without saying that acne, hirsutism and alopecia have a negative impact on body image, psychological health and quality of life. Women with hirsutism are more likely to suffer from significantly higher social fears, anxiety, and psychotic symptoms than normal women.[42] In addition to drugs and/or cosmetic measures, hirsute women may require specific psychotherapy. Hirsutism is more than just a cosmetic problem; successful treatment of hirsutism may enhance self-esteem.

Hirsutism is characterized by terminal hair growth in a male pattern of distribution, including the chin, upper lip, chest, upper and lower back, upper and lower abdomen, upper arm, thigh and buttocks. Treatment options include cosmetic and medical therapies. As drug therapies may take six to nine months or longer before any improvement of hirsutism is perceived, physical treatments including electrolysis, laser therapy, waxing and bleaching may be helpful while waiting for medical treatments to work.

Hirsutism has been shown to lead to psychological distress,[37] and may affect social wellbeing both within the family and in the community. Sonino et al found that Italian women with hirsutism were more likely to suffer from significantly higher social fears, anxiety, and psychotic symptoms than the control group.[37] They suggested in addition to drugs and/or cosmetic measures, hirsute women may require specific psychotherapy. Hirsutism is more than just a cosmetic problem to these women; successful treatment of hirsutism aids the woman's self-esteem. A study of 20 women with facial hirsutism found significant levels of depression that correlated with free testosterone concentrations more than with the degree of hirsutism.[40] This is a highly complex area as testosterone concentrations have also been equated with sexual wellbeing and so there are many factors which may interrelate.

Wilmott performed a study on the experiences of women with PCOS in the UK, and her findings supported the Italian study.[41] The UK PCOS sufferers also revealed feelings of freakiness, considering themselves to be 'hairy monsters and bearded ladies', and women who had irregular menses or dysfunctional bleeding felt abnormal as women, and that infertility was 'crushing' to their womanhood. Treatment for irregular periods and infertility via drugs made some feel artificial, fake or false compared with normal women. Wilmott argues that PCOS sufferers are not merely 'victims of dominant images of normal femininity, but the image of normal womanhood exerts power over them as it does for all women, and they perceive themselves much farther away from achieving the feminine ideal'.[41]

Long-term health

Concerns about increased risks of developing type 2 diabetes, cardiovascular disease, endometrial and breast cancer may lead to anxiety, depression and also concern for family members, because of the genetic links and a possible pre-existing tendency to disease within the family. This area has not been specifically quantified with respect to PCOS.

Depression

Depression in women with PCOS may be simply caused by the psychological stress of having this disorder. There may be neuro-endocrine disturbances, however, that adversely affect wellbeing. Shulman et al suggested that in women with hirsutism, depression was due to neuroendocrine abnormalities,[40] and Nappi et al reported that women with hypothalamic amenorrhea showed a secretory pattern of cortisol that was higher than in normal women.[43] In addition, the lack of naloxone or fenfluramine induced release of cortisol and a blunted response to corticotropin-releasing hormone. It is suggested that there may be impaired activity of some central pathways (particularly of endogenous opioids and serotonin), which affect the hypothalamic–pituitary–adrenal axis in amenorrheic women.

Women with bipolar disorders have been reported as having higher rates of obesity and menstrual disturbances.[44]

Sexual function

Psychosexual behavior in PCOS appears to be similar to that in women without PCOS. Gorzynski and Katz found in their sample group of PCOS women that they had a higher sexual drive, reflected in 'readiness to initiate, pursue, and dominate sexual activity' than in a control group.[45] Exposing women to exogenous (external) or endogenous (internal) sources of increased plasma androgens raises the possibility that some psychosexual behaviors can be at least modified during later developmental stages. Adamopoulos et al found contrasting evidence in their study; while the hirsute women had raised free testosterone levels, their sexual activity was comparable to the non-hirsute women of the reference group.[46] Treatment with cyproterone acetate (CA) combined with ethinyl estradiol (EE_2) reduced circulating androgen levels but had no effect on sexuality, except for increased coital frequency, which was put down to the psychosocial factors of improved self-image or attractiveness.

Sexual orientation has been studied extensively in psychology, and there is speculation that hormones are involved at some level, particularly testosterone. Homosexuality and bisexuality more often appear in women with congenital adrenal hyperplasia than in women with normal levels of androgens.[47] Gorzynski and Katz also referred to a form of postnatal androgenization called acquired adrenal hyperplasia, and it was suggested that these women are 'hypersexual'.[45] Whilst there is some evidence that lesbian women have a higher than expected prevalence of PCOS,[48] there is no hard evidence that PCOS leads to an increased rate of homosexual behaviors.

Ethnic issues

There appear to be significant ethnic variations in the prevalence and expression of PCOS. For example women from South Asia have a greater rate of insulin resistance than white Caucasian women, and hence are more likely to express symptoms of PCOS at a lower BMI. Women with dark hair from Mediterranean and South Asian countries are more likely to exhibit hirsutism, to a degree that may be considered as within the normal range. Women from East Asia, however, have little in the way of bodily hair despite the presence of dark head hair. There has been no formal assessment of psychological aspects and

quality of life issues for women with PCOS from different ethnic backgrounds.

Key points

- While research has been performed on some of the psychological aspects of problems such as obesity, acne and hirsutism – which in women will often include those with PCOS – there is little study of the psychopathology of women defined as having PCOS (by whatever criteria).
- A disease-specific questionnaire has been developed for PCOS (PCOSQ) and further work is currently being undertaken to further assess 'health-related quality of life' (HRQoL).
- Obesity and infertility appear to cause the greatest degree of distress for women with PCOS.
- Both anorexia nervosa and bulimia have been linked with PCOS, but an etiological link has never been satisfactorily explained.
- Many conditions co-exist with PCOS, such as pelvic pain, depression and altered mood. Little information is available specifically on causal or casual association.

References

1. Sonino N, Fava GA, Mani E, Bellurdo P, Boscaro M. Quality of life in hirsute women. Postgrad Med J 1993; 69:186–189.
2. Paulson JD, Haarmann BS, Salerno RL, Asmar P. An investigation of the relationship between emotional maladjustment and infertility. Fertil Steril 1988; 49:258–262.
3. Downey J, Yingling S, McKinney M, Husami N et al. Mood disorders, psychiatric syptoms and distress in women presenting for infertility evaluation. Fertil Steril 1989; 52:425–432.
4. Jones G, Kennedy S, Barnard A, Wong J. Development of an endometriosis quality-of-life instrument: the Endometriosis Health ProFile-30. Obstet Gynecol 2001; 98:258–264.
5. Naughton MJ, McBee WL. Health-related quality of life after hysterectomy. Clin Obstet Gynecol 1997; 40:947–957.

6. Cronin L, Guyatt G, Griffith L, Wong E et al. Development of a health-related quality-of-life questionnaire (PCOSQ) for women with polycystic ovary syndrome (PCOS). J Clin Endocrinol Metab 1998; 83:1976–1987.

7. Fayers PM, Machin D. Quality of life: assessment, analysis and interpretation. Chichester: Wiley, 2000.

8. Ware JE, Sherbourne EC. The MOS 36-Item Short Form Health Survey 1: conceptual framework and item selection. Med Care 1992; 30:473–483.

9. Epstein YM, Rosenberg HS. He does, she doesn't; she does, he doesn't: couple conflicts about infertility. In: Leiblum SR, ed. Infertility: psychological issues and counselling strategies. New York: Wiley, 1997:129–148.

10. Leiblum SR, Greenfeld DA. The course of infertility: immediate and long-term reactions. In: Leiblum SR (ed) Infertility: psychological issues and counselling strategies. New York: Wiley, 1997:83–102.

11. Fairburn CG, Beglin SJ. Studies of the epidemiology of bulimia nervosa. Am J Psychiatry 1990; 147:401–408.

12. Whitehouse AM, Cooper PJ, Vize CV et al. Prevalence of eating disorders in three Cambridge general practices: hidden and conspicuous morbidity. Br J Gen Pract 1992; 42:57–60.

13. Cooper PJ, Fairburn CG. Binge-eating and self-induced vomiting in the community. A preliminary study. Br J Psychiatry 1983; 142:139–144.

14. Patton GC, Selzer R, Coffey C, Carlin JB, Wolfe R. Onset of adolescent eating disorders: population based cohort study over 3 years. Br Med J 1999; 318:765–768.

15. Gupta MA, Gupta AK, Ellis CN, Voorhees JJ. Bulimia nervosa and acne may be related: a case report. Can J Psychiatry 1992; 37:58–61.

16. Fairburn CG. Eating Disorders. In: Oxford Textbook of Medicine, 1999:4212–4218.

17. Franks S. Polycystic ovary syndrome: a changing perspective. Clin Endocrinol (Oxf) 1989; 31:87–120.

18. Balen AH, Conway GS, Kaltsas G, Techatrasak K et al. Polycystic ovary syndrome: the spectrum of the disorder in 1741 patients. Hum Reprod 1995; 10:2107–2111.

19. Raphael FJ, Rodin DA, Peattie A, Bano G et al. Ovarian morphology and insulin sensitivity in women with bulimia nervosa. Clin Endocrinol (Oxf) 1995; 43:451–455.

20. Jahanfar S, Eden JA, Nguyent TV. Bulimia nervosa and polycystic ovary syndrome. Gynecol. Endocrinol. 1995; 9:113–117.

21. McCluskey S, Lacey JH, Pearce JM. Binge-eating and polycystic ovaries. Lancet 1992; 340:723.

22. McCluskey S, Evans C, Lacey JH, Pearce JM, Jacobs H. Polycystic ovary syndrome and bulimia [see comments]. Fertil Steril 1991; 5: 287–291.

23. McSherry JA. Bulimia nervosa and polycystic ovary syndrome: evidence for an occasional causal relationship. The Medical Therapist 1990; 6:10–11.

24. Michelmore KF, Balen AH, Dunger DB. Polycystic ovaries and eating disorders: are they related? Hum Reprod 2001; 16:765–769.

25. Michelmore KF, Balen AH, Dunger DB, Vessey MP. Polycystic ovaries and associated clinical and biochemical features in young women. Clin Endocrinol (Oxf) 1999; 51:779–786.

26. Fairburn CG, Cooper Z. The eating disorder examination (12th edn). In: Binge eating: nature, assessment and treatment. New York: Guilford Press, 1993:317–331.

27. Fairburn CG, Welch SL, Doll HA, Davies BA, O'Connor ME. Risk factors for bulimia nervosa. A community-based case-control study. Arch Gen Psychiatry 1997; 54:509–517.

28. Schweiger U, Poellinger J, Laessle R, Wolfram G et al. Altered insulin response to a balanced test meal in bulimic patients. Int J Eat Disord 1987; 6:551–556.

29. Blouin AG, Blouin J, Bushnik T, Braaten J et al. A double-blind placebo-controlled glucose challenge in bulimia nervosa: psychological effects. Biol Psychiatry 1993; 33:160–168.

30. Johnson WG, Jarrell MP, Chupurdia KM, Williamson DA. Repeated binge/purge cycles in bulimia nervosa: role of glucose and insulin. Int J Eat Disord 1994; 15:331–341.

31. Weingarten HP, Hendler R, Rodin J. Metabolism and endocrine secretion in response to a test meal in normal-weight bulimic women. Psychosom Med 1988; 50:273–285.

32. Morgan JF. Polycystic ovary syndrome [letter]. Br J Hosp Med 1997; 57:??

33. Jones GL, Benes K, Clark TL, Denham R et al. The polycystic ovary syndrome health-related quality of life questionnaire (PCOSQ): a validation. Hum Reprod 2004; 19:371–377.

34. Zondervan KT, Yudkin PL, Vessey MP. The community prevalence of chronic pelvic pain in women and associated illness behaviour. Br J Gen Pract 2001; 51:541–547.

35. Halligan S, Campbell D, Bartram CI, Rogers V et al. Transvaginal ultrasound examination of women with and without pelvic venous congestion. Clin Radiol 2000; 55:954–958.

36. Domar A, Broome A, Zuttermeister P, Seibel M, Friedman R. The prevalence and predictability of depression in infertile women. Fertil Steril 1992; 58:1158–1163.

37. Sonino N, Fava GA, Mani E, Belluardo P, Boscaro M. Quality of life of hirsute women. Postgrad Med J 1993; 69:186–189.

38. Paulson JD, Haarmann BS, Salerno RL, Asmar P. An investigation of the relationship between

emotional maladjustment and infertility. Fertil Steril 1988; 49:258–262.

39. Downey J, Yingling S, McKinney M, Husami N et al. Mood disorders, psychiatric symptoms and distress in women presenting for infertility evaluation. Fertil Steril 1989; 52:425–432.

40. Shulman LH, DeRogatis L, Speivogel R, Miller JL, Rose LI. Serum androgens and depression in women with facial hirsutism. J Am Acad Dermatol 1993; 27:178–181.

41. Wilmott J. The experiences of women with polycystic ovarian syndrome. Feminism and Psychology 2001; 101a.

42. Derogatis LR, Rose LL, Shulman LH, Lazarus LA. Serum androgens and psychopathology in hirsute women. J Psychosom Obstet Gynaecol 1993; 14:269–282.

43. Nappi RE, Petraglia F, Genazzani AD, D-Ambrogio G, Zara C, Genazzani AR. Hypothalamic amenorrhea: evidence for a central derangement of hypothalamic-pituitary-adrenal cortex axis activity. Fertil Steril 1993; 59:571–576.

44. Elmslie JL, Silverstone JT, Mann JL, Williams SM, Romans SE. Prevalence of overweight and obesity in bipolar patients. J Clin Psychiatry 2000; 61:179–184.

45. Gorzynski G, Katz JL. The polycystic ovary syndrome: psychosexual correlates. Arch Sex Behav 1977; 6:215–222.

46. Adamopoulos DA, Kampyli S, Georgiacodis F, Kapolla N, Abrahamian-Michalakis A. Effects of antiandrogen-estrogen treatment on sexual and endocrine parameters in hirsute women. Arch Sex Behav 1988; 17:421–429.

47. Meyer-Bahlburg-Heino FL, Dolezal C, Baker SW, Carlson AD, Obeid JS, New MI. Prenatal androgenization affects gender-related behaviour but not gender identity in 5–12 year old girls with congenital adrenal hyperplasia. Arch Sex Behav 2004; 33:97–104.

48. Agrawal R, Sharma S, Bekir J, Conway G, Balen AH et al. Prevalence of polycystic ovaries and polycystic ovary syndrome in lesbian women compared with heterosexual women. Fertil Steril 2004; 82:1352–7.

Chapter 7
The effects of obesity and diet

Introduction

There is a close association between obesity and polycystic ovary syndrome (PCOS). Women with PCOS are on average more obese than their non-PCOS counterparts with 50% having a body mass index (BMI) over 30 kg/m² .[1] Women with PCOS commonly misinterpret this relationship, supposing that PCOS status somehow leads to obesity. In fact, the causal relationship is more likely to be that obesity drives polycystic ovaries to be more clinically manifest. Thus, obesity must convert some women with occult polycystic ovary (PCO) morphology to clinically obvious PCOS. Obese women are therefore over-represented in clinics while the relatively asymptomatic lean women remain at home. Every physician treating women with PCOS has to become an expert in obesity management – as indeed does each obese woman with the syndrome.

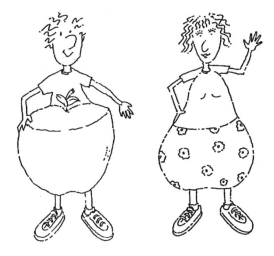

Figure 7.1

Cartoon of 'apple'- and 'pear'-shaped individuals. Reproduced from Health Canada.

Measuring obesity

Body fat is a continuous variable and the labels 'obese' or 'morbidly obese' obviously apply arbitrary cut-off criteria. These criteria are based on epidemiological risk analysis of health outcomes in relation to body weight. For simplicity, much of these data are based on body mass index as a crude adjustment of body weight for height where the BMI = weight (kg)/height (m)². BMI, however, has to be interpreted carefully as it does not take into account several important variables. First, is ethnicity. For instance, individuals from South Asia have a high incidence of insulin resistance and cardiovascular risk at a lower BMI than their Western counterparts.[2] Second, is fat distribution. Visceral or central fat is associated with a more adverse metabolic risk profile than subcutaneous fat. Consequently, measures of central fat such as waist circumference, are thought to correlate more closely with obesity risk than BMI (Figure 7.1). Visceral fat can also be measured by magnetic resonance imaging (MRI) or computed tomography (CT) scanning, but these tools are too expensive and time consuming for routine clinical application (Figure 7.2). Such scanning is used, however, as a precise measure of fat distribution in PCOS research. Alternatively, conductive impedance is applicable in the clinical setting but may not offer a great deal more information than waist circumference in everyday practice. Women with PCOS

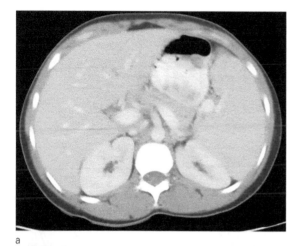

a

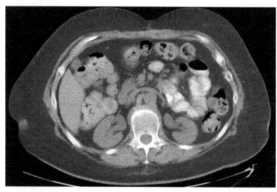

b

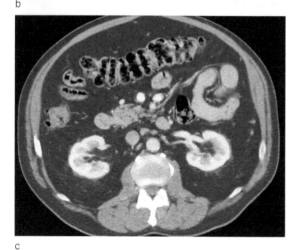

c

Figure 7.2

CT scans to demonstrate visceral fat distribution: a) Slim woman with little visceral fat; b) obese woman with subcutaneous and some visceral fat; c) obese woman with PCOS and significant visceral fat (dark grey).

Table 7.1 The metabolic syndrome (requires three to be present)

- Abdominal obesity >88 cm
- Triglycerides ≥150 mg/dl
- High density lipoprotein (HDL)-C <50 mg/dl
- Blood pressure ≥130/85 mmHg
- Abnormal oral glucose tolerance test: see Table 2.4

have been shown to have a raised waist to hip ratio, signaling an increased visceral fat mass.[3,4] In clinical practice it is important to standardize the measurement of hip and waist circumference and it is generally thought that a simple measure of waist circumference is sufficient to provide an assessment of 'metabolic risk'. A waist circumference of greater than 88 cm is a criterion for the metabolic syndrome (Table 7.1).

Determinants of obesity

Genetics

It is estimated that 30–40% of obesity is genetically determined. Several single gene defects have been identified as causes of obesity but these account for only a few per cent of the obese population.[5] Inheritance of obesity is likely to be polygenic, with influences both on energy expenditure and on control of appetite. On a practical level a genetic effect can be shown by the close association between the BMI of women with PCOS and that of their mothers. Furthermore, the mother's BMI is closely correlated with that of their partner who, of course, is not usually genetically related. Couples tend to match with respect to lifestyle preferences. In this way, obese women tend to have obese partners and so any genetic factors are pooled and passed on to their offspring.

Energy expenditure

One major factor influencing the accumulation of fat is the basal metabolic rate (BMR). The average

BMR is equivalent to 2200 kcal per day in women but of course there is a normal distribution around this mean and undoubtedly some women with PCOS have drawn the short straw and may have a lower than average BMR. There is no evidence that BMR is influenced by PCOS status or endocrine milieu: PCOS does not cause obesity.[6] The most obvious evidence against PCOS driving weight gain comes from the observation that after oophorectomy in obese women with PCOS, post-operative weight change does not occur.

BMR falls throughout life which is one reason for the common experience of weight gain in middle age. BMR also falls sharply at the end of linear growth – ages 18 to 20 when energy expended in growth vertically then abruptly stops and is translated in many to expansion of girth. Late adolescence is consequently a common 'problem age' for women with PCOS.

Last, exercise is a significant determinant of metabolic rate. Cardiovascular exercise not only results in short-term energy expenditure but also increases the BMR, leading to an additive boost to overall daily energy expenditure. Much of the current obesity epidemic is related to diminished activity, and exercise therefore must be at the forefront of management of obese women with PCOS. There is no clear evidence that one type of exercise is better than another in this respect although there is a current fashion to emphasize cardiovascular exercise of moderate duration rather then isometric or short-duration intense exercise.[7]

Energy intake

The endocrinology of satiety has exploded to be a major new field over the past few years. The discovery of leptin was followed by among others neuropeptide-Y (NPY), orexin, ghrelin, resistin and peptide YY (PYY). These peptides influence the sensation of satiety, food intake, or energy expenditure to different degrees. It is tempting to speculate that an abnormality of one of these peptides might be the mechanism of obesity in PCOS. Each of these has been measured in the circulation in women with PCOS, and no consistent disturbance of any of these components has emerged as an underlying mechanism of obesity.

Composition of diet

The fashions of effective weight loss diets come and go with advocates for the manipulation of various components in order to achieve 'a quick fix'. With a focus on the hyperinsulinemia of PCOS, the components of diet that are most potent in stimulating insulin release have become a particular target for women with the syndrome. In trying to construct a diet specific for hyperinsulinemia the first target would be refined sugar. Having removed sugar from the diet the next consideration is simple carbohydrates which are absorbed quickly and converted to glucose as measured by their glycemic index. Glucose itself is given the highest glycemic index. Carbohydrates with a low glycemic index usually have high fiber content allowing glucose to be retained within the lumen of the gut for slower release, leading to lower peak plasma glucose concentrations and therefore a lower insulin response. In taking this logic a step further many women find it effective to reduce carbohydrate intake altogether to the point where the body begins to metabolize adipose tissue leading to ketogenesis (which can be measured in the urine). This process is the basis of the Atkins diet.

While some studies support carbohydrate-restricted diets as a particularly effective means of weight loss,[8,9] others have found that low carbohydrate has little benefit over a low-fat diet in PCOS.[10] Clearly, the effect of specific diet manipulations on energy balance is small enough that a large number of women are required for a sufficiently powered study.

A second issue is timing of meals. The insulin excursion after a single large meal is greater than the accumulated insulin secretion from several small meals of equivalent calorie content. In other words, a 'grazer' will have a lower mean serum insulin concentration throughout the day compared with a 'binger'. In addition, skipping meals may reduce metabolic rate slightly and commencing calorie intake early in the day appears to reduce later intake.

There is some evidence to support women's claims that carbohydrate craving is more common in PCOS than expected. Carbohydrate craving, particularly for refined sugar, is well-recognized in the premenstrual phase of the menstrual cycle, and this is thought to be mediated in part by progesterone. It is notable that many women with PCOS and oligomenor-rhea describe feeling constantly premenstrual even in the absence of progesterone peaks from the corpus luteum. This observation raises the possibility that sugar craving could have an endocrine basis although the exact mediator in PCOS is unclear. Anecdotally, some women say that suppression of carbohydrate craving is one of the benefits of metformin.

Adipose tissue as an endocrine organ

Adipose tissue is the site of production of several peptides, many of which have the properties of a conventional endocrine messenger.[11] Here we consider the most prominent of these, leptin, interleukin-6 (IL-6), tumor necrosis factor alpha (TNFα) and adiponectin. As each of these peptides is characterized there is a flurry of papers that document measurements in women with PCOS. The usual pattern in the literature is that small studies often with poorly matched control groups appear first, probably using stored samples from earlier studies. There follow more considered prospective studies which often temper the initial findings. At the time of writing we are missing a fully integrated assessment of adipose endocrinology in women with PCOS.

Leptin is produced by adipocytes and circulat-ing levels correlate closely with BMI. The main target for leptin is the hypothalamus, where specific receptors mediate signaling to centers for appetite and reproduction. With respect to repro-duction, leptin signals both directly to the neurons of the gonadotropin-releasing hormone (GnRH) pulse generator and indirectly through adjacent neurons by suppressing neuropeptide Y synthesis (see Figure 4.16). In obese women with PCOS, one might wonder if high leptin levels could alter GnRH drive to the gonadotrophs. In fact, the leptin axis appears to be most important at low body weight whereby the lower leptin levels contribute to the state of hypo-gonadotrophic hypogonadism characteristic of weight-related amenorrhea. No consistent leptin abnormality has been found in PCOS.[12–14]

IL-6 is an adipokine which may play a key role in several of the mechanisms that contribute to the development of coronary heart disease (CHD),

insulin resistance and diabetes.[15] Furthermore, there are close associations between circulating levels of IL-6 and various risk factors for CHD, such as insulin resistance, high triglyceride and low HDL-cholesterol concentrations, and elevated blood pressure. IL-6 is a major regulator of the hepatic acute phase response mediating the release of C-reactive protein (CRP) and fibrinogen. Like leptin, IL-6 is released by adipose tissue, its levels increase with increasing fat mass,[16] and there is greater expression of IL-6 in the visceral fat compared with the subcutaneous fat. Although raised concentrations of IL-6 have been reported in PCOS,[17] others report no abnormal-ity.[18] In such studies, subjects must be matched not only by BMI but also by waist measurements as visceral fat is the main source of IL-6.[19]

TNFα is a cytokine which is made by many cell types of which the adipocyte is only one. TNFα secretion is stimulated by IL-1 and endotoxins. One of the actions of TNFα is to serine phospho-rylate insulin receptor substrate-1 (IRS-1), which is thought to be one of the mechanisms of insulin resistance in PCOS (see Chapter 4). In PCOS one study has reported TNFα to be raised,[20] but the significance of this observation is not yet clear.

Adiponectin is a peptide hormone made by adipocytes which has an inverse relationship with fat mass, unlike leptin, with obese individuals having lower circulating levels than lean individu-als. In PCOS, adiponectin shows the normal inverse correlation with BMI and is not closely related to insulin resistance.[21,22]

Adipose tissue as an endocrine modulator

In addition to hormone synthesis, adipose tissue is an active site of two major hormone conver-sions, the conversion of androgens to estrogens and the interconversion of cortisol and cortisone.

Relatively inert androgens are converted to estro-gens, predominantly estrone, through the mecha-nism of aromatization in adipose tissue. By this mechanism, the production rate of estrogen is related to fat mass.[23] This estrogen source from adipose tissue is the reason why menstrual dysfunc-tion is so common in obese women who are also the group who carry the risk for endometrial carci-noma driven by unopposed estrogen stimulation (see Chapter 9). Serum estrone concentrations are raised in PCOS, commensurate with obesity.[24]

The principal pathways of cortisol metabolism include irreversible inactivation by 5α-reductase (5α-R) and 5β-reductase (5β-R) in the liver, and reversible interconversion with cortisone by 11β-hydroxysteroid dehydrogenase (11β-HSD) in liver and adipose tissue. Increased peripheral cortisol metabolism either by increased 5α-R activity and thus increased inactivation of cortisol,[25] or impaired 11β-HSD activity and thus impaired regeneration of cortisol results in compensatory increase of adrenocorticotrophic hormone (ACTH) secretion via a decrease in the negative feedback signal,[26] maintaining normal serum cortisol levels at the expense of adrenal androgen excess. In support of this hypothesis, urinary metabolites of cortisol were found to be abnormal in women with PCOS and these effects seem to be independent of insulin resistance.[27]

Endocrinological associations of obesity

In addition to the active endocrine role of adipose tissue there are various endocrine changes in obesity that are related or, alternatively, are downstream events that may be relevant to obese women with PCOS. The most obvious of these is the association between insulin resistance and obesity.

The mechanisms by which obesity and insulin resistance are associated are complex.[28] One of the most prominent links is via the release of free fatty acids from adipocytes interfering with insulin action on hepatocytes. Insulin resistance can be acquired through obesity and also inherited. In women with PCOS, excessive phosphorylation of serine residues on the insulin receptor has been identified as a molecular defect in 50% of cases.[29]

The direct measurement of insulin sensitivity requires a measurement of the effectiveness of exogenous insulin in stimulating glucose uptake.[30,31] The classic method of measuring insulin resistance is with the glucose clamp. The glucose clamp is however an arduous method for anything other than research in small numbers of subjects, and for this reason other methods have been sought. For instance, the gradient of the fall in glucose after an insulin injection is proportional to insulin sensitivity and can be measured over 15 minutes. Even more simply, insulin resistance can be estimated from fasting insulin and glucose concentrations using various equations of which Homeostatic Model Assessment (HOMA) is probably the most widely used. Last, the assessment of insulin concentrations in the fasting state provides slightly different information compared with stimulated insulin after glucose ingestion, and for this reason an oral glucose tolerance test is often used.

Insulin resistance has various downstream effects that have been explored in PCOS. In particular, insulin resistance is associated with suppression of the production by the liver of sex hormone binding globulin (SHBG) and insulin-like growth factor binding protein 1 (IGFBP-1) – both of which may modulate sex steroid action in PCOS.

SHBG is a glycoprotein synthesized in the liver which has a high binding affinity for testosterone compared with estradiol. The synthesis of SHBG is stimulated by several factors of which the most potent are estrogens and thyroid hormone. SHBG synthesis is suppressed by androgens and insulin in particular.[32] Circulating SHBG concentrations therefore have an inverse relationship with body weight.[33] In PCOS, SHBG concentrations are low, commensurate with the degree of obesity and insulin resistance.[34] The lower circulating SHBG concentrations may increase the bioavailability of testosterone and thereby potentiate the androgenic manifestations of the syndrome.

Insulin has a complex relationship with the IGF axis culminating and an amplification of IGF stimulation of the ovary.[35] Serum insulin and IGF-1 concentrations are positively associated and insulin upregulates the IGF-1 receptor.[36] Furthermore, insulin is a potent suppressor of IGFBP-1 leading to an increase in the bioavailability of IGF-1. In this way, the hyperinsulinemia of obesity may stimulate ovarian function not only through the direct 'co-gonadotropin' effect of insulin but also indirectly via IGF-1 modulation.

NPY is the most abundant neuropeptide in the brain and is a member of a family of proteins that includes pancreatic polypeptide, PYY. NPY is a stimulator of feeding behavior. Circulating NPY levels have been shown to be raised in women with PCOS, but the degree to which this reflects its neurotransmitter activity is unclear.[37]

Ghrelin is synthesized in the lining of the stomach and signals to receptors in the hypothalamus, pituitary and adipose tissue. Ghrelin stimulates growth hormone secretion and takes part in the regulation of energy balance. Ghrelin stimulates the sensation of hunger through its action on hypothalamic feeding centers, with circulating levels of ghrelin increasing with fasting. Ghrelin levels have been reported to be low in obese women with PCOS,[38] but others find no difference.[39] Treatment with metformin results in an increase in circulating ghrelin levels.[40]

CRP is an acute phase reactant released by the liver in response to stimulation by IL-6 and TNFα. Like leptin and IL-6, serum CRP concentrations are closely associated with body fat. Recently Kelly et al have shown that PCOS women have significantly increased CRP concentrations relative to women without PCOS, and have proposed that chronic low-grade inflammation may account for the increased type II diabetes in these women.[41] In addition, CRP concentration falls in women with PCOS treated with metformin, suggesting that this treatment might have an anti-inflammatory mode of action.[42]

Targeting obesity in the management of PCOS

So fundamental is the link between obesity and PCOS, that lifestyle modification has become the most important first-line management in obese women with the syndrome.[43,44] An effective weight-loss program requires education and support with regard to both diet and exercise.[45] Almost universally, weight loss in women with PCOS has resulted in an improvement in the clinical features of the syndrome, and in most of the biochemical markers related to it. Lifestyle modification and metformin have been shown to improve fat distribution, insulin sensitivity, luteinizing hormone (LH) hypersecretion,[46] and androgen excess in women with PCOS.[47] These changes reflect themselves clinically with improvement in oligomenorrhea and anovulation as well as a modest benefit to hirsutism.[48] It is the improvement in insulin sensitivity that appears to be the prime mover in this sequence. For this reason, insulin-lowering agents and insulin sensitizers have become a major part of the treatment program for obese women with PCOS. Metformin, thiozoladindiones, and chiro-inositol have all been shown to improve clinical outcome in PCOS by reducing hyperinsulinemia.[49,50]

In constructing a treatment program for obese women with PCOS, it must be remembered that metformin is not a magic bullet, and that diet and exercise are more effective then metformin in the prevention of type 2 diabetes in an at-risk population.

Key points

- There is a close association between obesity and PCOS.
- Women with PCOS are on average more obese than their non-PCOS counterparts, with 50% having a body mass index over 30 kg/m^2.
- Rather than PCOS leading to obesity, obesity drives polycystic ovaries to be more clinically manifest.
- Visceral or central fat is associated with a more adverse metabolic risk profile than subcutaneous fat. Measurement of waist circumference therefore correlates more closely with metabolic risk than BMI.
- No consistent disturbance of any of the satiety peptides has emerged as an underlying mechanism of obesity in PCOS.
- While it appears logical to restrict carbohydrates and aim for a diet with a low glycemic index, there is little evidence that any one diet is better than another for women with PCOS.
- Carbohydrate craving, particularly for refined sugar, is well-recognized in the premenstrual phase of the menstrual cycle, and this is thought to be mediated in part by progesterone.

References

1. Norman RJ, Davies MJ, Lord J, Moran LJ. The role of lifestyle modification in polycystic ovary syndrome. Trends Endocrinol Metab 2002; 13:251–257.
2. Wijeyaratne CN, Balen AH, Barth JH, Belchetz PE. Clinical manifestations and insulin resistance (IR) in polycystic ovary syndrome (PCOS) among South Asians and Caucasians: is there a difference? Clin Endocrinol (Oxf) 2002; 57:343–350.
3. Rebuffe-Scrive M, Cullberg G, Lundberg PA, Lindstedt G, Bjorntorp P. Anthropometric variables and metabolism in polycystic ovarian disease. Horm Metab Res 1989; 21:391–397.

4. Pasquali R, Casimirri F, Venturoli S, Antonio M et al. Body fat distribution has weight-independent effects on clinical, hormonal, and metabolic features of women with polycystic ovary syndrome. Metabolism 1994; 43:706–713.

5. Damcott CM, Sack P, Shuldiner AR. The genetics of obesity. Endocrinol Metab Clin North Am 2003; 32:761–786.

6. Segal KR, Dunaif A. Resting metabolic rate and postprandial thermogenesis in polycystic ovarian syndrome. Int J Obes 1990; 14:559–567.

7. Racette SB, Schoeller DA, Kushner RF, Neil KM, Herling-Iaffaldano K. Effects of aerobic exercise and dietary carbohydrate on energy expenditure and body composition during weight reduction in obese women. Am J Clin Nutr 1995; 61:486–494.

8. Layman DK, Boileau RA, Erickson DJ, Painter JE et al. A reduced ratio of dietary carbohydrate to protein improves body composition and blood lipid profiles during weight loss in adult women. J Nutr 2003; 133:411–417.

9. Kasim-Karakas SE, Almario RU, Gregory L, Wong R et al. Metabolic and endocrine effects of a polyunsaturated fatty acid-rich diet in polycystic ovary syndrome. J Clin Endocrinol Metab 2004; 89:615–620.

10. Moran LJ, Norman RJ. The obese patient with infertility: a practical approach to diagnosis and treatment. Nutr Clin Care 2002; 5:290–297.

11. Guerre-Millo M. Adipose tissue hormones. J Endocrinol Invest 2002; 25:855–861.

12. Gennarelli G, Holte J, Wide L, Berne C, Lithell H. Is there a role for leptin in the endocrine and metabolic aberrations of polycystic ovary syndrome? Hum Reprod 1998; 13:535–541.

13. Jacobs HS, Conway GS. Leptin, polycystic ovaries and polycystic ovary syndrome. Hum Reprod Update 1999; 5:166–171.

14. Telli MH, Yildirim M, Noyan V. Serum leptin levels in patients with polycystic ovary syndrome. Fertil Steril 2002; 77:932–935.

15. Yudkin JS, Panahloo A, Stehouwer C, Emeis JJ et al. The influence of improved glycaemic control with insulin and sulphonylureas on acute phase and endothelial markers in type II diabetic subjects. Diabetologia 2000; 43:1099–1106.

16. Mohamed-Ali V, Goodrick S, Rawesh A, Katz DR et al. Subcutaneous adipose tissue releases interleukin-6, but not tumor necrosis factor-alpha, in vivo. J Clin Endocrinol Metab 1997; 82:4196–4200.

17. Amato G, Conte M, Mazziotti G, Lalli E et al. Serum and follicular fluid cytokines in polycystic ovary syndrome during stimulated cycles. Obstet Gynecol 2003; 101:1177–1182.

18. Escobar-Morreale HF, Villuendas G, Botella-Carretero JI, Sancho J, San Millan JL. Obesity, and not insulin resistance, is the major determinant of serum inflammatory cardiovascular risk markers in pre-menopausal women. Diabetologia 2003; 46:625–633.

19. Fried SK, Bunkin DA, Greenberg AS. Omental and subcutaneous adipose tissues of obese subjects release interleukin-6: depot difference and regulation by glucocorticoid. J Clin Endocrinol Metab 1998; 83:847–850.

20. Sayin NC, Gucer F, Balkanli-Kaplan P, Yuce MA et al. Elevated serum TNF-alpha levels in normal-weight women with polycystic ovaries or the polycystic ovary syndrome. J Reprod Med 2003; 48:165–170.

21. Orio F, Jr, Palomba S, Cascella T, Milan G et al. Adiponectin levels in women with polycystic ovary syndrome. J Clin Endocrinol Metab 2003; 88:2619–2623.

22. Ducluzeau PH, Cousin P, Malvoisin E, Bornet H et al. Glucose-to-insulin ratio rather than sex hormone-binding globulin and adiponectin levels is the best predictor of insulin resistance in nonobese women with polycystic ovary syndrome. J Clin Endocrinol Metab 2003; 88:3626–3631.

23. Pasquali R, Casimirri F. The impact of obesity on hyperandrogenism and polycystic ovary syndrome in premenopausal women. Clin Endocrinol (Oxf) 1993; 39:1–16.

24. Fox R, Corrigan E, Thomas PG, Hull MG. Oestrogen and androgen states in oligo-amenorrhoeic women with polycystic ovaries. Br J Obstet Gynaecol 1991; 98:294–299.

25. Stewart PM, Shackleton CH, Beastall GH, Edwards CR. 5 alpha-reductase activity in polycystic ovary syndrome. Lancet 1990; 335:431–433.

26. Rodin A, Thakkar H, Taylor N, Clayton R. Hyperandrogenism in polycystic ovary syndrome. Evidence of dysregulation of 11 beta-hydroxysteroid dehydrogenase. N Engl J Med 1994; 330:460–465.

27. Tsilchorozidou T, Honour JW, Conway GS. Altered cortisol metabolism in polycystic ovary syndrome: insulin enhances 5alpha-reduction but not the elevated adrenal steroid production rates. J Clin Endocrinol Metab 2003; 88:5907–5913.

28. Caro JF. Clinical review 26: insulin resistance in obese and nonobese man. J Clin Endocrinol Metab 1991; 73:691–695.

29. Dunaif A. Insulin resistance and the polycystic ovary syndrome: mechanism and implications for pathogenesis. Endocr Rev 1997; 18:774–800.

30. Ferrannini E, Mari A. How to measure insulin sensitivity. J Hypertens 1998; 16:895–906.

31. Scheen AJ, Lefebvre PJ. Assessment of insulin resistance in vivo: application to the study of type 2 diabetes. Horm Res 1992; 38:19–27.

32. Selby C. Sex hormone binding globulin: origin, function and clinical significance. Ann Clin Biochem 1990; 27:532–541.

33. Tchernof A, Despres JP. Sex steroid hormones, sex hormone-binding globulin, and obesity in men and women. Horm Metab Res 2000; 32:526–536.

34. Jayagopal V, Kilpatrick ES, Jennings PE, Hepburn DA, Atkin SL. The biological variation of testosterone and sex hormone-binding globulin (SHBG) in polycystic ovarian syndrome: implications for SHBG as a surrogate marker of insulin resistance. J Clin Endocrinol Metab 2003; 88:1528–1533.

35. Poretsky L, Cataldo NA, Rosenwaks Z, Giudice LC. The insulin-related ovarian regulatory system in health and disease. Endocrinol Rev 1999; 20:535–582.

36. Conway GS, Jacobs HS, Holly JM, Wass JA. Effects of luteinizing hormone, insulin, insulin-like growth factor-I and insulin-like growth factor small binding protein 1 in the polycystic ovary syndrome. Clin Endocrinol (Oxf) 1990; 33:593–603.

37. Baranowska B, Radzikowska M, Wasilewska-Dziubinska E, Kaplinski A et al. Neuropeptide Y, leptin, galanin and insulin in women with polycystic ovary syndrome. Gynecol Endocrinol 1999; 13:344–351.

38. Pagotto U, Gambineri A, Vicennati V, Heiman ML et al. Plasma ghrelin, obesity, and the polycystic ovary syndrome: correlation with insulin resistance and androgen levels. J Clin Endocrinol Metab 2002; 87:5625–5629.

39. Orio F, Jr, Lucidi P, Palomba S, Tauchmanova L et al. Circulating ghrelin concentrations in the polycystic ovary syndrome. J Clin Endocrinol Metab 2003; 88:942–945.

40. Schofl C, Horn R, Schill T, Schlosser HW et al. Circulating ghrelin levels in patients with polycystic ovary syndrome. J Clin Endocrinol Metab 2002; 87:4607–4610.

41. Kelly CC, Lyall H, Petrie JR, Gould GW et al. Low grade chronic inflammation in women with polycystic ovarian syndrome. J Clin Endocrinol Metab 2001; 86:2453–2455.

42. Morin-Papunen L, Rautio K, Ruokonen A, Hedberg P et al. Metformin reduces serum C-reactive protein levels in women with polycystic ovary syndrome. J Clin Endocrinol Metab 2003; 88:4649–4654.

43. Lefebvre P, Bringer J, Renard E, Boulet F et al. Influences of weight, body fat patterning and nutrition on the management of PCOS, Hum Reprod 1997; 12 (suppl 1):72–81.

44. Huber-Buchholz MM, Carey DG, Norman RJ. Restoration of reproductive potential by lifestyle modification in obese polycystic ovary syndrome: role of insulin sensitivity and luteinizing hormone. J Clin Endocrinol Metab 1999; 84:1470–1474.

45. Clark AM, Thornley B, Tomlinson L, Galletley C, Norman RJ. Weight loss in obese infertile women results in improvement in reproductive outcome for all forms of fertility treatment. Hum Reprod. 1998; 13:1502–1505.

46. Van Dam EW, Roelfsema F, Veldhuis JD, Helmerhorst FM et al. Increase in daily LH secretion in response to short-term calorie restriction in obese women with PCOS. Am J Physiol Endocrinol Metab 2002; 282:E865–E872.

47. Moghetti P, Castello R, Negri C, Tosi F et al. Metformin effects on clinical features, endocrine and metabolic profiles, and insulin sensitivity in polycystic ovary syndrome: a randomized, double-blind, placebo-controlled 6-month trial, followed by open, long-term clinical evaluation. J Clin Endocrinol Metab 2000; 85:139–146.

48. Lord JM, Flight IH, Norman RJ. Metformin in polycystic ovary syndrome: systematic review and meta-analysis. Br Med J 2003; 327:951–953.

49. Diamanti-Kandarakis E, Zapanti E. Insulin sensitizers and antiandrogens in the treatment of polycystic ovary syndrome. Ann NY Acad Sci 2000; 900:203–212.

50. Baillargeon JP, Iuorno MJ, Nestler JE. Insulin sensitizers for polycystic ovary syndrome. Clin Obstet Gynecol 2003; 46:325–340.

Chapter 8

Long-term sequelae of polycystic ovary syndrome: diabetes and cardiovascular disease

Introduction

Long-term sequelae of polycystic ovary syndrome (PCOS) are a major concern of affected women, and offer an opportunity for clinical intervention and prevention. The relationship between PCOS and many of its proposed sequelae, however, rest primarily on shared risk profiles until we have confirmation from epidemiological studies. The tendency in the literature and in clinical practice is to assume the worst and intervene. This chapter will examine a variety of sequelae in women with PCOS linked to insulin resistance, including diabetes and heart disease. The risk, however, is often implied based on case series or small inferential studies.

The basis for the concerns about long-term sequelae is that women with PCOS have a number of reproductive and metabolic abnormalities. The reproductive abnormalities, alluded to by its very name, led to the initial recognition of the syndrome in the early part of the 20th century. The metabolic abnormalities, above and beyond obesity, were not recognized until later when reduced sensitivity to insulin and compensatory hyperinsulinemia were noted in women with PCOS.[1,2] The metabolic profile noted in women with PCOS is similar to the insulin resistance syndrome, that is a clustering within an individual of hyperinsulinemia, mild glucose intolerance, dyslipidemia, and hypertension.[3] The insulin resistance syndrome (or 'syndrome X', or 'metabolic syndrome', see Table 7.1) has been identified as both a risk factor for developing type 2 diabetes and for developing cardiovascular disease.[5] It is this 'common soil' hypothesis of

insulin resistance as the primary risk factor for the simultaneous development of diabetes and cardiovascular disease that we will examine in detail during this chapter. The markers and sequelae of insulin resistance syndrome have expanded over time, and will be discussed in more detail below (Figure 8.1).

Insulin resistance is defined as a diminution in the biological responses to a given level of insulin.[6] In the presence of an adequate pancreatic reserve, normal circulating glucose levels are maintained at higher serum insulin concentrations. In the general population, cardiovascular risk factors include insulin resistance, obesity, glucose intolerance, hypertension, and dyslipidemia.[7–9] A prospective population-based study of 1462 women aged between 38 and 60 years was undertaken in Gothenberg, to examine cardiovascular risk factors in women.[10] After a 12-year follow up, they reported four independent risk factors for myocardial infarction in women which included increasing waist:hip ratio, raised serum triglyceride concentrations, diabetes and hypertension. Bengtsson and colleagues followed up the same cohort of women for a period of 20 years, and found that the two most important factors relating to cardiovascular mortality were central obesity and raised serum triglycerides.[11] Central obesity was a more important risk factor than obesity itself.

Two large American epidemiological studies on heart disease in women – the Framingham[12] and Lipid Research Clinic Follow Up Studies[13], demonstrated that the mortality from cardiovascular disease was closely related to the lipid fractions, namely elevated serum triglycerides and reduced high-density lipoprotein (HDL) cholesterol

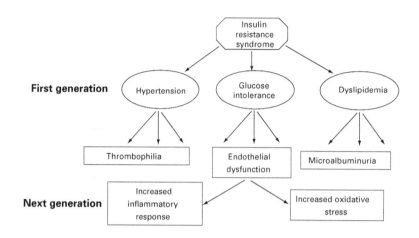

Figure 8.1

The insulin resistance syndrome or syndrome X, as originally described by Reaven,[3] was a cluster of signs consisting of hypertension, dyslipidemia, and glucose intolerance. Further study has yielded additional abnormalities. The number of potential markers has become dizzying.

levels.[12,13] Blass and colleagues analyzing this data, showed that in women with similarly elevated serum triglycerides, the mortality risk was significantly greater if, in addition, they had lower levels of HDL cholesterol.[13]

In 1988, Reaven described 'Syndrome X' or the insulin resistance syndrome.[14] It is characterized by the presence of compensatory hyperinsulinemia, secondary to resistance to insulin-mediated glucose uptake, resulting in varying degrees of glucose intolerance, dyslipidemia, central obesity and hypertension. It was suggested that the metabolic and hemodynamic abnormalities associated with syndrome X constitute a major role in the etiology/risk factors leading to coronary heart disease.[15]

The metabolic syndrome and polycystic ovary syndrome: separate and not equal

The current literature has so wedded the concepts of PCOS and insulin resistance syndrome (or syndrome X), that the two have become almost interchangeable.[16] PCOS is viewed as a diabetes and/or cardiovascular disease certainly in the minds of the physician, and increasingly also the patient. In such an environment there is substantial encouragement to publish supporting data, and there is a prolific literature identifying diabetes and cardiovascular disease risk factors

such as obesity, dyslipidemia, glucose intolerance, and occasionally hypertension in women with signs of PCOS.[17–22] But risk factors do not necessarily equate with disease and/or events.[23]

The metabolic syndrome X and PCOS remain distinct. When women with the metabolic syndrome are studied for reproductive stigmata of PCOS, they are no more likely to have polycystic ovaries (PCO) than other sections of the population are; only about half were found to have a history of oligomenorrhea (though oligomenorrhea was twice as common in the affected population as in the controls).[24] Nor do all women with PCOS have the metabolic syndrome. In some countries, obesity appears to be less common in women with PCOS. For instance, in England a large case series of over 1700 women reported a high percentage of non-obese women with PCOS (60%).[25] In the Netherlands, a follow-up case series on over 300 women with PCOS showed that 56% had a body mass index (BMI) <25 kg/m². While these case series are not a representative population sample, they suggest a less obese PCOS phenotype than commonly encountered in the US.[26–28]

Not all women with PCOS have documented insulin resistance found by invasive dynamic tests such at the euglycemic clamp or the frequently sampled intravenous glucose tolerance test. As many as 50% of obese women with PCOS may not have documented insulin resistance by intensive testing,[16,29] and this prevalence may be even lower in non-obese women with PCOS.[30,31] The clinical quantification of insulin resistance remains an imprecise science with no generally acknowledged guidelines or criteria.[32] Further, as discussed in more detail below, clinical hypertension is rarely noted in most women with PCOS, dyslipidemia is not invariably present, and the pattern of dyslipidemia is not always that of an insulin-resistant population. These caveats suggest that PCOS and the insulin resistance syndrome are not identical. Further we are just beginning to identify distinct racial effects and study the effect of the environment on PCOS.

Ethnic/racial effects

Insulin resistance has been found in women with PCOS of many racial and ethnic groups implying both that it is a universal characteristic and that a common defect may underlie its prevalence.[33-36] However, there are differences in the phenotype in PCOS according to ethnicity, although these have not been systematically studied. For example eastern Asian women have elevated circulating androgen levels without overt hirsutism,[33] and Latinos have been shown to have decreased insulin sensitivity compared with Caucasians.[34] In a large series examining the phenotypic characteristics of black and white individuals with PCOS, black people were noted to be significantly more heavy than white people, with other characteristics of the phenotype being similar, although this study did not look at glucose tolerance.[26] Black women have also been shown to have higher insulin levels than age- and weight-matched white individuals, and an increased risk for diabetes.[37]

The highest reported prevalence of PCO is 52% among South Asian immigrants in Britain, of whom 49.1% had menstrual irregularity.[38] Rodin et al demonstrated that South Asian women with PCO had a comparable degree of insulin resistance to that of established type 2 diabetes mellitus but no PCO in South Asian women, which was therefore independent of diabetes.[38] Nonetheless, there has been a paucity of data of the prevalence of PCOS among women of South Asian origin, among both migrant and native groups. Type 2 diabetes and insulin resistance have a high prevalence among indigenous populations in South Asia, with a rising prevalence among women. Insulin resistance and hyperinsulinemia are common antecedents of type 2 diabetes, with a high prevalence in South Asians. Type 2 diabetes also has a familial basis, inherited as a complex genetic trait that interacts with environmental factors, chiefly nutrition, commencing from fetal life. We are currently exploring the hypothesis that ethnic variations in the overt features of PCOS (i.e. symptoms of hyperandrogenism, menstrual irregularity, and obesity) in women of South Asian descent, are linked to the higher prevalence and degree of insulin resistance in South Asians. We have already found that South Asians with anovular PCOS have greater insulin resistance and more severe symptoms of the syndrome than anovular Caucasians with PCOS.[39] Furthermore, we have found that women from South Asia, living in the UK appear to express symptoms at an earlier age than their Caucasian British counterparts.

The question remains as to whether differences in expression of the syndrome are due to dietary and lifestyle factors, or genetic variations in hormone actions, such as polymorphisms in gonadotropin subunits or receptor function (affecting the expression of androgens, gonadotropins or insulin). Therefore ethnicity may contribute independently to a worsening risk for glucose intolerance.

Hyperhomocysteinemia and polycystic ovary syndrome

A moderately increased total plasma homocysteine (Hcy) concentration is associated with an increased risk of atherosclerosis.[40,41] Hcy is an essential intermediate in the transfer of activated methyl groups from tetrahydrofolate to S-adenylmethionine, in the synthesis of cysteine from methionine, and in the production of homocysteine thiolactone. An abnormal elevation of Hcy in plasma and urine is caused by an imbalance between Hcy production and metabolism, which can be of demographic, genetic, nutritional or metabolic etiology, and is associated with premature vascular disease.[42] Mild hyperhomocysteinemia has been demonstrated to induce sustained injury to the arterial endothelial cell that accelerates the development of thrombosis and atherosclerosis.[43] Normal concentrations of total plasma Hcy are in the range of 5–16 µmol/l, although 10 µmol/l is considered the desired upper limit, while there is an age-related rise and lower concentrations in women.[43]

Chambers and Kooner, while noting that almost 30% of patients with vascular disease have mild elevation of plasma Hcy, highlight that migrant South Asians living in the UK have increased mortality from coronary artery disease (CAD), which is not explained by conventional risk factors.[44] They postulate that reports of elevated Hcy concentrations among Asians could explain the observed difference in their atherosclerosis risk when compared with white Europeans.[44] Insulin resistance, the metabolic syndrome and diabetes mellitus being more prevalent in South Asians than in white Europeans, have also been linked to the observed increased risk of CAD among Asians.[45,46] Furthermore, insulin resistance and hyperinsulinemia play a central role in the multiple hormonal and metabolic derangement that occur in PCOS, and are recognized causes of premature CAD in women.[2,47] A recent report showed that migrant South Asians with PCOS present at a younger age, with more severe symptoms and greater insulin resistance than white Europeans with PCOS, which suggests that the degree of metabolic dysfunction in PCOS has an ethnic basis.[39] The even greater degree of insulin resistance among the indigenous South Asians than British Asians, excludes migration as being the sole explanation for the previously observed ethnic variation in the metabolic syndrome or PCOS.

There have been recent reports of elevated plasma Hcy in PCOS, although all studies were carried out predominantly on white European women.[48–50] Yarali et al demonstrated a significant elevation of plasma Hcy among PCOS subjects when compared with older BMI-matched controls.[48] Their finding correlated with echocardiographic evidence of diastolic dysfunction (considered as an early marker of CAD), plasma insulin, and uric acid concentrations in young women with PCOS, thus linking hyperhomocysteinemia with the insulin resistance of PCOS. Loverro et al reported a significantly greater mean plasma Hcy concentration in a group of 35 women with PCOS, when compared with age-matched controls.[49] A more recent report has been the first to demonstrate an ethnic difference in the elevation of Hcy in women with PCOS, which mirrors an ethnic variation in the degree of insulin resistance of PCOS.[51] Moreover, the signif-

icantly higher concentrations of plasma Hcy and insulin among normal Sri Lankan women of reproductive age, when compared with other control groups, supports the hypothesis of an inherent ethnic propensity to insulin resistance and hyperhomocysteinemia among the indigenous South Asians.

Randeva et al reported a significant decrease in plasma Hcy and waist:hip ratio among young overweight/obese PCOS women following six months of regular physical exercise.[50] Weight reduction and regular physical exercise are recognized interventions that help towards reducing the insulin resistance of the metabolic syndrome. Further evidence of a linear relationship between plasma Hcy and insulin concentrations includes a positive correlation reported among non-obese and obese pre-menopausal women,[52] in obese insulin-resistant middle-aged males,[53] and among adolescents with essential hypertension.[54] The Framingham Offspring Study of middle-aged men and women of European Caucasian mixed descent revealed a positive association between fasting plasma Hcy and some individual traits of the insulin resistance syndromes i.e., central obesity, and fasting insulin concentration.[55,56] Meigs et al propose that hyperhomocysteinemia and insulin resistance are directly linked by similar pathogenic effects on vascular endothelial cells, as well as the establishment of a vicious cycle of an elevated Hcy-induced insulin resistance, while hyperinsulinemia in turn leads to further accumulation of plasma Hcy.[56]

It is noteworthy that central obesity as determined by waist:hip ratio (WHR), an important component of the metabolic syndrome, showed a significant linear relationship with plasma Hcy in PCOS. This is particularly significant in the light of Sri Lankan women with PCOS, who were found to have the highest mean concentration of Hcy as well as the highest WHR for a given BMI.[51] A difference in central obesity is also attributed to one's ethnic origin, with Asians being identified to have a higher body fat percentage at a lower BMI.[57] These findings were of the greatest severity in the cohort of young Sri Lankan PCOS subjects, who were recruited in an identical manner to the UK-based recruitment of subjects, and are supported by the highest prevalence of glucose intolerance among Sri Lankan PCOS patients when compared with British Asians and white Europeans with PCOS. Nevertheless, the

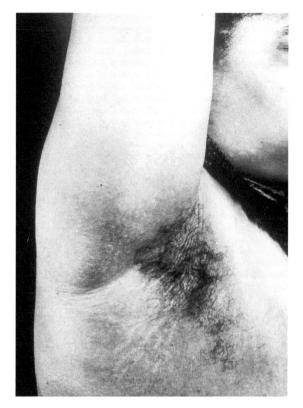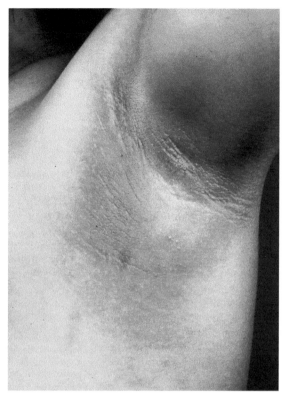

Figure 8.2

Acanthosis nigricans is a skin manifestation of hyperinsulism, secondary to hypertrophy and keratinisation. It is best visualized in skin creases, in particular the neck, elbows, knees and groin.

greater metabolic derangement observed in the indigenous Asians is likely to be explained by differing environmental influences.

Sri Lankan women have a high rate of literacy (90%) when compared with neighboring countries in the South Asian region, and a high rate of urbanization which is accompanied by an increase in the average age of marriage (27.5 years).[58,59] All of this supports the hypothesis of a change in lifestyle of a high-risk ethnic group influencing the degree of manifestation of the metabolic derangement of PCOS. No doubt further research into the degree of change in physical activity and quality of life by urbanization is required to confirm this. Nevertheless, there has been disparity in the finding of hyperhomo-cysteinemia among those at risk of CAD in two Indian-based studies,[60,61] while reports from Sri

Lanka revealed a significant elevation of plasma Hcy being associated with a three-fold risk of CAD,[62] and three-fold risk of hypertension,[63] and a more recent report of a highly significant independent association of hyperhomocysteine-mia with CAD.[64] The regional difference of Hcy elevation could be explained by dietary differ-ences, in that persons adhering to a vegetarian diet are far more common in India than in Sri Lanka. It has therefore been demonstrated for the first time that there is a consistent elevation of plasma total homocysteine concentration in three ethnic groups of women with PCOS when compared with ethnically matched controls, with the greatest elevation of plasma homocysteine corresponding to the highest degree of insulin resistance and central obesity observed in a cohort of young indigenous Sri Lankan women with PCOS.[51] These observations in young South Asian women bear major implications for their long-term risks of CAD and calls for urgent action towards early screening and primary prevention.

Environmental effects

Unfortunately there have been few studies that have looked extensively at the local environment and the effect of local dietary and activity standards on the expression of PCOS. A recent comparative study of women with PCOS in the US and in Sicily found women in the US had a significantly higher BMI, despite a similar caloric intake, and a similar dietary composition of protein, fat, and carbohydrate (though US women consumed a higher percentage of dietary fat).[65] The authors attributed the difference in BMI to a more sedentary lifestyle in the US compared with Sicily. The aforementioned findings of Wijeyeratne et al also demonstrate lifestyle and dietary influences on the expression of insulin resistance in women with PCOS.[51]

Diabetes and PCOS

Women with PCOS have been identified as having an increased risk for diabetes both by retrospective case-control and cohort studies as well as by prevalence studies in selected populations. Glucose intolerance rates approach 40% and undiagnosed diabetes approximates to 10% of women with PCOS, although these studies were performed in an obese population.[27,28] PCOS has been associated predominantly with type 2 diabetes (formerly called adult-onset diabetes or non-insulin dependent diabetes mellitus (NIDDM)), although there are occasional small series linking type 1 diabetes with stigmata of PCOS.[66] Women with PCOS have multiple factors that contribute to increased diabetes risk including insulin resistance, beta-cell dysfunction, obesity, and especially centripetal obesity, a family history of type 2 diabetes, and a personal history of gestational diabetes. Additionally there is some evidence to suggest that polycystic ovaries and chronic anovulation are risk factors.

Prevalence of glucose intolerance and diabetes in PCOS

Studies of large cohorts of women with PCOS in the US have demonstrated that the prevalence rates of glucose intolerance are as high as 40% in PCOS women when the less stringent World Health Organization (WHO) criteria are used (Figure 8.3).[27,28] These studies are of interest because they have shown nearly identical rates of impaired glucose tolerance and type 2 diabetes among a cohort that was diverse both ethnically and geographically, as well as from different investigational groups.

Undiagnosed diabetes approaches 10% in these cohorts. The majority of affected women are in their third and fourth decade of life, but we have encountered PCOS adolescents with impaired glucose tolerance or type 2 diabetes, and also lean individuals with glucose intolerance. Based on the prevalence of glucose intolerance in women in the US population (7.8% impaired glucose tolerance and 1.0% undiagnosed diabetes by WHO criteria in women aged

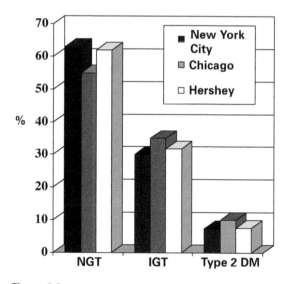

Figure 8.3

Percentage prevalence of glucose intolerance, either impaired glucose tolerance (IGT or 2-h glucose challenged glucose to a level of 140–199 mg/dl) or type 2 diabetes (glucose challenged glucose level of ≥200 mg/dl). NGT: normal glucose tolerance. From Ehrmann et al and Legro et al.[27,28]

20–44 years old),[67] the prevalence of glucose intolerance in PCOS (40%),[22,28] and on a population-based study of the prevalence of PCOS (~5%),[26] it can be extrapolated that PCOS contributes to approximately 20% of impaired glucose tolerance and 40% of type 2 diabetes in reproductive-aged women.

This would suggest that these abnormalities may represent a universal characteristic of women with PCOS, at least those diagnosed on the basis of hyperandrogenic chronic anovulation. Less stringent, more inclusive criteria (that is using the Rotterdam consensus definitions, 2004)[68] are more likely to include a group of metabolically normal women with lower prevalence rates of glucose intolerance. The inclusion of both ovulatory and anovulatory women may explain the failure of a previous large study of glucose tolerance in hyperandrogenic women to detect glucose intolerance using the more stringent National Diabetes Data Group (NDDG) criteria.[69]

Retrospective studies of diabetes in polycystic ovary syndrome

Retrospective studies looking at diabetes have generally noted an increased prevalence with age in women with PCOS. Studies from Scandinavia have shown increased rates of type 2 diabetes and hypertension compared with controls.[70] This study used a combination of ovarian morphology and clinical criteria to identify women with PCOS and found that 15% had developed diabetes compared with 2.3% of the controls.[70] A case-control study of PCOS in the US has shown persistent hyperinsulinemia and dyslipidemia as PCOS women age, although androgen levels tend to decline in older PCOS women.[71] In a thin Dutch population, however, the overall prevalence of self-reported diabetes by a telephone survey was 2.3%, in PCOS women aged 45–54 years (n = 32) and the prevalence of diabetes was four times higher (p <0.05) than in the age-matched female population.[72] The same findings have not been documented in every cohort of women with PCOS, for instance a retrospective study of mortality among women with polycystic ovaries found an increased, though non-significant risk of death due to diabetes (after adjustment for BMI, odds ratio was 2.2 (0.9–5. 2) for diabetes).[73]

Prospective studies of conversion to diabetes in polycystic ovary syndrome

Natural history supportive of significant worsening of glucose tolerance would support more aggressive identification and treatment of this disorder in PCOS women. To date there have been two small published studies of conversion rates to diabetes over time. Ehrmann reported in a follow-up study of 25 PCOS women, a significant increase in the mean 2-h glucose value over a three-year average period of follow up to 161 ± 9 mg/dl compared with the baseline 2-h value of 139 ± 6 mg/dl.[22] Recently Norman et al have also noted a trend towards worsening glucose tolerance in a study of 67 women who were followed up after an average time of 6.2 years.[74] All women followed prospectively had normal glucose tolerance (n = 54) or impaired glucose tolerance (IGT) (n = 13) at the start of the study. Conversion rate was high with 5/54 (9%) of normoglycemic women at baseline developing IGT, and a further 4/54 (8%) moving directly from normoglycemia to type 2 diabetes. For women with IGT at baseline, 7/13 (54%) had type 2 diabetes at follow up. A greater BMI at baseline was an independent significant predictor of conversion risk. These data support a worsening of glucose intolerance over time and the need for periodic screening. How often this should be is uncertain, but an educated guess would be every 3–5 years.

Risk factors for the development of diabetes in women with polycystic ovary syndrome

Insulin resistance in polycystic ovary syndrome

Burghen and colleagues made the first suggestion of a relationship between the hyperandrogenism of PCOS and hyperinsulinemia in 1980.[1] They found that the plasma insulin levels during an oral glucose tolerance test (OGTT) were elevated in eight obese subjects with PCOS, compared with controls. In addition there was a significant correlation between basal insulin measurements with both serum testosterone and androstenedione concentrations, and between insulin response during the OGTT and serum testosterone concentrations. Subsequently Chang et al showed the presence of hyperinsulinemia in non-obese PCOS subjects, in order to demonstrate that this was a feature specific to PCOS rather than secondary to obesity.[76] Since then there have been a large number of studies demonstrating the presence of insulin resistance and corresponding hyperinsulinemia in both obese and non-obese women with PCOS,[16,75–77] while others failed to demonstrate insulin resistance in non-obese women.[78–82] Obese women with PCOS have consistently been shown to be insulin resistant to a greater degree than their weight-matched controls. It appears that obesity and PCOS appear to have a synergistic effect on the degree and severity of the insulin resistance and subsequent hyperinsulinemia in this group of women. Robinson et al found that the insulin sensitivity varied depending upon the menstrual pattern.[83] They found that non-obese women with PCOS who were oligomenorrheic were more likely to be insulin resistant than those with regular cycles. Conway et al found that 30% of non-obese women with PCOS have a mild degree of insulin resistance,[84] while Falcone et al reported that 63% of their non-obese subjects

were insulin resistant.[85] There are differences of opinion in the literature concerning the interrelationship of insulin resistance and hyperandrogenemia. It is suggested that hyperinsulinemia results in raised ovarian androgens,[84] while others have failed to demonstrate a direct relationship.[16,80,86,87]

The increase in insulin resistance in women with PCOS compared with appropriate controls (~35–40%), is of a similar magnitude to that seen in type 2 diabetes and is independent of obesity, glucose intolerance, increases in waist–hip–girth ratio and differences in muscle mass (Figure 8.4).[88,89] The synergistic negative effect of obesity and PCOS on hepatic glucose production is an important factor in the pathogenesis of glucose intolerance in PCOS. Insulin resistance is thought to be the primary pathogenetic defect leading to the development of type 2 diabetes, and prospective population studies have identified it as an independent risk factor for type 2 diabetes.[90]

Beta-cell dysfunction in polycystic ovary syndrome and diabetes

One of the most common prevailing theories about the etiology of type 2 diabetes proposes that the primary pathogenetic defect is peripheral insulin resistance resulting in compensatory hyperinsulinemia. Over time there is beta-cell dysfunction leading to inadequate secretion of insulin, and ultimately to beta-cell exhaustion, and the development of frank type 2 diabetes (Figure 8.5). There is now a relatively substantial body of literature confirming beta-cell dysfunction in PCOS,[30,91] though as in diabetes, there is still considerable debate as to the primacy of the defects and their worsening over time.[92] Basal insulin levels are increased and insulin secretory response to meals has been shown to be reduced in PCOS women.[91,92] This dysfunction is also independent of obesity.[30] Beta-cell dysfunction, per se, is not thought to be an independent risk factor for cardiovascular disease.

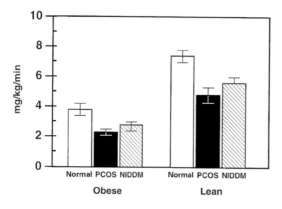

Figure 8.4

Insulin-mediated glucose disposal at steady-state insulin levels during hyperinsulinemic euglycemic clamp is decreased by 35–40% in PCOS women compared with age- and weight-matched control women. This decrease is similar in magnitude to that seen in type 2 diabetes (NIDDM). Error bars show standard error of mean (SEM). Figure is adapted from Dunaif, 1997.[89]

Chronic anovulation and diabetes

Chronic anovulation as evidenced by oligo- or amenorrhea has not been traditionally identified as a risk factor for diabetes. However there is emerg-

Table 8.1 Relative risks (RRs) for type 2 diabetes mellitus associated with menstrual cycle pattern at age 18–22 years in the Nurse's Health Study II (from Solomon et al, 2001)[4]

	Usual cycle length (days)				
	<21	21–25	26–31[a]	32–39	>40 or highly irregular
No. of cases	7	51	297	71	81
Person-years[b]	5,633	56,412	372,971	86,243	43,074
Age-adjusted RR (95% confidence interval)	1.55 (0.73–3.29)	1.18 (0.88–1.59)	1.0	1.04 (0.80–1.35)	2.40 (1.88–3.07)
Multivariate RR (95% confidence interval)[c]	1.50 (0.70–3.19)	1.18 (0.87–1.58)	1.0	1.03 (0.79–1.33)	2.08 (1.62–2.66)

[a]Referent.

[b]Person-years reflect follow-up time from return of baseline (1989) questionnaire.

[c]Adjusting for age (continuous), time period (3 categories), BMI at age 18 years (6 categories), smoking (current, past, never), family history of diabetes mellitus in a first-degree relative, physical activity level (quintiles of total metabolic expenditure), and duration of oral contraceptive use.

ing evidence that this symptom alone identifies a group of women at marked increased risk for type 2 diabetes. In a report involving over 100,000 women in the Nurses' Health Study II, a largely non-Hispanic white group, the authors have prospectively demonstrated a significant increase

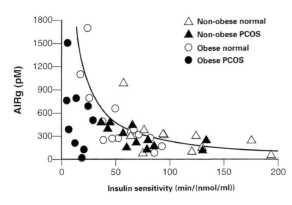

Figure 8.5

The relationship between insulin sensitivity determined by frequently sampled intravenous glucose tolerance test and first-phase insulin secretion to an intravenous glucose load (AIRg), a marker of beta-cell function. The majority of PCOS women fall below the normal curve determined in concurrently studied age- and weight-matched control women as well as normative data in the literature. This implies both defects in insulin sensitivity and compensatory beta-cell function. Adapted from Dunaif and Finegood, 1996.[30]

in the risk for type 2 diabetes in women with oligo- or amenorrhea. Women with a cycle length of 40 days or greater, including those with complete amenorrhea, had more than twice the risk for developing type 2 diabetes compared with women with regular menstrual cycles 21–39 days in length (Table 8.1).[93] In a clinical trial of insulin-sensitizing agents in women with PCOS, an increase in cycle length at baseline (i.e. decreased menstrual frequency) has been associated with a decreased likelihood of response.[94,95] Thus fewer menstrual cycles may identify a greater risk for diabetes or failure to respond to insulin-sensitizing therapy within the population of females with PCOS.

Hyperandrogenism and diabetes

The relationship between hyperandrogenism and diabetes is complex, and there does not appear to be a linear relationship between the degree of androgen excess and markers of insulin action. Nonetheless there is increasing evidence that hyperandrogenemia per se may reflect underlying metabolic dysfunction and a tendency to glucose intolerance. This is not only based on the classic association of diabetes with 'bearded ladies' (Figure 8.6),[96] but also on rare syndromes of marked elevated hyperandrogenemia, marked insulin resistance, and acanthosis nigricans, the

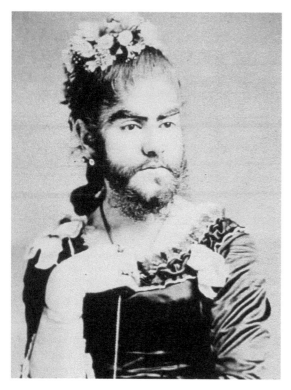

Figure 8.6

The relationship between diabetes and hyperandrogenism was first noted by the French physician Achard (with the help of Thiers) in 1921.[96]

HAIR-AN syndrome.[97] Small studies which show a marked reduction in testosterone levels in women after either spontaneous remission or pharmacologically induced hyperinsulinemia are intriguing and support a causal link between insulin resistance and hyperendrogenism.[98] Sisters of probands with PCOS who have isolated elevated testosterone levels are hyperinsulinemic.[100] Others have shown increased rates of glucose intolerance among first-degree male and female relatives of women with PCOS.[99,100]

Polycystic ovaries and diabetes

The bulk of evidence linking polycystic ovaries with diabetes is noted in follow-up studies of aging populations with a prior diagnosis of PCOS. Their meaning in terms of diabetes risk in a younger population is uncertain. Polycystic ovaries have been found in up to 30% of a random female population,[101] and their presence does not necessarily signal metabolic abnormalities such as glucose intolerance. Many women with polycystic ovaries appear endocrinologically normal, without hirsutism or irregular menses.[102] Nonetheless more intensive study of apparently normal females with polycystic ovaries have detected metabolic and reproductive abnormalities.[103,104] A high prevalence of polycystic ovaries has been detected among reproductive-aged females who present with type 2 diabetes.[105] Although the predictive value of the presence of polycystic ovaries is unknown, the preliminary data are suggestive that this is a possible predictive sign of metabolic dysfunction.

Obesity and diabetes

Obesity is one of the clearest risk factors for developing diabetes.[106] Even women of average weight (BMI 23–23.8 kg/m^2) were at substantial increased risk for diabetes (relative risk 3.6) when compared with thinner women (BMI <22).[106] It has been estimated that 50% of women with PCOS are obese.[107] However this can vary greatly between populations. In an English population of 1741 PCOS women, about 40% of patients were obese,[108] whereas in the US population obesity and morbid obesity is much more common – up to 80%.[22,28] Many studies have also identified a centripetal pattern of obesity in obese PCOS women, which may further contribute to diabetes risks in these women.[109] Although even approximately 10% of thin women with PCOS can have glucose intolerance, there is a stepwise increase in prevalence as BMI increases (Figure 8.7).[28]

Simple obesity is associated with greater deposition of gluteo-femoral fat while central obesity involves greater truncal abdominal fat distribution. Obesity is seen in 35–60% of women with PCOS.[25,110] Hyperandrogenism is associated with a preponderance of fat localized to truncal abdominal sites.[111] Women with PCOS have a greater truncal abdominal fat distribution as demonstrated by a higher waist:hip ratio.[79,111–113] The central distribution of fat in these studies, was independent of BMI and associated with higher plasma insulin and triglyceride concentrations, and reduced HDL cholesterol concentrations.[113]

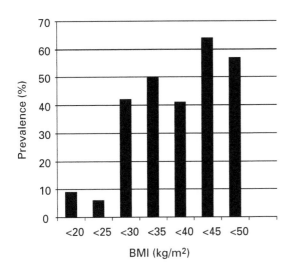

Figure 8.7

Increasing prevalence (%) of glucose intolerance by increasing BMI among 254 women with PCOS. Adapted from Legro et al, 1999.[28]

Family history of type 2 diabetes

Multiple studies have shown that a family history of diabetes significantly contributes to the risk of diabetes.[114,115] First-degree relatives of patients with type 2 diabetes are more likely to suffer stigmata of insulin resistance, including impaired glucose tolerance.[116] Diabetes risk is increased according to both the number of relatives affected with type 2 diabetes and the closeness of relation. In PCOS, a family history of diabetes has been found to further magnify the severity of insulin secretory defects compared with PCOS women without a family history.[117] A family history of diabetes increases the risk for glucose intolerance in a women with PCOS by 2–3-fold.[28]

This suggests that the pathogenesis of type 2 diabetes is similar in all of these groups. An underlying genetic defect conferring insulin resistance and, perhaps, beta-cell dysfunction interacts with environmental factors worsening insulin resistance.[118,119] Beta-cell function worsens and glucose intolerance supervenes.[118,119] This genetic predisposition may also contribute to varying risks of type 2 diabetes among different ethnic and racial populations.

Previous gestational diabetes

While a history of gestational diabetes is a clear risk factor for type 2 diabetes, it is uncertain how much the diagnosis of PCOS increases this risk. Both disorders again involve a marked reduction in peripheral insulin sensitivity.[120] In Latino women with a history of gestational diabetes mellitus, cumulative conversion rates as high as 80% over five years have been reported.[121] Clearly there may be independent and additive contributions of lifestyle and genetics in this case (see below). Women who present with gestational diabetes have a higher prevalence of polycystic ovaries detected postpartum,[122,123] and this can be associated with persistent postpartum glucose intolerance.[124] The impact of pre-existing glucose intolerance in a woman with PCOS is less certain, but probably increases risk.[125] Hyperinsulinemia may be an independent risk factor for developing gestational diabetes in women with PCOS,[126] but in other cases no additional risk of gestational diabetes has been detected.[127] This is an area of PCOS pathophysiology and epidemiology ripe for further study.

Polycystic ovary syndrome and cardiovascular disease

When approached by the more stringent requirement of cardiovascular events, i.e. increased mortality from cardiovascular disease (CVD), premature mortality from CVD, or an increased incidence of cardiovascular events (stroke and/or myocardial infarction), there is little published evidence to show that PCOS women are unduly affected. The increased cardiovascular risk ascribed to women with PCOS is almost entirely inferential, based on surrogate risk factors.[18,128] There are multiple potential reasons for the lack of published data confirming increased cardiovascular events in this group. Varying or age-specific diagnostic criteria have limited both clinical trials and long-term follow up of women with PCOS. This heterogeneity of diagnostic criteria is both confounding and confusing, when assessing CVD in women with PCOS. The lack of any measure of hyperinsulinemia and/or insulin resistance in any of the current diagnostic criteria diminishes recognition of the most plausible link between PCOS and CVD.

The study of women with PCOS has been characterized by small sample sizes, usually in a pre-menopausal reproductive age population, with limited follow up. There have been few large-scale epidemiological trials of such a young female population that could document relatively rare events such as stroke and myocardial infarction. The lack of a post-menopausal PCOS phenotype, or more importantly the fading of the reproductive phenotype with age,[129,130] inhibits the linking of past, seemingly irrelevant, reproductive problems with current CVD in older populations.

There is the additional confounding effect of treatment on future complications of PCOS. Long-term benefits may have possibly resulted from ovarian wedge resection or other forms of ovarian surgery. The current widespread use of insulin-lowering agents for women of all ages with PCOS may complicate ongoing or future studies of cardiovascular disease. Finally, the alternative hypothesis must always be entertained, that is that PCOS is not associated with an increased CVD risk (or an earlier presentation with disease).

Polycystic ovary syndrome and cardiovascular disease events

A large-scale epidemiological case-control study from the University of Pittsburgh, initiated in 1992 has identified cases with PCOS, primarily based on hyperandrogenic chronic anovulation (n >200), and concurrently recruited community-based controls (n >200).[131] The investigators have now followed this cohort for a decade. In preliminary data reported from the follow-up, there was an increased trend towards events/disease in the PCOS group compared with the control group. Among 126 Caucasian PCOS cases, there were two myocardial infarctions, four cases of angina pectoris, and two cases of surgical cardiac intervention (an angioplasty and a coronary bypass surgery). Among 142 controls of similar age there were no events. The odds ratio of a cardiovascular event in a woman with PCOS compared with a control was 5.91 (95% confidence interval (CI), 0.7–135.6).[132] One criticism of this study, that is not addressed in these preliminary data, but

which has consistently been controlled for in published analyses is the greater BMI in the PCOS group compared with controls. Nonetheless, the abnormal cardiovascular risk profile has persisted in women with PCOS, even after adjustment for differences in BMI, lipids, fat distribution, etc., compared with the reference population.

Another study from the Czech Republic with a much smaller case group (n = 28) noted a higher prevalence of self-reported CHD symptoms when compared with age-matched controls (n = 752) (21% of PCOS vs 5.2% of controls, p = 0.001).[133] This group used diagnostic criteria of both hyperandrogenic chronic anovulation and past histopathologic evidence of PCO to identify cases, but only 28 of 61 cases identified responded to the questionnaire. Within the University of Pittsburgh study, the presence or absence of PCO had little effect on their cardiovascular risk,[134] and the presence of PCO was primarily associated with increased incidence of reproductive abnormalities.

Polycystic ovary syndrome and increased subclinical cardiovascular disease

Several surrogate markers for atherosclerotic disease, including carotid wall thickness as determined by B-mode ultrasonography and coronary/aortic calcification as determined by electron beam computed tomography (EBCT) have been studied in women with PCOS.

Wild et al reported that in 102 women undergoing coronary angiography to evaluate the significance of chest pain, hirsutism and acne were found to be twice as common in those with CAD as in those without. In addition, an increased waist:hip ratio was associated with both hirsutism and CAD.[17] They concluded that altered fat distribution (android pattern) associated with classical manifestations of androgen excess (hirsutism and/or acne) may be an indicator of a greater risk for ischemic heart disease (IHD). Birdsall and colleagues reported the association between polycystic ovaries and extent of CAD in 143 women aged 60 years or younger, undergoing cardiac catheterization.[19] Polycystic ovaries were detected in 42% of the subjects by transabdominal or transvaginal scans. Women with polycystic ovaries had more coronary artery segments with greater than 50% stenosis, and showed a trend towards greater severity of IHD, than women with normal ovaries. By multivariate regression analysis the extent of CAD was found to be independently associated with polycystic ovaries (p = 0.032) as was family history of heart disease (p = 0.022). To summarize, those with more extensive disease (number of segments with >50% stenosis) were more likely to have polycystic ovaries on ultrasound scan, than those with less extensive coronary disease.

The incidence of CAD is strongly correlated with carotid atherosclerosis.[135] Early carotid atherosclerosis as assessed by ultrasonography has been reported to be associated with cardiovascular risk factors especially abnormal lipid profiles, in middle-aged and post-menopausal women. Guzick et al measured the intima to media thickness of the common and internal carotid vessels and carotid bulb to evaluate subclinical measures of atherosclerosis in 16 women with PCOS aged 40 years or more, and compared the measurements with 16 matched controls.[136] They found that the women with PCOS were more likely to have subclinical atherosclerosis of the carotid vessels. Although definitive evidence of a progression of carotid lesions from intima–media thickness to plaque formation, and to clinical events is lacking, increase in intima–media thickness has been viewed as early subclinical atherosclerosis before the occurrence of gross atheromatous plaque formation and blood flow alteration.[137] In this study, the presence of PCOS appeared to increase the risk of carotid atherosclerosis, although in view of the sample size the data must be interpreted with caution.

The University of Pittsburgh performed ultrasonography of the carotid arteries on 125 women with PCOS and 142 control women from their original cohort, and found a significantly higher prevalence of abnormal carotid plaque index in women with PCOS (7.2% vs 0.7% in controls).[138] Thus the vast majority of predominantly premenopausal women with PCOS (93%) had no evidence for subclinical carotid atherosclerosis. No difference was noted in the intima–media thickness between PCOS and controls until the age group 45–49 years, a difference which persisted and increased in the age group in the

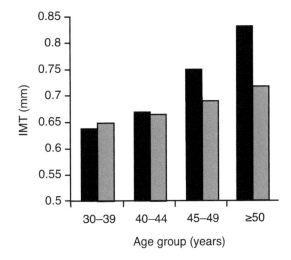

Figure 8.8

Mean intimal medial thickness (IMT) of the carotid artery in PCOS (cases, black bars) and controls (grey bars) by age (in 1999) from the University of Pittsburgh PCOS study. PCOS × age interaction p = 0.031. Adapted from Talbott et al, 2000.[138]

menopausal range (≥50 years) (Figure 8.8).[138] These data would suggest that an increased risk for subclinical atherosclerotic disease is not apparent until the perimenopause in women with PCOS.

Coronary artery calcification correlates with the degree of histopathologic atherosclerosis and has been found to predict actual events.[132] More recently, the University of Pittsburgh group has performed a pilot study of coronary and aortic calcification in a group of 32 women with PCOS and 30 controls. There was a significantly higher rate of detectable coronary artery calcification among PCOS women compared with controls (54% vs 24%, p <0.05), with no difference noted in the abdominal aorta (Table 8.2).[132] Another investigative group recently reported a higher prevalence of coronary artery calcification in women with PCOS.[139] Healthy, community-dwelling, ovulatory controls (n = 71) were matched by age and BMI to PCOS women (n = 36). Women with diabetes or known coronary heart disease were excluded. Coronary artery calcification was more prevalent in PCOS women (39%) than in matched

Table 8.2 Distribution of coronary and aortic calcification scores by electron beam computed tomography in PCOS cases and controls. Preliminary data from the University of Pittsburgh Study. Adapted from Talbott et al, 2001.[132]

Score	Coronary calcification		Aortic calcification	
	PCOS % (n)	Control % (n)	PCOS % (n)	Control % (n)
0	46 (13)	76 (22)	57 (16)	69 (20)
1–10	46 (13)	17 (5)	7 (2)	14 (4)
11–50	4 (1)	6 (2)	14.3 (4)	10 (3)
50–300	0	0	11 (3)	7 (2)
300+	4 (1)	0	11 (3)	0

Chi squared (any versus none) = 5.2 (p = 0.022 and 0.9 (p = 0.355) for coronary and aortic calcification, respectively.

controls (21%; odds ratio, 2.4; p = 0.05) or community-dwelling women (9.9%; odds ratio, 5.9; p <0.001).[139]

In 1992, Dahlgren and colleagues[140] extrapolated the findings of the Gothenberg study,[10] to ascertain the relative risk of IHD in a group of 33 women diagnosed clinically and histologically to have PCOS between 1956 and 1965. By risk model analysis it was calculated that the women with PCOS had a 7.4-fold greater risk of myocardial infarction than age-matched controls. Compared with the control group, the women with PCOS, aged 40 years or more, showed a marked increase in the prevalence of central obesity, higher basal serum insulin concentrations, as well as a seven-fold higher prevalence of diabetes and three-fold higher prevalence of hypertension. These findings were not altogether surprising – in 1921 Achard and Thiers had described the association between hyperandrogenism and diabetes in a paper entitled *The diabetes of bearded women*.[141] However, in another study, Pierpoint et al reported the mortality rate in 1028 women diagnosed as having PCOS between 1930 and 1979.[142] All the women were older than 45 years, and 770 women had been treated by wedge resection of the ovaries. Seven-hundred and eighty-six women were traced; the mean age at diagnosis was 26.4 years and average duration of follow up was 30 years. There were 59 deaths, of which 15 were from circulatory disease. Of these 15 deaths, 13 were from IHD. There were six

deaths from diabetes as an underlying or contributory cause, compared with the expected 1.7 deaths. The standard mortality rate both overall and for cardiovascular disease was not higher in the women with PCOS compared with the national mortality rates in women, although the observed proportion of women with diabetes as a contributory or underlying factor leading to death was significantly higher than expected (odds ratio 3.6; 95% CI 1.5–8.4). Thus, despite surrogate markers for cardiovascular disease, in this study no increased rate of death from cardiovascular disease could be demonstrated.

Polycystic ovary syndrome in younger women

At what stage do the risk factors for CVD become apparent in women with PCOS? The majority of studies that have identified the risk factors of obesity and insulin resistance in women with PCOS have investigated adult populations, commonly including women who have presented to specialist endocrine or reproductive clinics. However, PCOS has been identified in much younger populations. Dramusic et al examined 150 adolescent girls between the ages of 12 and 22 years who presented with menstrual disorders, and who displayed ultrasound features of polycystic ovaries.[143] Twenty-five (17%) were found to be overweight and 16 (11%) were considered to be obese. Evaluation of biochemical profiles confirmed hyperandrogenism and elevated LH in the majority (60%), but insulin resistance was not assessed.

A recent community-based study by Michelmore et al assessed the prevalence and associated features of polycystic ovaries in 230 young women aged 18–25 years.[101] In this population polycystic ovaries were identified in 30% and a high proportion of these women (80%) had one additional feature associated with PCOS. Of those with PCOS, 32% were overweight, but none displayed a pattern of central obesity. Hyperinsulinemia and insulin resistance were not identified in these women with PCOS, nor did they have elevated blood pressure.[101] These data emphasize the need for long-term prospective studies of young women with PCOS in order to clarify the natural history, and to determine which

Table 8.3 Circulating lipid and lipoprotein values in polycystic ovary syndrome women (not stratified by weight) from selected studies

Author	PCOS (n)	Total cholesterol mg/dl	LDL-C mg/dl	HDL-C mg/dl	TTG
Wild et al, 1985[150]	29[a]	209 ± 11	119 ± 12	43 ± 2[d]	122 ± 11[c]
Norman et al, 1995[151]	54	205 ± 31[c]	145 ± 27	46 ± 8	89 ± 27
Talbott et al, 1995[132]	206	195 ± 34[c]	118 ± 32[c]	51 ± 15[d]	129 ± 89[c]
Robinson et al, 1996[152]	54[a]	182 ± 6	120 ± 50	38 (32–44)[b]	97 (68–169)[b]
Mather et al, 2000[153]	57	193 ± 43[e]	116 ± 31[e]	43± 11[e]	169 ± 105[e]
Legro et al, 2001[146]	195	195 ± 39	127 ± 33	37 ± 11	174 ± 199

TTG = triglycerides; LDL = low-density lipoprotein; HDL = high-density lipoprotein. Values are mean ± standard deviation (SD).
[a]mean ± standard error (SE) or median where applicable;
[b]interquartile ranges;
[c]increased and p <0.05 compared to controls;
[d]decreased and p <0.05 compared to controls;
[e]analysis not performed.

women will be at risk of diabetes and cardiovascular disease later in life.

General risk factors for cardiovascular disease

The major modifiable cardiovascular disease risk factors are smoking, hypertension, dyslipidemia, obesity, diabetes, and physical inactivity. Little has been published on the prevalence of smoking in women with PCOS. Non-modifiable risk factors include age, sex, and family history of premature CVD. While hypertension appears as an integral part of the insulin resistance syndrome, women with PCOS have only occasionally been noted to have hypertension,[144,145] and large clinical studies of women with PCOS (based on hyperandrogenic chronic anovulation) have reported normal baseline blood pressures.[71,146] Increases in blood pressure when noted are usually mild and of questionable clinical significance.[130,147] This may be because hypertension is a late-developing consequence of insulin resistance and is not found in reproductive age women with PCOS.[148]

Obesity and cardiovascular disease

Obesity is common among women with PCOS and affected by a variety of factors, including genetics, physical activity, and diet. It has been estimated to affect over 50% of women with PCOS,[88] but this may underestimate its true prevalence in the US population. In a large multicenter clinical trial of 305 US women with PCOS, mean BMI in the four treatment groups varied from 35 to 38 kg/m²,[94] Body fat distribution, especially an android or centripetal fat distribution, has been independently associated with cardiovascular mortality (a stronger predictor than obesity alone),[149] and an android habitus is frequently found in women with PCOS (hyperandrogenic chronic anovulation).[28,94,132]

Dyslipidemia and cardiovascular disease

Dyslipidemia may be the most common metabolic abnormality in PCOS, although the type and extent of the findings have been variable. Prevalence of an abnormal lipid level (borderline or high) by National Cholesterol Education Program (NCEP) guidelines approaches 70%.[28] Thus a substantial portion of women with PCOS may have a completely normal circulating lipid profile and in larger published series of lipid levels in women with PCOS, mean levels, for the most part, fall within normal limits as determined by NCEP cut-offs (Table 8.3). However these mean levels may exceed those for age- and weight-matched women in the larger population.

Controlling for the confounder of obesity has become the standard for analysis of lipids in PCOS women with parallel analyses in both obese and non-obese groups, with more abnormal levels usually to be found in the obese groups.[154–160] Lifestyle factors for dyslipidemia and CVD, such as smoking, hypertension, and physical inactivity have only rarely been controlled for when examining a PCOS population.[146,153]

High-density lipoproteins (HDL) play an important role in lipid metabolism and as described by Blass et al, are the most important lipid parameter in predicting cardiovascular risk in women.[13] HDLs perform the task of 'reverse cholesterol transport'. That is, they remove excess lipids from the circulation and tissues to transport them to the liver for excretion, or transfer them to other lipoprotein particles. Cholesterol is only one component of HDL, a particle with constantly changing composition forming HDL3 then HDL2, as unesterified cholesterol is taken from tissue, esterified and exchanged for triglyceride with other lipoprotein species. Consequently measurement of a single constituent in a particle involved in a dynamic process gives an incomplete picture.

Rajkowha et al, performed a detailed study of HDL composition to help understand the processes that lead to the reduced concentrations previously reported in PCOS.[159] This study included measurements of HDL cholesterol, HDL triglycerides, HDL phospholipids, and apolipoprotein A-1 in all the subfractions (i.e. total HDL, HDL3 and HDL2). Obesity was the most important factor associated with elevated serum total triglyceride, cholesterol and phospholipid concentrations in both PCOS subjects and controls. In addition, obese women with PCOS had lower HDL cholesterol and phospholipid concentrations in all subfractions compared with obese controls. This was in the presence of normal quantities of the protein component of HDL – apolipoprotein A-1. These findings imply that the number of HDL particles was the same in obese PCOS subjects compared with obese controls, but the HDL particles were lipid-depleted, hence less effective in function. The only factor that appeared to have an independent influence on the HDL composition was the presence of PCOS, rather than obesity, or raised serum androgen or insulin concentrations.

Women with PCOS also show elevated levels of plasminogen activator inhibitor-I (PAI-1), which is a potent inhibitor of fibrinolysis in obese[160] and non-obese women with PCOS.[161] Plasma levels of PAI-1 correlate directly with serum insulin concentrations, and have been shown to be an important predictor of myocardial infarction.

The effect of aging on the pattern of dyslipidemia in PCOS is best addressed by the study from the University of Pittsburgh, which upon initiation involved an older PCOS population (in their fourth decade).[47] This study has been extended with repeat lipid phenotyping in the cohort and changes over time have been reported.[71] The subsequent report showed persistent lipid abnormalities in the PCOS population, but compared with the reference population these abnormalities tended to persist and plateau, but not worsen as they did in the control population (Figure 8.9).[71] These data were interpreted as increasing cardiovascular risk over a lifetime, given the prolonged exposure of women with PCOS from an early age to abnormal circulating lipid values. Another alternative interpretation is that the stability of the risk profile into and through the menopause in women with PCOS may offer them a favorable risk profile compared with the worsening levels in the control population.

Insulin resistance and cardiovascular disease

Insulin resistance and compensatory hyperinsulinemia have been implicated in a number of processes relating to the development of atherosclerosis. Insulin resistance, and its frequent but not invariant companion, compensatory hyperinsulinemia, have been associated with other distinct patterns of dyslipidemia. These include decreased levels of high-density cholesterol lipoprotein (HDL-C), increased levels of small dense low-density lipoprotein (LDL-C), and elevated levels of triglycerides.[3] Several studies have reported similar findings of decreased HDL-C/increased triglycerides in the lipid profiles in PCOS women.[21,47,132,151,156,157,158,163] The largest case series have noted comparative elevations in LDL-C in a PCOS population,[71,132,147,154] a finding not usually noted in insulin-resistant states,[166] but one that may be related to elevations in circulating androgens. Further multivariate analysis of the

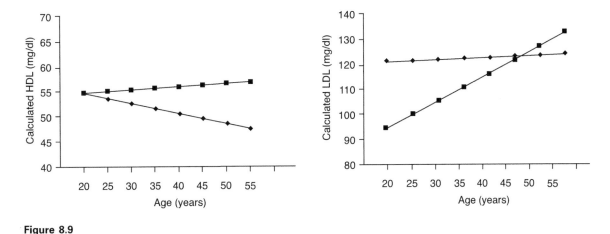

Figure 8.9

Calculated LDL-C and HDL-C by age, PCOS cases (diamonds) vs controls (squares) from the University of Pittsburgh PCOS study. Note the relative stability of LDL-C levels in women with PCOS. Adapted from Talbott et al, 1998.[71]

etiology of dyslipidemia in these larger series finds only a modest contribution of hyperinsulinemia.[71,147]

Low-density lipoprotein (LDL) subclasses are important predictors of CVD.[165] LDL particles are heterogeneous in size, density, and composition. Small dense LDL particles have been associated with an increased relative risk of CAD that ranges from 3–7-fold.[165] Multiple studies have shown a high prevalence of small LDL size in women with PCOS,[73,166] although not always significantly different from age- and weight-comparable controls.[21] Targeting and lowering LDL-C levels in at-risk groups has received greater attention in the National Cholesterol Education Program revised guidelines.[167]

Dyslipidemia represents just one aspect whereby insulin resistance may adversely affect cardiovascular risk. There has been a proliferation of reports identifying an increased cardiovascular risk profile based on a number of newer disease markers of insulin resistance in women with PCOS (based on varying diagnostic criteria), usually relative to controls. Space limitations prevent more extensive discussion of these, although a fuller discussion can be found in other reviews.[129,133] In summary, these abnormalities in women with PCOS include:

- decreased cardiac systolic flow velocity[18]
- diastolic dysfunction[168]
- endothelial dysfunction[169]
- increased vascular stiffness[170]
- low-grade chronic inflammation[171]
- increased oxidative stress[172]
- altered inflammatory markers (including homocysteine, C-reactive protein, etc.)[173]
- altered circulating divalent cations[174]
- altered hemostasis including impaired fibrinolysis[102]
- increased tissue plasminogen activator antigen.[175]

Hyperandrogenism and cardiovascular disease

Hyperandrogenism per se in women is not a recognized risk factor for cardiovascular disease, although it is tempting to cite as a possible reason for its importance the earlier onset of atherosclerosis in men compared with women. Hirsutism and acne, clinical signs of hyperandrogenism, have been identified as common features of women undergoing catheterization for CAD, and were associated with more severe disease.[176] There is little evidence in men of a relationship between androgenic alopecia and increased cardiovascular risk, and there is even less in women.[176] Iatrogenic hyperandrogenism in female to male trans-sexuals does not result in increased cardiovascular mortality.[177] Because rates of CVD are very low in pre-menopausal populations, only studies that either measure steroid levels or bank serum/urine for future assay can provide meaningful data, as CVD presents much later in these cohorts. In a nested case reference study, there was no evidence for increased urinary androgen excretion among pre-menopausal Dutch women in a breast cancer screening study who later developed CVD.[178] In case-control and prospective studies of post-menopausal populations, circulating androgen levels did not correlate with cardiovascular events.[179,180]

Biochemical hyperandrogenemia in a menopausal population is difficult to determine. Circulating androgen levels in the PCOS population normalize prior to menopause,[132] and there is a similar decline over the same period in all females.[182] There is also a decline in androgen production by the adrenal gland, as indicated by the declining levels of dehydroepiandrosterone (DHEAS) with age. However the circulating levels of more potent androgens such as androstenedione and testosterone are relatively stable during and after menopause, due to persistent androgen production by the ovaries.[182] Thus relative hyperandrogenism, given the absence of estrogen production by the ovary, is a distinguishing feature of all menopausal women. Hyperandrogenism in the menopause is accentuated by a decline in circulating sex hormone binding globulin (SHBG) due to its suppression by the lack of estrogen production,[183] and by the increased insulin resistance that may develop with increase in body weight, and possibly also with aging.[184] This loss in circulating SHBG, which preferentially binds androgens, leads to greater bioactivity of circulating androgens.

This phenomenon is demonstrated in several case-control studies of circulating androgens in women with clinical or subclinical signs of atherosclerosis, in which there is no difference in total testosterone between groups, but a significant depression in either circulating SHBG levels,[185] or increase in free testosterone levels in the affected group of women.[186] Again the mechanism behind this hyperandrogenemia, would not be endogenous overproduction of androgens, but decreased serum-binding capacity and therefore increased bioactivity. In summary, the evidence for an association between hyperandrogenism per se and cardiovascular disease in women is relatively weak.

Chronic anovulation and cardiovascular events

The etiology of anovulation represents a spectrum ranging from hypogonadotropic hypogonadism characterized by hypoestrogenism, to normogonadotropic hypergonadism with hyperandrogenism and chronic unopposed estrogens, i.e. PCOS. Ultimately with age, all women eventually experience menopause, a state of hypergonadotropic hypogonadism. These heterogeneous causes of anovulation confound studies linking menstrual history (and PCOS) to risk of CVD. Many studies do show that PCOS is the most common cause of anovulation (oligomenorrhea and amenorrhea).

Despite the above caveats, some of the best epidemiological studies of menstrual irregularity as a marker for chronic anovulation have shown an increased risk for cardiovascular events. The Dutch breast cancer screening study found a greater incidence of anovulatory cycles during the reproductive years (based on a mid-luteal urine sample), in women later developing cardiovascular disease.[182] Utilizing a prospective cohort design from the Nurse's Health Study,[186] 82,439 female nurses provided information in 1982 on prior menstrual regularity (at ages 20–35 years) and were followed through to 1996 for cardiovascular events. Incident reports of non-fatal myocardial infarction, fatal CHD, and non-fatal and fatal stroke were made and confirmed by review of medical records. Compared with women reporting a history of very regular menstrual cycles, women reporting usually irregular or very irregular cycles had an increased risk for non-fatal or fatal CHD (Table 8.4).[186] This increasing risk with increasing menstrual irregularity suggests a dose–response effect. Increased risks for CHD associated with prior cycle irregularity remained significant after adjustment for BMI and several other potential confounders, including family history of myocardial infarction and personal exercise history. There was a non-significant increase in overall stroke risk as well as in ischemic stroke risk associated with very irregular cycles. There was unfortunately no further characterization of the etiology of the oligomenorrhea, for instance, quantifying the amount of clinical or biochemical androgen excess among the study cohort, to make a diagnosis of the etiology of the anovulation.

Table 8.4 Relative risks (RRs with 95% confidence intervals (CI)) for coronary heart disease (CHD) as a function of menstrual cycle regularity at ages 20–35 years. Data from the Nurse's Health Study. Adapted from Solomon et al, 2002.[186]

	Menstrual cycle regularity ages 20–35 years				
	Regular	Usually regular	Usually irregular	Very irregular	p trend
Total CHD					
No. of cases	810	327	184	96	
Person-years	715,293	264,924	126,406	49,292	
Age-adjusted RR (95% CI)	1.0	1.02 (0.90–1.16)	1.25 (1.07–1.47)	1.67 (1.35–2.06)	<0.001
Multivariate[a] RR (95% CI)	1.0	1.02 (0.89–1.16)	1.22 (1.04–1.44)	1.53 (1.24–1.90)	<0.001
Non-fatal CHD					
No. of cases	562	210	132	60	
Age-adjusted RR (95% CI)	1.0	0.95 (0.81–1.11)	1.30 (1.07–1.60)	1.50 (1.15–1.96)	0.001
Multivariate[a] RR (95% CI)	1.0	0.96 (0.82–1.12)	1.27 (1.05–1.54)	1.38 (1.06–1.80)	0.005
Fatal CHD					
No. of cases	248	117	52	36	
Age-adjusted RR (95% CI)	1.0	1.17 (0.94–1.46)	1.16 (0.86–1.56)	2.04 (1.44–2.89)	0.001
Mutivariate[a] RR (95% CI)	1.0	1.12 (0.90–1.40)	1.11 (0.82–1.50)	1.88 (1.32–2.67)	0.005

[a]Adjusting for age, BMI, cigarette smoking, menopausal status/post-menopausal hormone use, parental history of myocardial infarction before age 60 years, parity, alcohol intake, aspirin use, multivitamin use, vitamin E supplement use, physical activity level, and history of oral contraceptive use.

Polycystic ovaries and cardiovascular events

Despite the periodic discordance between PCO and PCOS, many of the largest and best-designed studies of long-term health risks in women with PCOS, have been performed using ovarian morphology. In older women presently under study, ovarian morphology during their reproductive years may be retrieved from hospital records (i.e. pathology report, operative notes, etc., from a wedge resection/oophorectomy), and at least is not subject to the recall bias of a menstrual history in establishing a prior phenotype. But this method may also include a treatment bias if either wedge resection resulted in long-term benefits or a certain subgroup of women with PCOS were selected for wedge resection (for example those considered fit enough for surgery, possibly because of a more normal body weight). Indeed many of these women have experienced long-term resolution of their symptoms (infertility, anovulation, hirsutism),[187] and some researchers have theorized that there may have also been long-term reduction in their cardiovascular risk.[133] However this benefit is not supported by short-term studies of the metabolic effects of partial

ovarian destruction, which have shown little effect on insulin sensitivity and dyslipidemia.[188]

In a retrospective cohort study from the UK, over 800 women diagnosed with PCO, primarily by histopathology at the time of an ovarian wedge resection, were followed up after an average interval of 30 years after the procedure.[189] Observed death rates were compared with expected death rates using standardized mortality ratios. There was no increased death from cardiovascular-related causes, although there was an increased number of deaths due to complications of diabetes in the PCO group. In a follow-up study by the same investigative group of 345 of these women with PCO and 1060 age-matched control women, there was no increased long-term CHD mortality in the PCO group, although there was evidence of increased stroke-related mortality even after adjustment for BMI (Table 8.5).[73] In a cohort of women with proven CAD (n = 143 and age <60 years), PCO were noted in 42% of the women, and additionally their presence was associated with more severe coronary artery stenosis (OR 1.7; 95% CI 1.1–2.3 of >50% stenosis with PCO compared to normal ovaries).[190] While these studies are large in comparison with the average study of women with PCOS, they are

Table 8.5 Odds ratio (OR) and 95% confidence intervals (95% CI) for CHD, stroke/transient ischemic attack (TIA), diabetes, hypertension, and high cholesterol for PCO before and after adjusting for BMI from a retrospective cohort study of 319 women with PCO and 1060 age-matched controls from the UK. (Wild[73]).

Outcome	Model	OR	95% CI	p
CHD	PCOS	1.5	0.7–2.9	0.3
	PCOS, BMI	1.2	0.5–2.6	0.7
Cerebrovascular disease	PCOS	2.8	1.1–7.1	0.03
	PCOS, BMI	3.4	1.2–9.6	0.02
CHD and/or cerebrovascular disease	PCOS	1.9	1.1–3.3	0.03
	PCOS, BMI	1.7	0.9–3.2	0.09
Diabetes	PCOS	2.8	1.5–5.5	0.002
	PCOS, BMI	2.2	0.9–5.2	0.08
Hypertension	PCOS	1.4	1.0–2.0	0.04
	PCOS, BMI	1.4	0.9–2.0	0.1
High cholesterol	PCOS	2.9	1.6–5.2	<0.001
	PCOS, BMI	3.2	1.7–6.0	<0.001

small from the end-point of mortality, and their conclusions require support from additional studies.

Polycystic ovaries and cardiovascular risk factors

Polycystic ovaries per se in asymptomatic reproductive-age women have been associated with subtle alterations in endocrine function,[106] but there are scant data that this sign alone, without other stigmata of the syndrome, elevates cardiovascular risk. Some groups have found a high prevalence (approaching 40%) of PCO in postmenopausal women, and this was associated with mild changes in cardiovascular risks with elevations in circulating triglycerides, but no difference in cholesterol levels compared to controls.[191] The above-mentioned follow-up study of the UK cohort found a marked increase in the prevalence of cardiovascular risk factors in the PCO group, including hypertension, diabetes, hypercholesterolemia, hypertriglyceridemia, and an elevated waist-to-hip ratio.[73] A similar design

was used in a smaller Scandinavian cohort to identify an increased risk of diabetes and hypertension in the group with histopathologic evidence of PCO ($n = 32$), although the sample was too small to find a difference in events.[192]

A model was constructed based on risk factors in the Scandinavian case-control study to calculate the risk for myocardial infarction, and women with PCO were noted to have a seven-fold increased risk.[18] Not all studies of cardiovascular physiology support an adverse risk profile; one study reported beneficial internal carotid artery flow parameters consistent with reduced vascular tone in women with PCOS.[192] However articles of the latter sort are infrequent.

There are also data that polycystic ovary morphology recedes and disappears with age. Cohort studies of women with PCOS have shown significant decreases in the prevalence of PCO on ultrasound among women in their 30s and 40s compared with younger women with PCOS.[135,193] There are unfortunately no prospective cohort studies to adequately address the effect of age on PCO.

Family history of cardiovascular disease

Initial small studies of PCOS families reported clusters of cardiovascular disease in relatives.[194,195] More recent reports have reported clustering of cardiovascular risk factors such as hyperinsulinemia and dyslipidemia in family members.[100,102,196] Recently a survey of first-degree relatives reported a significantly increased prevalence of such cardiovascular risk factors as hyperglycemia and glucose intolerance.[197]

Implications for the diagnosis and evaluation of women with polycystic ovary syndrome

Insulin resistance is associated with reproductive abnormalities in women with PCOS including hyperandrogenemia, anovulation, and polycystic ovaries, as well as long-term risk for developing diabetes and probably also for cardiovascular

Table 8.6 Summary of diagnostic recommendations

- No test of insulin resistance is necessary to make the diagnosis of PCOS, nor is it needed to select treatments.
- Obese women with PCOS should be screened for the metabolic syndrome, including circulating lipids, and glucose intolerance with an oral glucose tolerance test.
- Further studies are necessary in non-obese women with PCOS to determine the utility of these tests, although they may be considered if additional risk factors for insulin resistance, such as a family history of diabetes, are present.

Table 8.7 Criteria for the metabolic syndrome in women with PCOS. Three of five symptoms qualify for the syndrome

Risk factor	Cut-off
1. Abdominal obesity in women	>88 cm (>35 in)
2. Triglycerides	≥150 mg/dl
3. HDL-C in women	<50 mg/dl
4. Blood pressure	≥130/≥85 mmHg
5. Fasting and 2-h glucose from oral glucose tolerance test	110–126 mg/dl and/or 2-h glucose 140–199 mg/dl

(For Glucose Tolerance Test see Table 2.4.)

disease. Insulin resistance, defined as decreased insulin-mediated glucose utilization, is commonly found in the larger population (10–25%), when sophisticated dynamic studies of insulin action are performed.[198] However the criteria for selecting abnormal cut-off points vary. Insulin resistance in women with PCOS appears even more common (50%), both absolutely (primarily in obese women), and relatively (in lean women).[88] Currently there are scant data that markers of insulin resistance predict response to treatment.[94,95] Therefore the role of these markers in selecting and following the response to specific treatments is uncertain.

The failure of tests to universally document insulin resistance in women with PCOS may be related to the insensitivity of the tests, or to the heterogeneity of PCOS with a wide variation in insulin sensitivity. There is currently no validated clinical test for detecting insulin resistance in the population. Dynamic invasive study procedures such as a euglycemic clamp or frequently sampled glucose tolerance test, due to their intensive utilization of time and resources, are primarily of research interest. While a number of tests exist that utilize fasting levels of insulin and glucose to create models that have varying degrees of correlation with more dynamic tests, there are multiple flaws that limit their widespread clinical use. These include changes in beta-cell function with the development of diabetes, which alter the sensitivity of the tests, normal physiological fluctuation in insulin levels, and the lack of a standardized universal insulin assay. There is no role for any test or clinical marker of insulin resistance in the diagnosis of PCOS.

The diagnostic recommendations are summarized in Table 8.6.

Other consensus conferences have recommended against screening for insulin resistance in both the general population and at-risk populations, because of these concerns and also because of concerns about the predictive value of these tests for developing clinical events, and the lack of clear treatments for abnormal results.[32] These groups have instead defined a metabolic syndrome, that includes components associated with the insulin resistance syndrome, including centripetal obesity, hypertension, fasting hyperglycemia and dyslipidemia (Table 8.7).[168]

Other groups have recommended adding a glucose tolerance test to these fasting blood tests and also examining the 2-h glucose level after a 75 g oral glucose load for glucose intolerance (OGTT) (see Table).[200,201] This is especially prudent in women with PCOS as they are likely to have normal fasting glucose levels (Figure 8.10).[27] IGT has long been recognized as a strong risk factor for diabetes, and recent studies have shown that progression to diabetes in this group is delayed by both lifestyle and pharmacological intervention.[202–204] Additionally IGT identifies a group at risk for excess mortality, especially in women.[205,206] Given the high prevalence of IGT and type 2 diabetes as diagnosed by the OGTT among obese women with PCOS, it is prudent to screen obese women (BMI >30 kg/m²) with PCOS with an OGTT.[27,28] Further studies of the prevalence of stigmata of the metabolic syndrome are

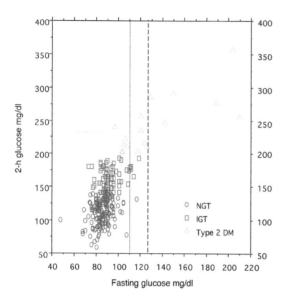

Figure 8.10

Scattergram of fasting blood glucose levels versus 2-h glucose-stimulated levels in 254 PCOS women. Points on the graph are coded to reflect the WHO status based on OGTT. The dotted vertical line is the threshold for impaired fasting glucose (IGT 110 mg/dl) by the 1997 ADA criteria and the dashed vertical line (126 mg/dl) is the threshold for type 2 diabetes (Type 2 DM) by the same criteria. NGT: normal glucose tolerance; IGT, impaired glucose tolerance. Most PCOS women, regardless of WHO OGTT status have normal fasting glucose levels. Adapted from Legro et al, 1999.[28]

necessary in lean women with PCOS, as well as in other racial populations to identify further high-risk groups for the stigmata of insulin resistance.

Implications for treatment

The treatment of PCOS appears to be evolving from a primarily symptom-oriented treatment approach, that often focused alternatively on either suppression of the ovaries (for hirsutism and menstrual disorders), or stimulation of the ovaries (for infertility), to one that improves insulin sensitivity.[207] Multiple studies have shown that improving insulin sensitivity, be it from lifestyle modifications or from pharmacological

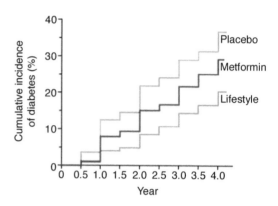

Figure 8.11

Cumulative incidence of diabetes according to Study Group in the Diabetes Prevention Program. The diagnosis of diabetes was based on the criteria of the American Diabetes Association (type 2 diabetes with fasting plasma glucose ≥126 mg/dl). The incidence of diabetes differed significantly among the three groups ($p < 0.001$ for each comparison).

intervention can result in lowered circulating androgens (primarily mediated through increased SHBG and less bioavailable androgen, but also through decreased total testosterone), spontaneous ovulation, and spontaneous pregnancy.

The Diabetes Prevention Program is a model for the potential prevention or at least delay in the development of frank diabetes in women with PCOS. This study enrolled men and women at risk for diabetes (based on the presence of IGT) and showed that lifestyle interventions had a more profound effect at preventing diabetes than did the use of metformin (approximately a two-fold greater benefit), and both were superior to the placebo arm (Figure 8.11).[204] However long-term studies documenting decreases in sequelae such as cardiovascular disease with improvements in insulin sensitivity are lacking in the PCOS population.

Diet/weight loss

The gold standard for improving insulin sensitivity in obese PCOS women should be weight loss, diet, and exercise. Obesity has become epidemic in our society and contributes substantially to reproductive and metabolic abnormalities in PCOS. Unfortunately there are no effective medical treatments that result in permanent weight loss and it is estimated that 90–95% of patients who experience a weight decrease will relapse.[207] Bariatric surgery may be an effective surgical option for the morbidly obese woman with PCOS, but there has been little study of this intervention in this population.

Multiple studies in PCOS women have shown that weight loss can improve the fundamental aspects of the endocrine syndrome of PCOS – it can lower circulating androgen levels and cause spontaneous resumption of menses.[208–211] These changes have been reported with a weight loss as small as 5% of the initial weight.[212,213] Other benefits that have been reported include decreased circulating insulin levels.[213,214] The decrease in unbound testosterone levels after weight loss may be largely mediated through increases in SHBG.[212,213]

The type of diet that best improves insulin sensitivity and results in weight loss has received much attention in the popular press, and the consensus opinion is that high-protein, low-carbohydrate diets are the best. Although we know that weight loss is of benefit in treating PCOS, the ideal diet composition for this management is unclear. Isocaloric diets have been shown to have vastly different effects, depending on the composition of the diet.[13] High-carbohydrate diets have resulted in the highest insulin secretion rates in women.[13] Diets higher in protein and fat result in proportionately lower secretion rates, well below those of a standard diet.[215] There have also been several studies to suggest that in mild type 2 diabetes, without vascular compromise, a high-protein diet (50%) can result in significant improvement in glucose and insulin responses to an OGTT.[216] Similar results have been noted in obese, hyperinsulinemic individuals.[217] There is also widespread popular support found in diet books, websites, and participant testimonials to the benefit of a high-protein diet in the treatment of PCOS. However, the effects of diets of varying composition on weight loss, as well as on reproductive and metabolic abnormalities, have been infrequently studied as primary treatment in women with PCOS.[218]

One concern about high-protein diets in a population prone to insulin resistance is the potentially high protein stress on kidney function,[219] as well as the adverse effects of the increased fat content often found in diets on the high prevalence of dyslipidemia typically seen in this population.[28] Finally we do not know the long-term effects of these diets, especially if they can achieve maintenance of the initial weight loss. A recent well-designed randomized study has shown that while hypocaloric high-protein diets can result in greater initial weight loss (up to 6 months), there is no benefit over longer periods (12 months).[220] Randomized trials of varying hypocaloric diets have shown significant improvements in the PCOS phenotype with weight loss, but no significant differences between the composition of the diet. These studies have been plagued by high dropout rates. They suggest however that hypocaloric diets per se have a significant benefit in treating PCOS.

Exercise is a promising treatment, but there have, unfortunately been few studies of the effect of exercise alone on insulin action in PCOS women.[209] It is reasonable to assume that exercise would have the same beneficial effects in PCOS women as in women with type 2 diabetes.[225] The goal of the lifestyle intervention in the Diabetes Prevention Program was not only to lose and maintain 7% of weight but also to exercise for 150 minutes a week.[203]

Pharmacological treatment to improve insulin sensitivity

Drugs developed initially to treat type 2 diabetes have also been utilized to treat PCOS (Figure 8.12).[222] None of these agents is currently Food and Drug Administration (FDA) approved for the treatment of PCOS or for related symptoms such as anovulation, hirsutism, or acne. These include metformin,[223–225] thiazolidinediones, and an experimental insulin sensitizer drug D-*chiro*-inositol.[226]

Metformin

Metformin is one of the most commonly used drugs to treat PCOS and most studies using pharmacological insulin sensitizers in women with PCOS have used it. Metformin has consistently showed an insulin-lowering effect and that

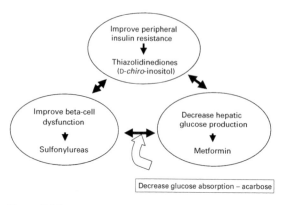

Figure 8.12

The pharmacological treatment of type 2 diabetes has been borrowed to treat women with PCOS. The major targets are to improve peripheral insulin sensitivity (primarily in the skeletal muscle), suppress hepatic gluconeogenesis, and to improve beta-cell insulin secretory function. This latter strategy is rarely utilized in normoglycemic women with PCOS due to the increased risk of hypoglycemia.

may be its prime mechanism of action. Metformin was approved for the treatment of type 2 diabetes by the FDA in 1994, but was used clinically for close to 20 years before that in other parts of the world.[227] Metformin is a biguanide that works primarily by suppressing hepatic gluconeogenesis, but it also improves insulin sensitivity in the periphery. Gastrointestinal symptoms (diarrhea, nausea, vomiting, abdominal bloating, flatulence, and anorexia) are the most common reactions to metformin and approximately 30% more frequent in women treated with metformin compared with placebo-treated patients. There is a small risk of lactic acidosis among women taking this medication, which may be triggered by exposure to intravenous iodinated radiocontrast agents in susceptible individuals. This most commonly occurs in patients with poorly controlled diabetes and impaired renal function.

Metformin is pregnancy category B with no known human teratogenic risk and no known embryonic lethality in humans. There have been no reported abnormalities associated with its use during pregnancy in women with diabetes,[227-229] or in women with marked hyperandrogenism during pregnancy,[230] or in the small number of PCOS women who have conceived during treatment.[231-233] Some clinicians advocate its use during early pregnancy to reduce the miscarriage rate, but the documentation for this claim is poor, consisting primarily of case series (see Chapter 14).[234,235]

Comparison: metformin versus placebo or no treatment (biochemical outcomes)
Outcome: fasting insulin (mIU/l)

Study	Treatment n	Mean (SD)	Control n	Mean (SD)	Weighted mean difference (95% CI fixed)	Weight %	Weighted mean difference (95% CI fixed)
Fleming 2002	25	16.80 (9.70)	37	18.40 (12.30)		24.8	−1.60 (−7.09 to 3.89)
Jakubowicz 2001	26	13.17 (11.90)	22	46.01 (30.49)		4.1	−32.84 (−46.38 to −19.30)
Kocak 2002	27	21.30 (29.70)	28	22.30 (29.10)		3.1	−1.00 (−16.55 to 14.55)
Moghetti 2000	11	10.20 (7.30)	12	21.30 (13.51)		9.7	−11.10 (−19.88 to −2.32)
Nestler 1996	11	9.00 (6.63)	13	31.00 (18.02)		6.7	−22.00 (−32.55 to −11.45)
Ng 2001	8	7.10 (1.90)	7	9.30 (5.70)		38.3	−2.20 (−6.62 to 2.22)
Pasquali 2000	10	21.60 (31.20)	8	19.00 (14.40)		1.6	2.60 (−19.6 to 24.36)
Vandermolen 2001	11	10.40 (6.97)	14	14.40 (15.71)		8.8	−4.00 (−13.20 to 5.20)
Yarali 2002	16	16.40 (32.71)	16	12.20 (7.00)		2.8	4.20 (12.19 to 20.59)
Total (95% CI)	145		157			100.0	−5.37 (−8.11 to −2.63)

Test for heterogeneity: $\chi^2 = 33.00$, df = 8 $p = 0.0001$
Test for overall effect: $z = 3.84$ $p = 0.0001$

−100   −50   0   50   100
Favors controls   Favors treatment

Figure 8.13

Effect of metformin on fasting insulin levels from a meta-analyis of the effects of metformin in women with PCOS. df = degrees of freedom. Adapted from Lord et al, 2003.[236]

Studies of longer duration treatment with metformin in PCOS, suggest long-term improvement in ovulatory function in about half of the patients,[94] but there has not been any long-term study of diabetes and cardiovascular risk factors. A recent meta-analysis of the effects of metformin in PCOS showed a significant lowering of insulin levels (Figure 8.13),[236] implying a beneficial effect on these long-term sequelae through this mechanism. There was also a slight but significant lowering of LDL-C levels, with no effect on HDL-C and total triglyceride (TTG) levels. These results are somewhat puzzling as LDL-C is usually not associated with either insulin resistance or therapy with insulin sensitizers. Several studies with metformin have shown decreases in markers associated with both insulin resistance and cardiovascular disease such as PAI-1 and CRP levels.[237,238]

Thiazolidinediones

Thiazolidinediones are PPAR-γ (peroxisome proliferator activating receptor) agonists and are thought to improve insulin sensitivity through a post-receptor mechanism and include troglitazone, rosiglitazone, and pioglitazone. Troglitazone has subsequently been removed from the worldwide market due to hepatotoxicity. In a large multicenter trial, troglitazone has been shown to have a dose–response effect in improving ovulation and hirsutism.[95] This appeared to be mediated through decreases in hyperinsulinemia and decreases in free testosterone levels. There was however no effect on circulating lipid levels during this trial, implying that thiazolidinediones may not normalize dyslipidemia in women with PCOS (Figure 8.14),[239] and there was also a trend towards a dose-related weight increase.

Newer thiazolidinediones such as rosiglitazone and pioglitazone appear to be safer in terms of hepatotoxicity, but have also been associated with embryotoxicity in animal studies (both are pregnancy category C) and little has appeared on their effects in PCOS women. Liver function should be monitored on a regular basis when using these medications. Combination treatment with other medications, primarily metformin, has been shown to further improve insulin sensitivity and glycemic control in type 2 diabetes, but the effect on women with PCOS is not clearly delin-

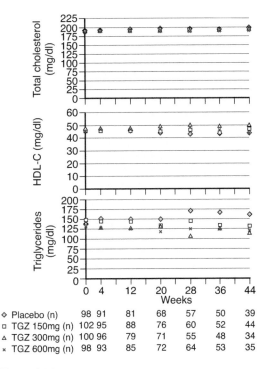

	0	4	12	20	28	36	44
◇ Placebo (n)	98	91	81	68	57	50	39
□ TGZ 150mg (n)	102	95	88	76	60	52	44
△ TGZ 300mg (n)	100	96	79	71	55	48	34
× TGZ 600mg (n)	98	93	85	72	64	53	35

Figure 8.14

Data from the troglitazone in PCOS study, a randomized, multicenter, dose ranging study of the effects of troglitazone (TGZ) in women with PCOS. Mean levels of circulating lipids, total cholesterol, HDL-C, and TTG according to treatment arm, and the number of women present in the study (see table) at varying time points in the study. Adapted from Legro et al, 2003.[239]

eated. Preliminary studies show a beneficial effect on ovulation and reproductive abnormalities,[244–246] but little has been published on metabolic effects in women with PCOS.

D-*chiro*-inositol

A deficiency of the D-*chiro*-inositol phosphoglycan mediator of the action of insulin may result in resistance to insulin. Some of the actions of insulin may involve low-molecular weight inositol phosphoglycan mediators. Although different species have been identified, an inositol phosphoglycan molecule containing D-*chiro*-inositol and galactosamine is known to have a role in activating key enzymes that control insulin action. This led to an initial trial in women with PCOS, that showed beneficial effects on insulin sensitivity

---

Key points

- Long-term metabolic abnormalities, above and beyond obesity, are related to reduced sensitivity to insulin and compensatory hyperinsulinemia in women with PCOS.
- Ethnicity may contribute independently to a worsening risk for glucose intolerance, with South Asian women in the UK, for example, being more at risk than their white Caucasian counterparts.
- The features of the insulin resistance syndrome ('metabolic syndrome' or 'syndrome X') are common in overweight women with PCOS.
- Intermenstrual interval correlates with degree of insulin resistance, the risk for type 2 diabetes and a reduced likelihood of response to insulin-sensitizing therapy.
- Women who present with gestational diabetes have a higher prevalence of polycystic ovaries detected postpartum. Hyperinsulinemia may be an independent risk factor for developing gestational diabetes in women with PCOS, but some studies have not demonstrated an additional risk of gestational diabetes.
- Subclinical and clinical atherosclerotic disease has been described in women with PCOS at a greater rate than in women with normal ovaries, although this is not apparent until the perimenopause.

---

and improved ovulation rates.[226] Administration of D-*chiro*-inositol (1200 mg/day) to 22 obese PCOS patients for 6–8 weeks was reported to significantly reduce the insulin curve during an OGTT from 13,417 ± 11,572 to 5158 ± 6714 U/ml/min. Diastolic and systolic blood pressure dropped by 4 mmHg and plasma triglycerides decreased from 184 ± 19 to 110 ± 13 mg/dl. The women showed a significant reduction in plasma testosterone and 19 of 22 ovulated during therapy. No side-effects have yet been reported. However subsequent phase II studies were negative and led the sponsoring company to stop clinical development of the product. It is unlikely therefore that this drug will ever receive widespread use in women with PCOS.

Acarbose

Acarbose is a synthetic disaccharide that inhibits glucosidase activity of intestinal villi. It therefore slows digestion of complex carbohydrates and the more readily absorbed mono- and disaccharides. Inhibition of this enzyme causes a reduction in glucose absorption and therefore a decrease in post-prandial hyperglycemia. There are little data in the literature on the effects of acarbose in PCOS. In hyperinsulinemic hyperandrogenic premenopausal women treated with acarbose, a significant reduction in post-prandial hyperglycemia, hyperinsulinemia, and androgen levels

was observed.[243] Acarbose therapy (300 mg/day for 3 months) also had beneficial effects on acne, circulating androgen and insulin levels in hyperinsulinemic PCOS patients.[244]

Summary

Insulin resistance is key to the pathophysiology of many aspects of PCOS. Obesity and a number of markers for cardiovascular disease (e.g. disturbed lipid profile, raised blood pressure) are common in women with PCOS. The risk of developing cardiovascular disease and diabetes is related to insulin resistance and obesity, although it is more difficult to prove a causal link between PCOS per se and disease events.

References

1. Burghen GA, Givens JR, Kitabchi AE. Correlation of hyperandrogenism with hyperinsulinism in polycystic ovarian disease. J Clin Endocrinol Med 1980; 50:113–116.

2. Dunaif A, Graf M, Mandeli J, Laumas V, Dobrjansky A. Characterization of groups of hyperandrogenic women with acanthosis nigricans, impaired glucose tolerance, and/or hyperinsulinemia. J Clin Endocrinol Metab 1987; 65:499–507.

3. Reaven GM. Banting lecture. Role of insulin resis-

tance in human disease. Diabetes 1988; 37:1595–1607.

4. Solomon CG, Hu FB, Dunaif A, Rich-Edwards J et al. Long or highly irregular menstrual cycles as a marker for risk of type 2 diabetes mellitus. JAMA 2001; 286:2421–2426.

5. Stern MP. Diabetes and cardiovascular disease. The 'common soil' hypothesis. Diabetes 1995; 44:369–374.

6. Moller DE, Flier JS. Insulin resistance- mechanisms, syndromes, and implications. N Engl J Med 1991; 325:938–949.

7. Pyorola K. Relationship of glucose tolerance and plasma insulin to the incidence of coronary heart disease: Results from two population studies in Finland. Diabetes Care 1979; 2:131–141.

8. Ducimetiere P, Eschwege E, Papoz L, Richard JL et al. Relationship of plasma insulin levels to the incidence of myocardial and coronary heart disease mortality in a middle aged population. Diabetologica 1980; 19:205–210.

9. Zavaroni I, Bonora E, Pagliara M et al. Risk factors for coronary artery disease in healthy persons with hyperinsulinaemia and normal glucose tolerance. N Engl J Med 1989; 320:702–706.

10. Lapidus L. Ischaemic heart disease, stroke and total mortality in women; results from a prospective population study in Gothenberg, Sweden. Acta Med Scand supp 1986; 705:1–42.

11. Bengtsson C, Bjorkelund C, Lapidus L, Lissner L. Association of serum lipid concentration and obesity with mortality in women. 20 year follow up of participants in prospective population study in Gothenberg, Sweden. Br Med J 1993; 307:1385–1388.

12. Posner BM, Cupples LA, Franz MM, Gagnon DR. Diet and heart disease risk factors in adult American men and women: the Framingham Offspring-Spouse nutrition studies. Int J Epidemiol 1993; 22:1014–1025.

13. Blass KM, Newschaffer CJ, Klag MJ, Bush TL. Plasma lipoprotein levels as predictor of cardiovascular death in women. Arch Intern Med 1993; 153:2209–2216.

14. Reaven GM. Role of insulin resistance in human disease. Diabetes 1988; 37:1595–1607.

15. Laws A, Reaven GM. Insulin resistance and risk factors for coronary heart disease. Baillieres Clin Endocrinol Metab 1993; 7:1063–1078.

16. Dunaif A, Segal KR, Futterweit W, Dobrjansky A. Profound peripheral insulin resistance independent of obesity in polycystic ovary syndrome. Diabetes 1989; 38:1165–1174.

17. Wild RA, Aplebaum-Bowden D, Demers LM. Lipoprotein lipids in women with androgen excess: independent associations with increased insulin and androgen. Clin Chem 1990; 36:283–289.

18. Dahlgren E, Janson PO, Johansson S, Lapidus L, Oden A. Polycystic ovary syndrome and risk for myocardial infarction. Evaluated from a risk factor model based on a prospective population study of women. Acta Obstet Gynecol Scand 1992; 71:599–604.

19. Prelevic GM, Beljic T, Balint-Peric L, Ginsburg J. Cardiac flow velocity in women with the polycystic ovary syndrome. Clin Endocrinol (Oxf) 1995; 43:677–681.

20. Birdsall MA, Farquhar CM, White HD. Association between polycystic ovaries and extent of coronary artery disease in women having cardiac catheterisation. Ann Intern Med 1997; 126:32–35.

21. Legro RS, Blanche P, Krauss RM, Lobo RA. Alterations in low-density lipoprotein and high-density lipoprotein subclasses among Hispanic women with polycystic ovary syndrome: influence of insulin and genetic factors. Fertil Steril 1999; 72:990–995.

22. Wild RA. Long-term health consequences of PCOS. Hum Reprod Update 2002; 8:231–241.

23. Temple R. Are surrogate markers adequate to assess cardiovascular disease drugs? JAMA 1999; 282:790–795.

24. Korhonen S, Hippelainen M, Niskanen L, Vanhala M, Saarikoski S. Relationship of the metabolic syndrome and obesity to polycystic ovary syndrome: a controlled, population-based study. Am J Obstet Gynecol 2001; 184:289–296.

25. Balen AH, Conway GS, Kaltsas G, Techatrasak K et al. Polycystic ovary syndrome: the spectrum of the disorder in 1741 patients. Hum Reprod 1995; 10:2107–2111.

26. Knochenhauer ES, Key TJ, Kahsar-Miller M, Waggoner W et al. Prevalence of the polycystic ovary syndrome in unselected black and white women of the Southeastern United States: a prospective study. J Clin Endocrinol Metab 1998; 83:3078–3082.

27. Ehrmann DA, Barnes RB, Rosenfield RL, Cavaghan MK, Imperial J. Prevalence of impaired glucose tolerance and diabetes in women with polycystic ovary syndrome. Diabetes Care 1999; 22:141–146.

28. Legro RS, Kunselman AR, Dodson WC, Dunaif A. Prevalence and predictors of risk for type 2 diabetes mellitus and impaired glucose tolerance in polycystic ovary syndrome: a prospective, controlled study in 254 affected women. J Clin Endocrinol Metab 1999; 84:165–169.

29. Legro RS, Finegood D, Dunaif A. A fasting glucose to insulin ratio is a useful measure of insulin sensitivity in women with polycystic ovary syndrome. J Clin Endocrinol Metab 1998; 83:2694–2698.

30. Dunaif A, Finegood DT. Beta-cell dysfunction independent of obesity and glucose intolerance in the polycystic ovary syndrome. J Clin Endocrinol Metab 1996; 81:942–947.

31. Gennarelli G, Holte J, Berglund L, Berne C et al. Prediction models for insulin resistance in the polycystic ovary syndrome. Hum Reprod 2000; 15:2098–2102.

32. American Diabetic Association. Consensus Development Conference on Insulin Resistance: 5–6 November 1997. Diabetes Care 1998; 21:310–314.

33. Carmina E, Koyama T, Chang L, Stanczyk FZ, Lobo RA. Does ethnicity influence the prevalence of adrenal hyperandrogenism and insulin resistance in polycystic ovary syndrome? Am J Obstet Gynecol 1992; 167:1807–1812.

34. Dunaif A, Sorbara L, Delson R, Green G. Ethnicity and polycystic ovary syndrome are associated with independent and additive decreases in insulin action in Caribbean–Hispanic women. Diabetes 1993; 42:1462–1468.

35. Osei K, Schuster DP. Ethnic differences in secretion, sensitivity, and hepatic extraction of insulin in black and white Americans. Diabet Med 1994; 11:755–762.

36. Norman RJ, Mahabeer S, Masters S. Ethnic differences in insulin and glucose response to glucose between white and Indian women with polycystic ovary syndrome. Fertil Steril 1995; 63:58–62.

37. Palaniappan LP, Carnethon MR, Fortmann SP. Heterogeneity in the relationship between ethnicity, bmi, and fasting insulin. Diabetes Care 2002; 25:1351–1357.

38. Rodin DA, Bano G, Bland JM, Taylor K, Nussey SS. Polycystic ovaries and associated metabolic abnormalities in Indian subcontinent asian women. Clin Endocrinol 1998; 49:91–99.

39. Wijeyaratne CN, Balen AH, Barth JH, Belchetz PE. Clinical manifestations and insulin resistance (IR) in polycystic ovary syndrome (PCOS) among South Asians and Caucasians: is there a difference? Clin Endocrinol (Oxf) 2002; 57:343–350.

40. Hankey GJ, Eikelboom JW. Homocysteine and vascular disease. Lancet 1999; 354:407–413.

41. Medina MA, Amores-Sánchez MI. Homocysteine: an emergent cardiovascular risk factor? Eur J Clin Invest 2000; 30:754–762.

42. Medina MA, Urdiales JL, Amores-Sánchez MI. Roles of homocysteine in cell metabolism – old and new functions. Eur J Biochem 2001; 268: 3871–3882.

43. Harker LA, Slichter SJ, Scott CR, Ross R. Homocysteinaemia: vascular injury and arterial thrombosis. N Engl J Med 1974; 291:537–543.

44. Chambers JC, Kooner JS. Homocysteine: a novel risk factor for coronary heart disease in UK Indian Asians. Heart 2001; 86:121–122.

45. McKeigue PM, Ferrie JE, Pierpoint T et al. Association of early onset coronary heart disease in South Asian men with glucose intolerance and hyperinsulinaemia. Circulation 1993; 87:152–161.

46. Bhopal R, Unwin N, White M et al. Heterogeneity of coronary heart disease risk factors in Indian, Pakistani, Bangladeshi and European origin populations: cross sectional study. Br Med J 1999; 319:215–220.

47. Talbott E, Guzick D, Clerici A, Berga S et al. Coronary heart disease risk factors in women with polycystic ovary syndrome. Arterioscler Thromb Vasc Biol 1995; 15:821–826.

48. Yarali H, Yldirir A, Aybar F, Kabacki G et al. Diastolic dysfunction and increased serum homocysteine concentrations may contribute to increased cardiovascular risk in patients with polycystic ovary syndrome. Fertil Steril 2001; 76:511–515.

49. Loverro G, Lorusso F, Mei L, Depalo R et al. The plasma homocysteine levels are increased in polycystic ovary syndrome. Gynecol Obstet Invest 2002; 53:157–162.

50. Randeva HS, Lewandowski KC, Drzewoski J, Brooke-Wavell K et al. Exercise decreases plasma total homocysteine in overweight young women with polycystic ovary syndrome. J Clin Endocrinol Metab 2002; 87:4496–4501.

51. Wijeyaratne CN, Pathmakumara A, Warnakulasuriya AM, Gunawardhare AUA et al. Plasma homocysteine in polycystic ovary syndrome: does it correlate with insulin resistance and ethnicity? Clin Endocrinol (Oxf) 2004; 60:560–567.

52. De Pergola G, Pannacciulli N, Zamboni M, Minnena A et al. Homocysteine plasma levels are independently associated with insulin resistance in normal weight, overweight and obese pre-menopausal women. Diabetes Nutr Metab 2001; 14:253–258.

53. Sanchez-Margalet V, Valle M, Ruz FJ, Gascon F, Mateo J, Goberna R. Elevated plasma total homocysteine levels in hyperinsulinaemic obese subjects. J Nutr Biochem 2002; 13:75–79.

54. Kahleova R, Palyzova D, Zvara K, Zvarova J et al. Essential hypertension in adolescents: association with insulin resistance and with metabolism of homocysteine and vitamins. Am J Hypertens 2002; 15:857–864.

55. The Framingham Offspring Study. Diabetes Care 2001; 24:1403–1410

56. Meigs JB, Jacques PF, Selhub J, Singer DE et al. Fasting plasma homocyteine levels in the insulin resistance syndrome. Diabetes Care 2001; 24:1403–1410.

57. Deurenberg P, Deurenberg-Yap M, Guricci S. Asians are different from Caucasians and from each other in their body mass index/body fat per cent relationship. Obes Rev 2002; 3:141–146.

58. Annual Health Bulletin, DHS, Ministry of Health, Sri Lanka, 2001.

59. Central Bank of Sri Lanka, Annual Report 2001.

60. Deepa R, Velmurugan K, Saravanan G, Karkuzhali

K, Dwarakanath V. Absence of association between serum homocysteine levels and coronary artery disease in south Indian males. Indian Heart J 2001; 53:44–47.

61. Refsum H, Yajnik CS, Gadkari M, Schneede J et al. Hyperhomocysteinemia and elevated methylmalonic acid indicate a high prevalence of cobalamin deficiency in Asian Indians. Am J Clin Nutr 2001; 74:233–241.

62. Mendis S, Athauda SB, Takashi K. Association between hyperhomocysteinaemia and ischaemic heart disease in Sri Lankans. Int J Cardiol 1997; 62:221–225.

63. Mendis S, Athauda SB, Naser M, Takashi K. Association between hyperhomocysteinaemia and hypertension in Sri Lankans. J Int Med Res 1999; 27:38–44.

64. Mendis S, Ranatunga P, Jayatilleke M, Wanninayake S, Wickremasinghe R. Hyperhomocysteinaemia in Sri Lankan patients with coronary artery disease. Ceylon Med J 2002; 47:89–92.

65. Carmina E, Legro RS, Stamets K, Lowell J, Lobo RA. Difference in body weight between American and Italian women with polycystic ovary syndrome: influence of the diet. Hum Reprod 2003; 18:2289–2293.

66. Escobar-Morreale HF, Roldan B, Barrio R, Alonso M et al. High prevalence of the polycystic ovary syndrome and hirsutism in women with type 1 diabetes mellitus. J Clin Endocrinol Metab 2000; 85:4182–4187.

67. Harris MI, Hadden WC, Knowler WC, Bennett PH. Prevalence of diabetes and impaired glucose tolerance and plasma glucose levels in US, population aged 20–74 yr. Diabetes 1987; 36:523–534.

68. The Rotterdam ESHRE/ASRM-sponsored PCOS consensus workshop group: Fauser B, Tarlatzis B, Chang J, Azziz R et al. Revised 2003 consensus on diagnostic criteria and long-term health risks related to polycystic ovary syndrome (PCOS). Hum Reprod 2004; 19:41–47.

69. Falsetti L, Eleftheriou G. Hyperinsulinemia in the polycystic ovary syndrome- a clinical, endocrine, and echographic study in 240 patients. Gynecol Endocrinol 1996; 10:319–326.

70. Dahlgren E, Johansson S, Lindstedt G, Knutsson F et al. Women with polycystic ovary syndrome wedge resected in 1956 to 1965: a long-term follow-up focusing on natural history and circulating hormones. Fertil Steril 1992; 57:505–513.

71. Talbott E, Clerici A, Berga SL, Kuller L et al. Adverse lipid and coronary heart disease risk profiles in young women with polycystic ovary syndrome: results of a case-control study. J Clin Epidemiol 1998; 51:415–422.

72. Elting MW, Korsen TJ, Bezemer PD, Schoemaker J. Prevalence of diabetes mellitus, hypertension and cardiac complaints in a follow-up study of a dutch PCOS population. Hum Reprod 2001; 16:556–560.

73. Wild S, Pierpoint T, McKeigue P, Jacobs H. Cardiovascular disease in women with polycystic ovary syndrome at long-term follow-up: a retrospective cohort study. Clin Endocrinol (Oxf) 2000; 52:595–600.

74. Norman RJ, Masters L, Milner CR, Wang JX, Davies MJ. Relative risk of conversion from normoglycaemia to impaired glucose tolerance or non-insulin dependent diabetes mellitus in polycystic ovarian syndrome. Hum Reprod 2001; 16:1995–1998.

75. Chang RJ, Nakamura RM, Judd HI, Kaplan SA. Insulin resistance in nonobese patients with polycystic ovary syndrome. J ClinEndocrinol Metab 1983; 57:356–359.

76. Conway GS, Jacobs HS, Holly JM, Wass JA. Effects of luteinizing hormone, insulin, insulin like growth factor and insulin like growth factor small binding protein in polycystic ovary syndrome. Clin Endocrinol (Oxf) 1990; 33:593–603.

77. Jialal I, Naiker P, Reddi K, Moodley J, Joubert SM. Evidence for insulin resistance in nonobese patients with polycystic ovarian disease. J Clin Endocrinol Metab 1987; 64:1066–1069.

78. Ovesen P, Moller J, Ingerslev HJ et al. Normal basal and insulin stimulated fuel metabolism in lean women with polycystic ovary syndrome. J Clin Endocrinol Metab 1993; 77:1636–1640.

79. Holte J, Bergh T, Berne C, Berglund L, Lithell H. Enhanced early insulin response to glucose in relation to insulin resistance in women with polycystic ovary syndrome and normal glucose tolerance. J Clin Endocrinol Metab 1994; 78:1052–1058.

80. Rajkhowa M, Bicknell J, Jones M, Clayton RN. Insulin sensitivity in obese and nonobese women with polycystic ovary syndrome- relationship to hyperandrogenaemia. Fertil Steril 1994; 61:605–611.

81. Dale PO, Tomb T, Vaolir S, Abyholm T. Body weight, hyperinsulinaemia and gonadotrophin levels in the polycystic ovary syndrome: evidence of two distinct populations. Fertil Steril 1992; 58:487–491.

82. Antilla L, Ding YQ, Ruuitiaianen K, Erkkola R et al. Clinical features and circulating gonadotrophin, androgen, and insulin interactions in women with features of polycysatic ovary syndrome. Fertil Steril 1991; 55:1057–1061.

83. Robinson S, Kiddy D, Gelding SV, Willis D et al. The relation of insulin sensitivity to menstrual pattern in women with hyperandrogenism and polycystic ovaries. Clin Endocrinol (Oxf) 1993; 39:351–355.

84. Conway GS, Honour JW, Jacobs HS. Heterogeneity of the polycystic ovary syndrome – clinical, endocrine and ultrasound features in 556 patients. Clin Endocrinol (Oxf) 1989; 30:459–470.

85. Falcone T, Finegood DT, Fantus G, Morris D. Androgenous response to endogenous insulin secretion during frequently sampled intravenous glucose tolerance test in normal and hyperandrogenic women. J Clin Endocrinol Metab 1990; 71:1653–1657.

86. Toscano V, Bianchi P, Balducci R, Gugliemi R et al. Lack of linear relationship between hyperinsulinaemia and hyperandrogenaemia in polycystic ovary syndrome. Clin Endocrinol (Oxf) 1992; 36:197–202.

87. Weber RFA, Pache TD, Jacobs ML, Docter R et al. The relationship between clinical manifestations of polycystic ovary syndrome and beta cell function. Clin Endocrinol (Oxf) 1993; 38:295–300.

88. Dunaif A, Segal KR, Futterweit W, Dobrjansky A. Profound peripheral insulin resistance, independent of obesity, in polycystic ovary syndrome. Diabetes 1989; 38:1165–1174.

89. Dunaif A. Insulin resistance and the polycystic ovary syndrome: mechanism and implications for pathogenesis. Endocr Rev 1997; 18:774–800.

90. Martin BC, Warram JH, Krolewski AS, Bergman RN et al. Role of glucose and insulin resistance in development of type 2 diabetes mellitus: results of a 25-year follow-up study [see comments]. Lancet 1992; 340:925–929.

91. O'Meara NM, Blackman JD, Ehrmann DA, Barnes RB et al. Defects in beta-cell function in functional ovarian hyperandrogenism. J Clin Endocrinol Metab 1993; 76:1241–1247.

92. Pimenta W, Korytkowski M, Mitrakou A, Jenssen T et al. Pancreatic beta-cell dysfunction as the primary genetic lesion in NIDDM, Evidence from studies in normal glucose-tolerant individuals with a first-degree NIDDM relative [see comments]. JAMA 1995; 273:1855–1861.

93. Solomon CG, Rich-Edwards JW, Dunaif A et al. Abnormal menstrual cycle length predicts subsequent diabetes mellitus. Am J Epidemiol 1998; 11(suppl):S237.

94. Moghetti P, Castello R, Negri C, Tosi F et al. Metformin effects on clinical features, endocrine and metabolic profiles, and insulin sensitivity in polycystic ovary syndrome: a randomized, double-blind, placebo-controlled 6-month trial, followed by open, long-term clinical evaluation. J Clin Endocrinol Metab 2000; 85:139–146.

95. Azziz R, Ehrmann D, Legro RS, Whitcomb RW et al. and PCOS/Troglitazone Study Group. Troglitazone improves ovulation and hirsutism in the polycystic ovary syndrome: a multicenter, double blind, placebo-controlled trial. J Clin Endocrinol Metab 2001; 86:1626–1632.

96. Jeffcoate W, Kong MF. Diabete des femmes a barbe: a classic paper reread. Lancet 2000; 356:1183–1185.

97. Barbieri RL. Hyperandrogenism, insulin resistance and Acanthosis nigricans. 10 years of progress. J Reprod Med 1994; 39:327–336.

98. Legro RS, Bentley-Lewis R, Driscoll D, Wang SC, Dunaif A. Insulin resistance in the sisters of women with polycystic ovary syndrome: association with hyperandrogenemia rather than menstrual irregularity. J Clin Endocrinol Metab 2002; 87:2128–2133.

99. Colilla S, Cox NJ, Ehrmann DA. Heritability of insulin secretion and insulin action in women with polycystic ovary syndrome and their first degree relatives. J Clin Endocrinol Metab 2001; 86:2027–2031.

100. Yildiz BO, Yarali H, Oguz H, Bayraktar M. Glucose intolerance, insulin resistance, and hyperandrogenemia in first degree relatives of women with polycystic ovary syndrome. J Clin Endocrinol Metab 2003; 88:2031–2036.

101. Michelmore KF, Balen AH, Dunger DB, Vessey MP. Polycystic ovaries and associated clinical and biochemical features in young women. Clin Endocrinol (Oxf) 1999; 51:779–786.

102. Polson DW, Adams J, Wadsworth J, Franks S. Polycystic ovaries – a common finding in normal women. Lancet 1988; 1:870–872.

103. Carmina E, Wong L, Chang L, Paulson RJ et al. Endocrine abnormalities in ovulatory women with polycystic ovaries on ultrasound. Hum Reprod 1997; 12:905–909.

104. Chang PL, Lindheim SR, Lowre C, Ferin M et al. Normal ovulatory women with polycystic ovaries have hyperandrogenic pituitary-ovarian responses to gonadotropin-releasing hormone-agonist testing. J Clin Endocrinol Metab 2000; 85:995–1000.

105. Conn JJ, Jacobs HS, Conway GS. The prevalence of polycystic ovaries in women with type 2 diabetes mellitus. Clin Endocrinol (Oxf) 2000; 52:81–86.

106. Colditz GA, Willett WC, Stampfer MJ, Manson JE et al. Weight as a risk factor for clinical diabetes in women. Am J Epidemiol 1990; 132:501–513.

107. Franks S. Polycystic ovary syndrome [published erratum appears in N Engl J Med 1995; 333:1435]. Review: N Engl J Med 1995; 333:853–861.

108. Goldzieher JW. Polycystic ovarian disease. Fertil Steril 1981; 35:371–394.

109. Wild RA. Obesity, lipids, cardiovascular risk, and androgen excess. Am J Med 1995; 98:27S–32S.

110. Jacobs HS. Polycystic ovaries and polycystic ovary syndrome. Gynaecol Endocrinol 1987; 1:113–131.

111. Evans DJ, Hoffman DG, Kalkhoff RK, Kissebah AH. Relationship of androgenic activity to body fat topography fat cell morphology and metabolic aberrations in premenopausal women. J Clin Endocrinol Metab 1983; 57:304–310.

112. Rebuffe-Scrive M, Culberg G, Lundberg PA et al. Anthropometric variables and metabolism in polycystic ovarian disease. Horm Metab Res 1989; 21:391–397.

113. Talbott E, Guzick D, Clerici A, Berga S et al. Coronary heart disease risk factors in women with polycystic ovary syndrome. Arterioscler Thromb Vasc Biol 1995; 15:821–826.

114. Fernandez-Castaner M, Biarnes J, Camps I, Ripolles J et al. Beta-cell dysfunction in first-degree relatives of patients with non-insulin-dependent diabetes mellitus. Diabet Med 1996; 13:953–959.

115. Alford FP, Henriksen JE, Rantzau C, Vaag A et al. Impact of family history of diabetes on the assessment of beta-cell function. Metab Clin Exp 1998; 47:522–528.

116. Stewart MW, Humphriss DB, Berrish TS, Barriocanal LA et al. Features of syndrome X in first-degree relatives of NIDDM patients. Diabetes Care 1995; 18:1020–1022.

117. Ehrmann DA, Sturis J, Byrne MM, Karrison T et al. Insulin secretory defects in polycystic ovary syndrome. Relationship to insulin sensitivity and family history of non-insulin-dependent diabetes mellitus. J Clin Invest 1995; 96:520–527.

118. DeFronzo RA, Ferrannini E. Insulin resistance. A multifaceted syndrome responsible for NIDDM, obesity, hypertension, dyslipidemia, and atherosclerotic cardiovascular disease. Diabetes Care 1991; 14:173–194.

119. Saad MF, Knowler WC, Pettitt DJ, Nelson RG et al. A two-step model for development of non-insulin-dependent diabetes. Am J Med 1991; 90:229–235.

120. Kjos SL, Buchanan TA. Gestational diabetes mellitus. N Engl J Med 1999; 341:1749–1756.

121. Kjos SL, Peters RK, Xiang A, Henry OA et al. Predicting future diabetes in Latino women with gestational diabetes. Utility of early postpartum glucose tolerance testing. Diabetes 1995; 44:586–591.

122. Anttila L, Karjala K, Penttila RA, Ruutiainen K, Ekblad U. Polycystic ovaries in women with gestational diabetes. Obstet Gynecol 1998; 92:13–16.

123. Kousta E, Cela E, Lawrence N, Penny A et al. The prevalence of polycystic ovaries in women with a history of gestational diabetes. Clin Endocrinol (Oxf) 2000; 53:501–507.

124. Koivunen RM, Juutinen J, Vauhkonen I, Morin-Papunen LC et al. Metabolic and steroidogenic alterations related to increased frequency of polycystic ovaries in women with a history of gestational diabetes. J Clin Endocrinol Metab 2001; 86:2591–2599.

125. Harris MI. Gestational diabetes may represent discovery of pre-existing glucose intolerance. Diabetes Care 1988; 11:402–411.

126. Lanzone A, Caruso A, Di Simone N, De Carolis S et al. Polycystic ovary disease. A risk factor for gestational diabetes? J Reprod Med 1995; 40:312–316.

127. Vollenhoven B, Clark S, Kovacs G, Burger H, Healy D. Prevalence of gestational diabetes mellitus in polycystic ovarian syndrome (PCOS) patients pregnant after ovulation induction with gonadotrophins. Aust NZ J Obs Gynaecol 2000; 40:54–58.

128. Wild RA. Polycystic ovary syndrome: a risk for coronary artery disease? Am J Obs Gynecol 2002; 186:35–43.

129. Elting MW, Korsen TJ, Rekers-Mombarg LT, Schoemaker J. Women with polycystic ovary syndrome gain regular menstrual cycles when ageing. Hum Reprod 2000; 15:24–28.

130. Winters SJ, Talbott E, Guzick DS, Zborowski J, McHugh KP. Serum testosterone levels decrease in middle age in women with the polycystic ovary syndrome. Fertil Steril 2000; 73:724–729.

131. Talbott E, Guzick D, Clerici A, Berga S et al. Coronary heart disease risk factors in women with polycystic ovary syndrome. Arterioscl Thromb Vasc Biol 1995; 15:821–826.

132. Talbott EO, Zborowski JV, Sutton-Tyrrell K, McHugh-Pemu KP, Guzick DS. Cardiovascular risk in women with polycystic ovary syndrome. Obs Gynecol Clin North Am 2001; 28:111–133.

133. Cibula D, Cifkova R, Fanta M, Poledne R et al. Increased risk of non-insulin dependent diabetes mellitus, arterial hypertension and coronary artery disease in perimenopausal women with a history of the polycystic ovary syndrome. Hum Reprod 2000; 15:785–789.

134. Loucks TL, Talbott EO, McHugh KP, Keelan M et al. Do polycystic-appearing ovaries affect the risk of cardiovascular disease among women with polycystic ovary syndrome? Fertil Steril 2000; 74:547–552.

135. Handa N, Matsumoto M, Meade H et al. Ultrasonic evaluation of early carotid atherosclerosis . Stroke 1990; 21:1567–1572.

136. Guzick DS, Talbott EO, Sutton-Tyrell K, Herzog HC et al. Carotid atherosclerosis in women with polycystic ovary syndrome : initial results from case control study. Am J Obstet Gynaecol 1996; 174:1224–1229.

137. O'Leary DH, Polka JF, Wolfson SK et al. Use of sonography to evaluate carotid atherosclerosis in the elderly. Stroke 1991; 22:115–163.

138. Talbott EO, Guzick DS, Sutton-Tyrrell K, McHugh-Pemu KP et al. Evidence for association between polycystic ovary syndrome and premature carotid atherosclerosis in middle-aged women. Arterioscl Thromb Vasc Biol 2000; 20:2414–2421.

139. Christian RC, Dumesic DA, Behrenbeck T, Oberg AL et al. Prevalence and predictors of coronary artery calcification in women with polycystic ovary syndrome. J Clin Endocrinol Metab 2003; 88:2562–2568.

140. Dahlgren E, Janson PO, Johansson S, Lapidus L, Oden A. Polycystic ovary syndrome and risk for

myocardial infarction. Evaluated from a risk factor model based on a prospective population study of women. Acta Obstet Gynaecol Scand 1992; 71:599–604.

141. Achard C, Thiers J. Le virilsme pilaire et son associationa le insufisance glycolytique (diabetes a femmes de barbes) Bull Acad Natl Med (Paris) 1921; 86:51–66.

142. Pierpoint T, McKeigue PM, Issacs AJ, Wild SJ, Jacobs HS. Mortality in women with polycystic ovary syndrome at long term follow up. J Clin Epidemiol 1998; 51:581–586.

143. Dramusic V, Goh VH, Rajan U, Wong YC, Ratnam SS. Clinical, endocrinologic, and ultrasonographic features of polycystic ovary syndrome in Singaporean adolescents. J Pediatr Adolesc Gynecol 1997; 10:125–132.

144. Zimmermann S, Phillips RA, Dunaif A, Finegood DT et al. Polycystic ovary syndrome: lack of hypertension despite profound insulin resistance. J Clin Endocrinol Metab 1992; 75:508–513.

145. Sampson M, Kong C, Patel A, Unwin R, Jacobs HS. Ambulatory blood pressure profiles and plasminogen activator inhibitor (PAI-1) activity in lean women with and without the polycystic ovary syndrome. Clin Endocrinol (Oxf) 1996; 45:623–629.

146. Legro RS, Kunselman AR, Dunaif A. Prevalence and predictors of dyslipidemia in women with polycystic ovary syndrome. Am J Med 2001; 111:607–613.

147. Holte J, Gennarelli G, Berne C, Bergh T, Lithell H. Elevated ambulatory day-time blood pressure in women with polycystic ovary syndrome: a sign of a pre-hypertensive state? Hum Reprod 1996; 11:23–28.

148. Dahlgren E, Janson PO. Polycystic ovary syndrome – long-term metabolic consequences. Int J Gynaecol Obstet 1994; 44:3–8.

149. Folsom AR, Kaye SA, Sellers TA, Hong CP et al. Body fat distribution and 5-year risk of death in older women JAMA 1993; 269:483–487 [published erratum appears in JAMA 1993; 269:1254].

150. Wild RA, Painter PC, Coulson PB, Carruth KB, Ranney GB. Lipoprotein lipid concentrations and cardiovascular risk in women with polycystic ovary syndrome. J Clin Endocrinol Metab 1985; 61:946–951.

151. Norman RJ, Hague WM, Masters SC, Wang XJ. Subjects with polycystic ovaries without hyperandrogenaemia exhibit similar disturbances in insulin and lipid profiles as those with polycystic ovary syndrome. Hum Reprod 1995; 10:2258–2261.

152. Robinson S, Henderson AD, Gelding SV, Kiddy D et al. Dyslipidaemia is associated with insulin resistance in women with polycystic ovaries. Clin Endocrinol (Oxf) 1996; 44:277–284.

153. Mather KJ, Kwan F, Corenblum B. Hyperinsulinemia in polycystic ovary syndrome corre-lates with increased cardiovascular risk independent of obesity. Fertil Steril 2000; 73: 150–156.

154. Graf MJ, Richards CJ, Brown V, Meissner L et al. The independent effects of hyperandrogenaemia, hyperinsulinaemia, and obesity on lipid and lipoprotein profiles in women. Clin Endocrinol (Oxf) 1990; 33:119–131.

155. Slowinska-Srzednicka J, Zgliczynski S, Wierzbicki M, Srzednicki M et al. The role of hyperinsulinemia in the development of lipid disturbances in nonobese and obese women with the polycystic ovary syndrome. J Endocrinol Invest 1991; 14:569–575.

156. Conway GS, Agrawal R, Betteridge DJ, Jacobs HS. Risk factors for coronary artery disease in lean and obese women with the polycystic ovary syndrome. Clin Endocrinol (Oxf) 1992; 37:119–125.

157. Holte J, Bergh T, Berne C, Lithell H. Serum lipoprotein lipid profile in women with the polycystic ovary syndrome: relation to anthropometric, endocrine and metabolic variables. Clin Endocrinol (Oxf) 1994; 41:463–471.

158. Robinson S, Henderson AD, Gelding SV, Kiddy D et al. Dyslipidaemia is associated with insulin resistance in women with polycystic ovaries. Clin Endocrinol (Oxf) 1996; 44:277–284.

159. Rajkhowa M, Neary RH, Knmptala P, Game FL et al. Altered composition of high density lipoproteins in women with polycystic ovary syndrome. J Clin Endocrinol Metab 1997; 82:3389–3394.

160. Atiomo WU, Bates SA, Condon JE, Shaw S et al. The plasminogen activator system in women with polycystic ovary syndrome. Fertil Steril 1998; 69: 236–241.

161. Sampson M, Kong C, Patel A, Unwin R, Jacobs HS. Ambulatory blood pressure profiles and plasminogen activator inhibitor (PAI-1) in lean women with and without polycystic ovary syndrome. Clin Endocrinol (Oxf) 1996; 45:623–629.

162. Wild RA, Bartholomew MJ. The influence of body weight on lipoprotein lipids in patients with polycystic ovary syndrome. Am J Obstet Gynecol 1988; 159:423–427.

163. Laakso M. Dyslipidaemias, insulin resistance and atherosclerosis. Ann Med 1992; 24:505–509.

164. Gardner CD, Fortmann SP, Krauss RM. Association of small low-density lipoprotein particles with the incidence of coronary artery disease in men and women [see comments]. JAMA 1996; 276:875–881.

165. Austin MA, Breslow JL, Hennekens CH, Buring JE et al. Low-density lipoprotein subclass patterns and risk of myocardial infarction. JAMA 1988; 260:1917–1921.

166. Dejager S, Pichard C, Giral P, Bruckert E et al. Smaller LDL particle size in women with polycystic ovary syndrome compared to controls. Clin Endocrinol (Oxf) 2001; 54:455–462.

167. Expert Panel on Detection, Evaluation and Treatment of High Blood Cholesterol in Adults. Executive summary of the third report of the national cholesterol education program (NCEP) expert panel on detection, evaluation, and treatment of high blood cholesterol in adults (adult treatment panel iii) [See comments]. JAMA 2001; 285:2486–2497.

168. Yarali H, Yildirir A, Aybar F, Kabakci G et al. Diastolic dysfunction and increased serum homocysteine concentrations may contribute to increased cardiovascular risk in patients with polycystic ovary syndrome. Fertil Steril 2001; 76:511–516.

169. Paradisi G, Steinberg HO, Hempfling A, Cronin J et al. Polycystic ovary syndrome is associated with endothelial dysfunction. Circulation 2001; 103:1410–1415.

170. Kelly CJ, Speirs A, Gould GW, Petrie JR et al. Altered vascular function in young women with polycystic ovary syndrome. J Clin Endocrinol Metab 2002; 87:742–746.

171. Kelly CC, Lyall H, Petrie JR, Gould GW et al. Low grade chronic inflammation in women with polycystic ovarian syndrome. J Clin Endocrinol Metab 2001; 86:2453–2455.

172. Loverro G, Lorusso F, Mei L, Depalo R et al. The plasma homocysteine levels are increased in polycystic ovary syndrome. Gynecol Obstet Invest 2002; 53:157–162.

173. Muneyyirci-Delale O, Nacharaju VL, Dalloul M, Jalou S et al. Divalent cations in women with PCOS: implications for cardiovascular disease. Gynecol Endocrinol 2001; 15:198–201.

174. Kelly CJ, Lyall H, Petrie JR, Gould GW et al. A specific elevation in tissue plasminogen activator antigen in women with polycystic ovarian syndrome. J Clin Endocrinol Metab 2002; 87:3287–3290.

175. Wild RA, Grubb B, Hartz A, Van Nort JJ et al. Clinical signs of androgen excess as risk factors for coronary artery disease. Fertil Steril 1990; 54:255–259.

176. Rebora A. Baldness and coronary artery disease: the dermatologic point of view of a controversial issue. Arch Dermatol 2001; 137:943–947.

177. van Kesteren PJ, Asscheman H, Megens JA, Gooren LJ. Mortality and morbidity in transsexual subjects treated with cross-sex hormones. Clin Endocrinol (Oxf) 1997; 47:337–342.

178. Gorgels WJ, Blankenstein MA, Collette HJ, Erkelens DW. Urinary sex hormone excretions in premenopausal women and coronary heart disease risk: a nested case-referent study in the DOM-cohort. J Clin Epidemiol 1997; 50:275–281.

179. Price JF, Lee AJ, Fowkes FG. Steroid sex hormones and peripheral arterial disease in the Edinburgh Artery Study. Steroids 1997; 62:789–794.

180. Barrett-Connor E, Goodman-Gruen D. Prospective study of endogenous sex hormones and fatal cardiovascular disease in postmenopausal women [comment]. Br Med J 1995; 311:1193–1196.

181. Davis SR, Burger HG. Clinical review 82: androgens and the postmenopausal woman [comment]. J Clin Endocrinol Metab 1996; 81:2759–2763.

182. Tchernof A, Despres JP. Sex steroid hormones, sex hormone-binding globulin, and obesity in men and women. Horm Metab Res 2000; 32:526–536.

183. Ferrannini E, Vichi S, Beck-Nielsen H, Laakso M et al. Insulin action and age. European Group for the Study of Insulin Resistance (EGIR). Diabetes 1996; 45:947–953.

184. Reinecke H, Bogdanski J, Woltering A, Breithardt G et al. Relation of serum levels of sex hormone binding globulin to coronary heart disease in postmenopausal women. Am J Cardiol 2002; 90:364–368.

185. Phillips GB, Pinkernell TH, Jing TY. Relationship between serum sex hormones and coronary artery disease in postmenopausal women. Arterioscler Thromb Vasc Biol 1997; 17:695–701.

186. Solomon CG, Hu FB, Dunaif A, Rich-Edwards JE et al. Menstrual cycle irregularity and risk for future cardiovascular disease. J Clin Endocrinol Metab 2002; 87:2013–2017.

187. Donesky BW, Adashi EY. Surgically induced ovulation in the polycystic ovary syndrome: wedge resection revisited in the age of laparoscopy. Fertil Steril 1995; 63:439–463.

188. Lemieux S, Lewis GF, Ben-Chetrit A, Steiner G, Greenblatt EM. Correction of hyperandrogenemia by laparoscopic ovarian cautery in women with polycystic ovarian syndrome is not accompanied by improved insulin sensitivity or lipid-lipoprotein levels. J Clin Endocrinol Metab 1999; 84:4278–4282.

189. Pierpoint T, McKeigue PM, Isaacs AJ, Wild SH, Jacobs HS. Mortality of women with polycystic ovary syndrome at long-term follow-up. J Clin Epidemiol 1998; 51:581–586.

190. Birdsall MA, Farquhar CM, White HD. Association between polycystic ovaries and extent of coronary artery disease in women having cardiac catheterization. Ann Intern Med 1997; 126:32–35.

191. Birdsall MA, Farquhar CM. Polycystic ovaries in pre and post-menopausal women. Clin Endocrinol (Oxf) 1996; 44:269–276.

192. Lakhani K, Constantinovici N, Purcell WM, Fernando R, Hardiman P. Internal carotid artery haemodynamics in women with polycystic ovaries. Clin Sci 2000; 98:661–665.

193. Bili H, Laven J, Imani B, Eijkemans MJ, Fauser BC. Age-related differences in features associated with polycystic ovary syndrome in normogonadotrophic oligo-amenorrhoeic infertile women of reproductive years. Eur J Endocrinol 2001; 145:749–755.

194. Givens JR, Wiser WL, Coleman SA, Wilroy RS et al. Familial ovarian hyperthecosis: A study of two families. Am J Obstet Gynecol 1971; 110:959–972.

195. Wilroy RS, Jr, Givens JR, Wiser WL, Coleman SA et al. Hyperthecosis: an inheritable form of polycystic ovarian disease. Birth Defects: Original Article Series 1975; 11:81–85.

196. Norman RJ, Masters S, Hague W. Hyperinsulinemia is common in family members of women with polycystic ovary syndrome. Fertil Steril 1996; 66:942–947.

197. Yildiz BO, Yarali H et al. Glucose intolerance, insulin resistance and hypoandrogenemia in first degree relatives of women with polycystic ovary syndrome. J Clin Endocrinol Metab 2003; 88:2041–2046.

198. Ferrannini E, Natali A, Capaldo B, Lehtovirta M et al. Insulin resistance, hyperinsulinemia, and blood pressure: role of age and obesity. European Group for the Study of Insulin Resistance (EGIR). Hypertension 1997; 30:1144–1149.

199. Bloomgarden ZT. American Association of Clinical Endocrinologists (AACE) consensus conference on the insulin resistance syndrome: 25–26 August 2002, Washington, DC. Diabetes Care 2003; 26:933–939.

200. Bloomgarden ZT, American Association of Clinical Endocrinologists (AACE) consensus conference on the insulin resistance syndrome: 25–26 August 2002, Washington, DC. Diabetes Care 2003; 26:1297–1303.

201. Chiasson JL, Gomis R, Hanefeld M, Josse RG et al. The stop-NIDDM trial: an international study on the efficacy of an alpha-glucosidase inhibitor to prevent type 2 diabetes in a population with impaired glucose tolerance: rationale, design, and preliminary screening data. Study to prevent non-insulin-dependent diabetes mellitus. Diabetes Care 1998; 21:1720–1725.

202. Buchanan TA, Xiang AH, Peters RK, Kjos SL et al. Preservation of pancreatic beta-cell function and prevention of type 2 diabetes by pharmacological treatment of insulin resistance in high-risk hispanic women. Diabetes 2002; 51:2796–2803.

203. Knowler WC, Barrett-Connor E, Fowler SE, Hamman RF et al. Diabetes Prevention Program Research Group. Reduction in the incidence of type 2 diabetes with lifestyle intervention or metformin. N Engl J Med 2002; 346:393–403.

204. Anonymous. Glucose tolerance and mortality: comparison of WHO and American Diabetes Association diagnostic criteria. The Decode Study Group. European Diabetes Epidemiology Group. Diabetes epidemiology: collaborative analysis of diagnostic criteria in Europe [see comments]. Lancet 1999; 354:617–621.

205. Tominaga M, Eguchi H, Manaka H, Igarashi K et al. Impaired glucose tolerance is a risk factor for cardiovascular disease, but not impaired fasting glucose. The funagata diabetes study [see comments]. Diabetes Care 1999; 22:920–924.

206. Nestler JE. Role of hyperinsulinemia in the pathogenesis of the polycystic ovary syndrome, and its clinical implications. Semin Reprod Endocrinol 1997; 15:111–122.

207. Rosenbaum M, Leibel RL, Hirsch J. Obesity [see comments]. N Engl J Med 1997; 337:396–407.

208. Guzick DS, Wing R, Smith D, Berga SL, Winters SJ. Endocrine consequences of weight loss in obese, hyperandrogenic, anovulatory women. Fertil Steril 1994; 61:598–604.

209. Jaatinen TA, Anttila L, Erkkola R, Koskinen P et al. Hormonal responses to physical exercise in patients with polycystic ovarian syndrome. Fertil Steril 1993; 60:262–267.

210. Okajima T, Koyanagi T, Goto M, Kato K. Hormonal abnormalities were improved by weight loss using very low calorie diet in a patient with polycystic ovary syndrome [in Japanese]. Fukuoka Igaku Zasshi 1994; 85:263–266.

211. Clark AM, Ledger W, Galletly C, Tomlinson L et al. Weight loss results in significant improvement in pregnancy and ovulation rates in anovulatory obese women. Hum Reprod 1995; 10:2705–2712.

212. Franks S, Kiddy D, Sharp P, Singh A et al. Obesity and polycystic ovary syndrome. Ann NY Acad Sci 1991; 626:201–206.

213. Kiddy DS, Hamilton-Fairley D, Bush A, Short F et al. Improvement in endocrine and ovarian function during dietary treatment of obese women with polycystic ovary syndrome. Clin Endocrinol (Oxf) 1992; 36:105–111.

214. Kiddy DS, Hamilton-Fairley D, Seppala M, Koistinen R et al. Diet-induced changes in sex hormone binding globulin and free testosterone in women with normal or polycystic ovaries: correlation with serum insulin and insulin-like growth factor-I. Clin Endocrinol (Oxf) 1989; 31:757–763.

215. Nuttall FQ, Gannon MC, Wald JL, Ahmed M, Plasma glucose and insulin profiles in normal subjects ingesting diets of varying carbohydrate, fat, and protein content. J Am Coll Nutr 1985; 4:437–450.

216. Seino Y, Seino S, Ikeda M, Matsukura S, Imura H. Beneficial effects of high protein diet in treatment of mild diabetes. Hum Nutr Appl Nutr 1983; 37A(3):226–230.

217. Baba NH, Sawaya S, Torbay N, Habbal Z et al. High protein vs high carbohydrate hypoenergetic diet for the treatment of obese hyperinsulinemic subjects. Int J Obes Relat Metab Disord 1999; 23:1202–1206.

218. Pasquali R, Gambineri A, Biscotti D, Vicennati V et al. Effect of long-term treatment with metformin

added to hypocaloric diet on body composition, fat distribution, and androgen and insulin levels in abdominally obese women with and without the polycystic ovary syndrome. J Clin Endocrinol Metab 2000; 85:2767–2774.

219. Skov AR, Toubro S, Bulow J, Krabbe K et al. Changes in renal function during weight loss induced by high vs low-protein low-fat diets in overweight subjects. Int J Obes Relat Metab Disord 1999; 23:1170–1177.

220. Foster GD, Wyatt HR, Hill JO, McGuckin BG et al. A randomized trial of a low-carbohydrate diet for obesity [comment]. N Engl J Med 2003; 348:2082–2090.

221. Braun B, Zimmermann MB, Kretchmer N. Effects of exercise intensity on insulin sensitivity in women with non-insulin-dependent diabetes mellitus. J Appl Physiol 1995; 78:300–306.

222. De Leo V, la Marca A, Petraglia F. Insulin-lowering agents in the management of polycystic ovary syndrome. Endocrinol Rev 2003; 24:633–667.

223. Velazquez EM, Mendoza S, Hamer T, Sosa F, Glueck CJ. Metformin therapy in polycystic ovary syndrome reduces hyperinsulinemia, insulin resistance, hyperandrogenemia, and systolic blood pressure, while facilitating normal menses and pregnancy. Metabolism 1994; 43:647–654.

224. Nestler JE, Jakubowicz DJ. Lean women with polycystic ovary syndrome respond to insulin reduction with decreases in ovarian p450c17 alpha activity and serum androgens. J Clin Endocrinol Metab 1997; 82:4075–4079.

225. Nestler JE, Jakubowicz DJ, Evans WS, Pasquali R. Effects of metformin on spontaneous and clomiphene-induced ovulation in the polycystic ovary syndrome. N Engl J Med 1998; 338:1876–1880.

226. Nestler JE, Jakubowicz DJ, Reamer P, Gunn RD, Allan G. Ovulatory and metabolic effects of D-chiro-inositol in the polycystic ovary syndrome. N Engl J Med 1999; 340:1314–1320.

227. Coetzee EJ, Jackson WP. Metformin in management of pregnant insulin-independent diabetics. Diabetologia 1979; 16:241–245.

228. Coetzee EJ, Jackson WP. Pregnancy in established non-insulin-dependent diabetics. A five-and-a-half year study at groote schuur hospital. S Afr Med J 1980; 58:795–802.

229. Callahan TL, Hall JE, Ettner SL, Christiansen CL et al. The economic impact of multiple-gestation pregnancies and the contribution of assisted-reproduction techniques to their incidence [see comments]. N Engl J Med 1994; 331:244–249.

230. Sarlis NJ, Weil SJ, Nelson LM. Administration of metformin to a diabetic woman with extreme hyperandrogenemia of nontumoral origin: management of infertility and prevention of inadvertent masculinization of a female fetus. J Clin Endocrinol Metab 1999; 84:1510–1512.

231. Velazquez EM, Mendoza SG, Wang P, Glueck CJ. Metformin therapy is associated with a decrease in plasma plasminogen activator inhibitor-1, lipoprotein(a), and immunoreactive insulin levels in patients with the polycystic ovary syndrome. Metabolism 1997; 46:454–457.

232. Diamanti-Kandarakis E, Kouli C, Tsianateli T, Bergiele A. Therapeutic effects of metformin on insulin resistance and hyperandrogenism in polycystic ovary syndrome. Eur J Endocrinol 1998; 138:269–274.

233. Vandermolen DT, Ratts VS, Evans WS, Stovall DW et al. Metformin increases the ovulatory rate and pregnancy rate from clomiphene citrate in patients with polycystic ovary syndrome who are resistant to clomiphene citrate alone. Fertil Steril 2001; 75:310–315.

234. Glueck CJ, Phillips H, Cameron D, Sieve-Smith L, Wang P. Continuing metformin throughout pregnancy in women with polycystic ovary syndrome appears to safely reduce first-trimester spontaneous abortion: a pilot study. Fertil Steril 2001; 75:46–52.

235. Jakubowicz DJ, Iuorno MJ, Jakubowicz S, Roberts KA, Nestler JE. Effects of metformin on early pregnancy loss in the polycystic ovary syndrome. J Clin Endocrinol Metab 2002; 87:524–529.

236. Lord JM, Flight IH, Norman RJ. Metformin in polycystic ovary syndrome: systematic review and meta-analysis. BMJ 2003; 327:951–953.

237. Morin-Papunen L, Rautio K, Ruokonen A, Hedberg P et al. Metformin reduces serum C-reactive protein levels in women with polycystic ovary syndrome. J Clin Endocrinol Metab 2003; 88:4649–4654.

238. Velazquez E, Acosta A, Mendoza SG. Menstrual cyclicity after metformin therapy in polycystic ovary syndrome. Obstet Gynecol 1997; 90:392–395.

239. Legro RS, Azziz R, Ehrmann D, Fereshetian AG et al. Minimal response of circulating lipids in women with polycystic ovary syndrome to improvement in insulin sensitivity with troglitazone. J Clin Endocrinol Metab 2003; 88:5137–5144.

240. Cataldo NA, Abbasi F, McLaughlin TL, Lamendola C, Reaven GM. Improvement in insulin sensitivity followed by ovulation and pregnancy in a woman with polycystic ovary syndrome who was treated with rosiglitazone. Fertil Steril 2001; 76:1057–1059.

241. Romualdi D, Guido M, Ciampelli M, Giuliani M et al. Selective effects of pioglitazone on insulin and androgen abnormalities in normo- and hyperinsulinaemic obese patients with polycystic ovary syndrome. Hum Reprod 2003; 18:1210–1218.

242. Ghazeeri G, Kutteh WH, Bryer-Ash M, Haas D, Ke RW. Effect of rosiglitazone on spontaneous and clomiphene citrate-induced ovulation in women

with polycystic ovary syndrome. Fertil Steril 2003; 79:562–566.

243. Geisthovel F, Frorath B, Brabant G. Acarbose reduces elevated testosterone serum concentrations in hyperinsulinaemic premenopausal women: a pilot study. Hum Reprod 1996; 11:2377–2381.

244. Ciotta L, Calogero AE, Farina M, De Leo V et al. Clinical, endocrine and metabolic effects of acarbose, an alpha-glucosidase inhibitor, in PCOS patients with increased insulin response and normal glucose tolerance. Hum Reprod 2001; 16:2066–2072.

Chapter 9

Long-term sequelae of polycystic ovary syndrome: gynecological cancer

Introduction

Women with polycystic ovary syndrome (PCOS) have been reported to be at increased risk of a number of gynecological neoplasias, including endometrial, breast, and ovarian cancer. The data supporting an increased risk is almost entirely inferential, based primarily on small case series or shared risk factors. The level of evidence supporting an association between diabetes and cardiovascular disease with PCOS, for example, is much stronger (flawed as it is), than that linking women with PCOS with gynecological disease (see Chapter 8). One of the difficulties in exploring the association between these cancers and PCOS, is that they remain primarily diseases of post-menopausal women and present long after PCOS has faded. Only a fraction of cancer cases present in pre-menopausal women, where a concurrent diagnosis of PCOS may exist.

The basis for the concerns about long-term sequelae is that women with PCOS have a number of reproductive and metabolic abnormalities. The reproductive abnormalities include chronic anovulation, prolonged exposure to estrogen, progesterone deficiency, and androgen excess, which may contribute to an increased risk for gynecological cancers in which the hormonal milieu is an important contributor to etiology and prognosis.

Endometrial cancer is currently thought to be perhaps the best example of a hormone-dependent neoplasia. Endometrial cancer is thought to arise from prolonged exposure to estrogen, without the benefits of progesterone, a condition known as 'unopposed estrogen'.[1] Estrogen is a clear mitogen on the endometrium and leads to proliferation of both the glandular and stromal components. Women with PCOS have been shown to be normestrogenic, perhaps even hyper-estrogenic with elevated levels of estrone.[2] Testosterone is the precursor for estrogen biosynthesis and so even in the absence of normal folliculogenesis, steroid production continues, and furthermore testosterone is converted to estrone in the peripheral fat. Progestins act as an antimitogenic, antiproliferative hormone on the endometrium and cause differentiation of the endometrium. Thus, in relation to the mitogenic effects of estrogen on the lining of the uterus, progestins may be viewed as an estrogen antagonist. Hyperplasia of the endometrium is an intermediary step on the road to endometrial cancer and is marked by overgrowth and crowding of the glandular component of the endometrium. According to the 1994 World Health Organization (WHO) classification, there are two groups of hyperplasia: simple endometrial hyperplasia and atypical hyperplasia.[3] Atypical hyperplasia is more likely to develop into or co-exist with endometrial carcinoma.[4] The hormonal treatment of both forms of hyperplasia with progestin therapy is identical although follow up is traditionally more vigilant with atypical hyperplasia, and surgical therapy, i.e. hysterectomy is often suggested for women who no longer desire fertility.[5]

More recently, insulin resistance and hyperinsulinemia have been implicated as contributory agents to a variety of neoplasias. Smaller studies of women with endometrial cancer ($n = 10$ cases and $n = 32$ cases) have shown increased fasting and glucose-stimulated insulin levels compared with controls.[6,7] Another study found a similar result among women with endometrial cancers ($n = 18$) both in relation to controls and women with other hormone-dependent neoplasias such as

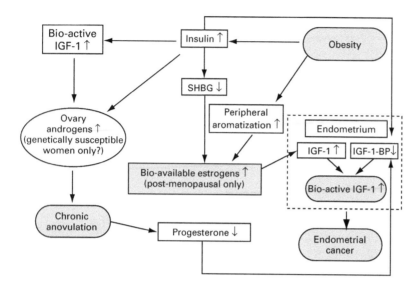

Figure 9.1

Mechanisms through which hormonal factors and insulin resistance contribute to increased risk for endometrial cancer. From Kaaks et al, 2002.[11]

breast cancer.[8] A variety of mechanisms has been proposed.

Insulin is a powerful mitogenic influence on a variety of tissues including endometrium and breast epithelium, and this proliferative effect may contribute to the appearance of oncogenes and transformation of benign tissue. In vitro studies of cancer cell lines have shown that insulin is mitogenic, and most cell cultures of tumor cells require the presence of insulin in order to survive.[9] Studies of endometrial cancer lines have shown that the insulin receptor is expressed in a variety of cell lines, and that there is increased expression in poorly differentiated cell lines, specifically estrogen receptor-negative cell lines HEC-1-A and HEC-1-B.[10] This suggests that insulin may play a role in the development of estrogen receptor-negative endometrial cancers – cancers that usually are more aggressive and have a poorer prognosis.

Insulin may also stimulate steroidogenesis in these tissues, through mechanisms increasing expression of key enzymes such as aromatase, and increasing the bioavailability of sex steroids and potent growth factors (such as insulin-like growth factor-1 (IGF-1)) through suppression of binding proteins such as sex hormone binding globulin (SHBG) and IGF1 binding protein (IGF-1-BP) (Figure 9.1).[11]

Breast and endometrial cancer: shared risk factors

There are a number of shared risk factors for breast and endometrial cancer, and many of these overlap with the PCOS phenotype (Table 9.1). Both cancers are viewed as the classic hormone-dependent-influenced cancers, which undergo a transformation from benign through to pre-malignant and then to malignant tissue over time. They are also associated with a number of reproductive factors associated with prolonged exposure to sex

Table 9.1 Shared risk factors for endometrial and breast cancer

- Prolonged gynecological age
  - early menarche/late menopause
- Nulliparity
- Obesity
  - diet high in animal fat
- Estrogen replacement therapy
- Prior or family history of breast/endometrial cancer
- Caucasian
- Age
- Prior irradiation
- Pre-malignant progressive changes
  - hyperplasia to atypical hyperplasia + atypia to malignancy

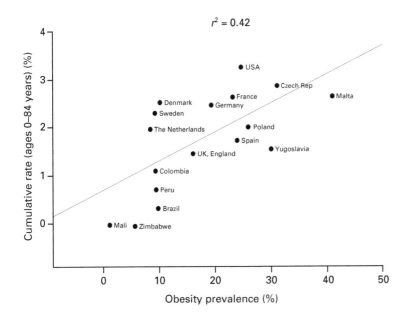

Figure 9.2

Increasing prevalence of endometrial cancer as the rate of obesity increases. From Akhmedkhanov et al.[18]

steroids, which include a long menstrual life as indicated by increased risk with earlier menarche and late menopause.[12,13] The association of PCOS with premature pubarche and early awakening of the adrenal gland may eventually be another risk factor.[14] Nulliparity is an additional risk factor. Iatrogenic exposure to estrogen replacement therapy may be an additional shared risk factor.

Familial clustering suggesting a genetic influence has been noted with both cancers, and in some studies the presence of one is a risk factor for the development of the other as a secondary cancer.[15] Lifestyle further contributes to risk. Obesity is a risk factor for both endometrial and breast cancer, and diets high in fat correlate with an increased risk.[16,17] Thus it is no surprise that countries with higher rates of obesity and fat consumption also experience the highest rates of endometrial cancer (Figure 9.2).[18] A sedentary lifestyle is an additive risk factor, and exercise is associated with a dose and duration response reduction in risk.[19,20]

Breast and endometrial cancer: unique and disparate risk factors

It is simplistic however to lump together breast and endometrial cancers as related disorders as

they also have many unique and disparate risk factors (Table 9.2). One of these is the response to tamoxifen, which is used as adjuvant or preventive therapy for breast cancer, but is associated with an increased endometrial cancer risk.[21,22] Also while the addition of progestin to estrogen replacement therapy appears to increase the risk of breast cancer in post-menopausal women,[23] it is protective against the development of endometrial cancer.[24] Progestins may thus have opposite effects on cancer risk. Progesterone deficiency, which characterizes PCOS, may therefore partially

Table 9.2 Unique risk factors for breast and endometrial cancer

Breast	Endometrium
• Tamoxifen benefit	• Tamoxifen risk
• No diabetes effect	• Diabetes risk
• Progestin risk	• Progestin benefit
• Early childbearing benefit	• Chronic anovulation risk
• Breastfeeding benefit	• No breastfeeding effect
• Oral contraceptive pill risk	• Oral contraceptive pill benefit
• Induced abortion risk	• Induced abortion benefit
• Alcohol risk	• Alcohol benefit

Table 9.3 Summary of publications linking women with PCOS to endometrial cancer. The majority are small case series, usually uncontrolled. From Hardiman et al, 2003[33]

Authors	Study design	Subjects	Findings	Comments
Speert 1949[50]	Case series	14 women under 40 years with endometrial carcinoma	8 with cystic and 1 with sclerotic ovaries	No controls
Dockerty et al, 1951[51]	Case series	36 women under 40 years with endometrial carcinoma	14 with cystic ovaries (no histology in 8)	No controls
Jackson and Dockerty, 1957[29]	(a) Case series; (b) Cross-sectional	(a) 'many thousands' of endometrial cancer cases; (b) 27 women with polycystic ovaries on biopsy	(a) 16 women with PCOS; (b) None had endometrial carcinoma	No evidence of association
Ramzy and Nizker, 1979[52]	Case control	15 ovaries from cases of endometrial cancer, 25 from women with PCOS, 21 from controls	Ovaries from endometrial carcinoma cases more similar to the normal than to polycystic ovaries	No evidence of association
Coulam et al, 1983[30]	Retrospective cohort	1270 women with chronic anovulation	SMR for endometrial carcinoma 3.1	No data for women with PCOS
Gallup & Stock, 1984[53]	Case series	111 cases of endometrial cancer	PCO in 31.2% of women under 40; 2.3% over 40	No controls
Escobedo, 1991[55]	Case-control	399 cases of endometrial carcinoma; 3040 controls	Odds ratio for endometrial carcinoma 4.2 for 'ovarian factor' infertility	No data for women with PCOS
Dahlgren et al, 1991[56]	Case-control	147 cases of endometrial cancer; 409 controls	↑ hirsuitism in cases with endometrial cancer	No data for PCOS
Ho et al, 1997[57]	Retrospective cohort	116 patients with endometrial hyperplasia	Prevalence of endometrial carcinoma not ↑ in cases with polycystic ovaries	No evidence of association
Pierpoint et al, 1998[58]	Retrospective cohort	786 women with PCOS	Mortality from 'miscellaneous cancers' not ↑	No data for endometrial cancer
Wild et al, 2000[59]	Retrospective cohort	345 surviving women from Pierpoint cohort	Odds ratio for endometrial cancer 5.3	Obesity a possible confounder

SMR: standardized mortality ratio.

protect against the development of breast cancer, while increasing endometrial cancer risk.

Neither diabetes nor chronic anovulation have been identified as risk factors for breast cancer.[25] Hypertension has been identified as a risk factor for endometrial cancer, but not breast cancer. Another disparate risk factor is alcohol consumption, which has a dose–response relationship with breast cancer,[26] but is associated with an apparent decrease in endometrial cancer.[27]

Endometrial cancer and polycystic ovary syndrome

Cancer of the endometrium is the most common cancer of the lower genital tract and is the fourth most common cancer diagnosed in women.[28] However only 4% of cases occur in women under 40 years of age. Women with PCOS have often been noted to have an especially high risk of developing endometrial cancer and often at an early age.[29-32] The long-term risk of endometrial hyperplasia and endometrial carcinoma due to chronic anovulation and unopposed estrogen has long been suggested. The multi-factorial nature of the syndrome combined with its heterogeneous presentation makes it difficult to ascertain which factors (i.e. hyperinsulinemia, elevated serum concentrations of growth factors, obesity or genetic predisposition) cause the most significant risk with respect to the development of cancer. Furthermore the majority of publications refer to case series or case reports or are inferential, being based on stigmata of PCOS such as hirsutism, obesity, and anovulation (Table 9.3).[33]

Chronic anovulation is associated with endometrial cancer.[30] In case series, women with PCOS have been over-represented in those developing endometrial cancer and often do so at an early age.[29,31,32] The fact that endometrial cancer is not noted in reference to a post-menopausal PCOS population reflects our difficulty in making the diagnosis after ovarian failure and cessation of menses.[34] A Scandinavian study looked at a group of both pre-menopausal and post-menopausal women with endometrial carcinoma, and found hirsutism and obesity in both affected groups more often than in controls.[35] In the younger group, they additionally noted a recent history of anovulation and infertility, two of the most common presenting complaints of women with PCOS (in addition to hirsutism and obesity).[36]

Endometrial hyperplasia has also often been noted in association with anovulation and infertility.[32,37,38] The risk of developing endometrial cancer has been shown to be adversely influenced by a number of factors including obesity, long-term use of unopposed estrogens, nulliparity and infertility.[35,39,40] In fact the relative risk of endometrial cancer is 1.6 in women with a menarche before the age of 12 years and 2.4 in women with their menopause after the age of 52 years.[41] Women with endometrial carcinoma have fewer births compared with controls,[41] and it has also been demonstrated that infertility per se gives a relative risk of 2.[42] Hypertension and type II diabetes mellitus have long been linked to endometrial cancer, with relative risks of 2.1 and 2.8 respectively – conditions that are now known also to be associated with PCOS.[41]

The association between PCOS and endometrial adenocarcinoma has been reported for many years. A report of 16 cases by Jackson et al indicated ages ranging from 27 to 48 years, a high rate of prolonged amenorrhea, obesity, hypertension, and nulliparity in 13 of the 15 married women.[43] A study by Coulam et al examined the risk of developing endometrial carcinoma in a group of 1270 patients who were diagnosed as having 'chronic anovulation syndrome'.[44] The defining characteristics of this group included pathological or macroscopic evidence of the Stein–Leventhal syndrome, or a clinical diagnosis of chronic anovulation. This study identified the excess risk of endometrial cancer to be 3.1 (95% confidence interval (CI), 1.1–7.3) and proposed that this might be due to abnormal levels of unopposed estrogen. Other authors have expanded this theory by suggesting that hyperandrogenism and hyperinsulinemia may further increase the potential for neoplastic change in the endometrium through their effects on levels of SHBG, IGF-1, and circulating estrogens.[45,46]

In a study of 97 women under the age of 36 years with adenomatous or atypical adenomatous hyperplasia, 25% were found to have typical polycystic ovaries confirmed by biopsy. The mean age of the 24 women in this group was 25.7 years and all were nulliparous (23 were married). In 12 patients, the diagnosis of polycystic ovaries was made at the time of hysterectomy (at which time two were found to have carcinoma). Treatment was by wedge resection of the ovaries in the other 12 patients, of whom eight had follow-up endometrial curettage and only three had persistent hyperplasia (one of which progressed to adenocarcinoma). One patient was found on initial curettage to have focal adenocarcinoma, which regressed after wedge biopsy, following which a normal pregnancy resulted from clomifene citrate treatment. The other patients all had problems with infertility; some were treated with clomifene citrate although results were poor.[47]

In a large case-control study, increased endometrial cancer risk was noted in women with lower levels of SHBG,[48] and elevated insulin levels,[49] both biochemical stigmata noted in women with PCOS. There are no systematic prospective studies of the prevalence of endometrial hyperplasia/neoplasia in a population with PCOS, or conversion rates over time. These data are summarized in Table 9.3. The true risk of endometrial cancer in women with PCOS thus is difficult to ascertain.

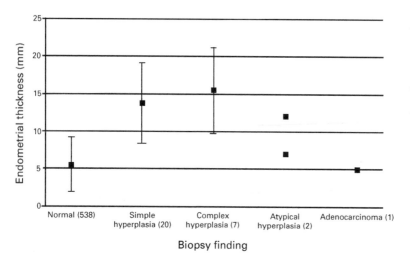

Figure 9.3

Endometrial thickness on transvaginal ultrasound examination according to the histopathological diagnosis in 477 women who participated in the PEPI study (Postmenopausal Estrogen/Progestin Interventions trial). Error bars inndicate SD. From Langer et al, 1997.[64]

Screening for endometrial hyperplasia and cancer in women with polycystic ovary syndrome

The prevalence of endometrial hyperplasia in a pre-menopausal population has not been determined in large cross-sectional studies. Endometrial hyperplasia may be a precursor of adenocarcinoma, with cystic glandular hyperplasia progressing in maybe 0.4% of cases, and adenomatous hyperplasia in up to 18% of cases over a time period of 2–10 years, although a precise estimate of rate of progression is impossible to determine.[60] The prevalence of endometrial hyperplasia and endometrial cancer in an asymptomatic population has not been well studied. There is one screening study of the endometrium available in a random population of 2586 American women, which included women of reproductive age and menopausal women.[61] This study found that the prevalence of endometrial hyperplasia was 8/1000 and for endometrial carcinoma was 7/1000.

There is currently no screening test for endometrial cancer, and patients are chosen for biopsy based on risk factors, or a presenting complaint of post-menopausal or dysfunctional uterine bleeding. Ultrasonography has been found to be a useful screening tool for endometrial pathology in a post-menopausal symptomatic population that is experiencing bleeding, the most common presenting complaint. An endometrial thickness of less than 5 mm is rarely associated with endometrial carcinoma.[62] The positive predictive value of an endometrial thickness >5 mm in this population approaches 30%.[62] In a similar population, the mean thickness of the endometrium measured by ultrasonography was significantly elevated in cases of endometrial hyperplasia and endometrial carcinoma (12–14 mm) compared with a benign endometrium.[63] The PEPI (Postmenopausal Estrogen/Progestin Intervention Trials) correlated ultrasound thickness of the endometrium in 448 asymptomatic women participating in a hormone replacement trial and found a high sensitivity for ultrasound in detecting pathology, but a poor predictive value (9% with endometrium >5 mm) due to the low prevalence of pathology.[64] However ultrasound had a high negative predictive value as there was little overlap noted between normal variants and pathology when the endometrial thickness exceeded 8–10 mm (Figure 9.3).[64] While these data are not completely applicable to a hypogonadal pre-menopausal population, they serve as a useful comparison.

There are few data available on the prevalence of endometrial hyperplasia in pre-menopausal women. In population-based studies the prevalence of endometrial hyperplasia in a pre-menopausal population is well under 1%. In a study of 97 women under the age of 36 years with

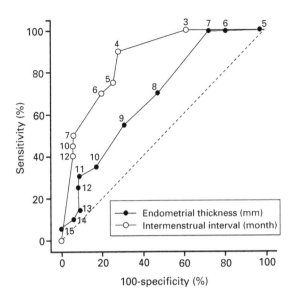

Figure 9.4

Receiver operating characteristic curves for endometrial thickness and intermenstrual interval. The closer the ROC plot is to the upper left corner, the higher the overall accuracy of the test. When the variable under study cannot distinguish between the two groups, the area under the ROC curve is equal to 0.5. From Cheung, 2001.[65]

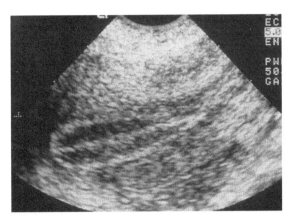

Figure 9.5

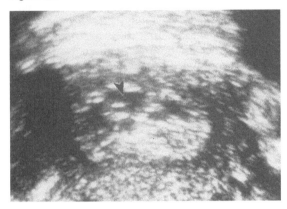

Figure 9.6

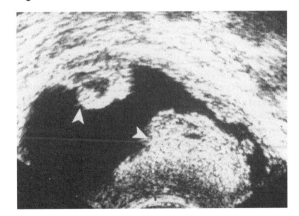

Figure 9.7

Figures 9.5–9.7

Ultrasound illustrations of normal endometrium (Figure 9.5), cystic hyperplasia (Figure 9.6) and endometrial adenocarcinoma (Figure 9.7).

adenomatous or atypical adenomatous hyperplasia, 25% were found to have typical polycystic ovaries confirmed by biopsy.[60] In one small study of 36 pre-menopausal women with PCOS, the rate of endometrial hyperplasia was an astounding 64%.[65] The author examined the predictive value of sonographic endometrial thickness (primary objective) and the menstrual history with other clinical characteristics (secondary objective) for proliferative endometrium and endometrial hyperplasia, by logistic regression analysis. Their predictive value was further examined by receiver operating characteristic (ROC) curve analysis (Figure 9.4). Endometrial thickness less than 7 mm or intermenstrual interval less than 3 months (corresponding to more than four menstrual periods yearly) were associated with proliferative endometrium only. The endometrial thickness correlated positively with endometrial hyperplasia (p = 0.018) and, together with the average intermenstrual interval, was a significant predictor of endometrial hyperplasia (p <0.001) (Figures 9.5–9.7).[65]

Prevention and treatment of endometrial hyperplasia/cancer

It is generally accepted that for women with PCOS who experience symptoms of amenorrhea, or oligomenorrhea, the induction of artificial withdrawal bleeds to prevent endometrial hyperplasia is prudent management. Indeed we consider it important that women with PCOS shed their endometrium at least every 2–3 months. An alternative is to use a progesterone-releasing intrauterine system (Mirena IUS®). For those with oligo-/amenorrhea who do not wish to use cyclical hormone therapy or a Mirena® coil, we recommend an ultrasound scan to measure endometrial thickness and morphology every 6–12 months (depending upon menstrual history). An endometrial thickness greater than 10 mm in an amenorrheic woman warrants an artificially induced bleed, which should be followed by a repeat ultrasound scan and endometrial biopsy if the endometrium has not been shed. Also any women who experiences a period of persistent vaginal bleeding after a prolonged period of amenorrhea should be evaluated by endometrial sampling.

The rationale for these recommendations is largely empiric. The frequency of induced cycles as well as the type of cyclic oral progestin therapy that prevents endometrial cancer in women with PCOS is unknown. Extrapolating from the post-menopausal hormone replacement literature, monthly treatments for a minimum of 10 days and perhaps longer are optimal.[66] Oral contraceptives in the larger population have been associated with a significant reduction in endometrial cancer risk (≥50% decrease), a benefit that persists for at least 10 years after stopping.[67–69] No differences were detected in a retrospective case-control study on the effect of the type of progestin on endometrial cancer risk, and even low-dose formulations were effective.[70] There are no studies to address the hypothesis of additional benefit in a PCOS population.

Some authors have also reported conservative management of endometrial adenocarcinoma in women with PCOS. The rationale is that cancer of the endometrium often presents at an early stage, is well differentiated, of low risk of metastasis and therefore is not perceived as being life-threatening.[71,72] Furthermore, these women are young and usually desirous of fertility. Fechner and Kaufman reported four cases of well-differentiated carcinoma in women aged 21–34 years, of whom two had a hysterectomy; one had a wedge resection, a subsequent regular menstrual cycle and no recurrence after 12 years – although she remained nulliparous; the fourth, aged 21 years, was treated with both wedge resection and clomifene citrate but eventually required hysterectomy for metromenorrhagia two years later – at which time there was still a superficial adenocarcinoma.[73] The authors suggest that if the histology indicates a well-differentiated lesion a conservative approach is acceptable, while poorly differentiated adenocarcinoma in a young woman has a worse prognosis and warrants hysterectomy.[73] Farhi et al agree with this suggestion, and used a combination of curettage and high-dose progestogens in three patients, one of whom later bore two children; nevertheless, seven of the ten patients that they reported required hysterectomy.[72] Others have also advocated a conservative approach, for example Muechler et al went as far as to induce ovulation with human menopausal gonadotropins in a woman who had a well-differentiated adenocarcinoma treated with medroxyprogesterone acetate for 6 months, following which there was persistent adenomatous hyperplasia but no malignancy.[74] The patient conceived twice, had a miscarriage of twins and then a successful singleton pregnancy, following which a hysterectomy was performed (histology again showed adenomatous hyperplasia but no malignancy).[74] Another case employed the use of hysteroscopically guided biopsy and endometrial curettage with clips applied to the fallopian tubes, in order to prevent retrograde spread of tumorous cells.[75] In this case, laparoscopic ovarian diathermy was used to reduce ovarian activity and follow-up treatment was first with progestins and then the combined oral contraceptive pill.[75]

In general, however, the literature on women with PCOS and endometrial hyperplasia or adenocarcinoma suggests that this group of patients has a poor prognosis for fertility. This may be because of the factors that predisposed to the endometrial pathology – chronic anovulation combined often with severe obesity – or secondary to the endometrial pathology disrupting potential embryonic implantation. Case studies and small series of cases treated successfully without recourse to hysterectomy may be

Table 9.4 Studies of breast cancer risk in polycystic ovary syndrome. From Solomon, 1999[84]

Study	Design	Findings	Comments
Coulam et al, 1983[30]	Retrospective cohort; 1270 women with chronic anovulation versus population incidence rates	RRs associated with PCOS: pre-menopausal, 1.3 (0.3–3.2); peri-menopausal, 0.9 (0.2–2.5); post-menopausal, 3.6 (1.2–8.3)	Only 698 person-years of follow up in post-menopausal group; not adjusted for other confounders
Gammon & Thompson, 1991[78]	Case-control study: 4730 breast cancer cases; 4688 controls, 20–54 years old	OR associated with PCOS: age-adjusted, 0.52 (0.32–0.87); multivariate, 0.47 (0.26–0.85)	PCOS reported by 23 cases, 44 controls; menopausal status did not affect results; PCOS self-reported, not validated
Anderson et al, 1997[79]	Prospective cohort (Iowa Women's Health Study) 55–69 years old at study entry; 472 women reporting PCOS	RR associated with PCOS: age-adjusted, 1.2 (0.7–2.0); multivariate, 1.0 (0.6–1.9)	Physician diagnosis of PCOS reported by 472, not validated; majority of these women reported regular cycles
Pierpont et al, 1998[58]	Retrospective cohort; SMR calculated for 786 PCOS cases (versus national rates) over mean 30 years' follow up	SMR for breast cancer associated with PCOS: 1.48 (0.79–2.54)	Not adjusted for confounders; non-fatal disease not assessed

RR = relative risk; OR = odds ratio; SMR = standardized mortality ratio.

subject to publication bias and may not represent widespread medical opinion.[76] There are fewer examples of published failure of conservative therapy. Thus a more traditional and radical surgical approach is suggested as the safest way to prevent progression of the cancer.[77]

Breast cancer and polycystic ovary syndrome

There is no consistent association reported between PCOS and breast cancer (Table 9.4). The study by Coulam et al calculated a relative risk (RR) of 1.5 (95% CI = 0.75–2.55) for breast cancer in their group of women with chronic anovulation, which was not statistically significant.[30] After stratification by age however, the RR was found to be 3.6 (95% CI = 1.2–8.3) in the post-menopausal age group. Conversely Gammon and Thompson reported a reduced risk of breast cancer in women with PCOS, finding an odds ratio of 0.52 (95% CI = 0.32–0.87).[78] This study

however is difficult to interpret as the prevalence of PCOS as identified by a self-assessed questionnaire was found to be only 0.49% in their 4697 cases and only 0.94% in the 4657 controls. These prevalence rates fall well below estimates expected for the normal population, and indicate that the method used to determine the presence of PCOS was not sufficiently sensitive.

Similar comments could be applied to the work by Anderson et al who designed a large prospective study to examine the development of breast carcinoma in post-menopausal women.[79] The prevalence of PCOS in their cohort of 34,835 women was found to be only 1.35%, and they determined that PCOS was not associated with an increased risk of breast carcinoma in this cohort. In this series, although women with PCOS were 1.8 times as likely to report benign breast disease as control women (p <0.01), they were not more likely to develop breast carcinoma (RR = 1.2; 95% CI = 0.7–2). Adjustment for age at menarche, age at menopause, parity, oral contraceptive use, body mass index (BMI), waist-to-hip ratio, and family history of breast carcinoma lowered the RR to 1 (95% CI = 0.6–1.9.). Thus, despite the high-risk profiles of some women with PCOS, these results do not suggest that the syndrome per se is associated with an increased risk of post-menopausal breast carcinoma.[79]

More recently Pierpoint et al reported a series of 786 women with PCOS in the UK who were traced from hospital records after histological diagnosis of polycystic ovaries between 1930 and 1979.[58] Mortality was assessed from the national registry of deaths and standardized mortality rates (SMR) calculated for patients with PCOS compared with the normal population. The average follow-up period was 30 years. The SMR for all neoplasms was 0.91 (95% CI = 0.60–1.32) and for breast cancer 1.48 (95% CI = 0.79–2.54). In fact breast cancer was the leading cause of death in this cohort.

Based on this conflicting literature, it is premature to recommend either alternative screening strategies or preventive strategies for breast cancer in women with PCOS.

Ovarian cancer and polycystic ovary syndrome

In recent years there has been much debate about the risk of ovarian cancer in women with infertility, particularly in relation to the use of drugs to induce superovulation for assisted conception procedures. Inherently the risk of ovarian cancer appears to be increased in women who have multiple ovulations – that is those who are nulliparous (possibly because of infertility), with an early menarche and late menopause. Thus it may be that inducing multiple ovulations in women with infertility will increase their risk,[80] a notion that is by no means proven.

Women with PCOS who are oligo-/anovulatory might therefore be expected to be at low risk of developing ovarian cancer if it is lifetime number of ovulations rather than pregnancies that is critical. Ovulation induction to correct anovulatory infertility aims to induce unifollicular ovulation and so, in theory, should raise the risk of a woman with PCOS to that of a normal ovulating woman. The polycystic ovary, however, is notoriously sensitive to stimulation and it is only in recent years with the development of high-resolution transvaginal ultrasonography that the rate of

unifollicular ovulation has attained acceptable levels.[81] The use of clomifene citrate and gonadotropin therapy for ovulation induction in the 1960s, 1970s and 1980s resulted in many more multiple ovulations (and indeed multiple pregnancies) than in more recent times, and these women might therefore present with an increased rate of ovarian cancer when they reach the age of greatest risk.

Another line of argument supporting an increased risk of ovarian cancer in women with PCOS suggests that, although affected women are relatively anovulatory, their ovaries are undergoing constant follicular recruitment, though the follicles arrest at an early stage. This constant turnover of follicles, especially with subcapsular follicles which may interact with the overlying epithelium, may contribute to an increased risk for epithelial cancer of the ovary. Some argue that the animal model of a luteinizing hormone (LH)-hypersecreting mouse, which has a hyperandrogenic phenotype and an increased risk for ovarian tumors, may also be applicable to women with PCOS.[82]

This however is poorly supported in the literature on humans. There are a few studies that have addressed the possibility of an association between polycystic ovaries in women and ovarian cancer. The results are conflicting, and generalizability is limited due to problems with the study designs. Coulam et al showed no increased risk of ovarian carcinoma in their group of anovulatory women.[30] Schildkraut et al however suggested that PCOS conferred a RR of 2.5 (95% CI = 1.1–5.9) for epithelial ovarian cancer in their case-control study.[83] The prevalence of PCOS as determined by questionnaire was found to be 1.5% in cases, and 0.6% in controls. The authors acknowledge that the small number of women with PCOS limits the interpretation of their findings, and that consideration must be given to the possibility of recall bias in subjects affected with ovarian cancer. In the large UK study of Pierpoint et al the standardized mortality rate for ovarian cancer was 0.39 (95% CI = 0.01–2.17).[58]

Summary

PCOS is common, and the criteria used for its diagnosis are varied, although becoming more

---

Key points

- Women with PCOS have been reported to be at increased risk for a number of gynecological neoplasias, including endometrial, breast, and ovarian cancer. The data supporting an increased risk are almost entirely inferential, based primarily on small cases series, or shared risk factors.
- Ultrasonography has been found to be a useful screening tool for endometrial pathology in a post-menopausal symptomatic population – an endometrial thickness of less than 5 mm is rarely associated with endometrial carcinoma. The mean thickness of the endometrium was significantly elevated in cases of endometrial hyperplasia and endometrial carcinoma (12–14 mm) compared with a benign endometrium. Normative data in pre-menopausal women are more variable and less well quantified. An endometrial thickness of less than 7 mm or an intermenstrual interval less than 3 months are associated with proliferative endometrium only.
- The induction of artificial withdrawal bleeds to prevent endometrial hyperplasia is prudent management. An alternative is to use a progesterone-releasing intrauterine system (Mirena IUS®).
- There is no consistent association reported between PCOS and breast cancer. Based on conflicting literature, it is premature to recommend either alternative screening strategies or preventative strategies for breast cancer in women with PCOS.
- An association between PCOS and ovarian cancer seems unlikely.

---

unified in the literature. Epidemiological studies often incorporate patients with infertility or ovarian dysfunction, which may result in imprecision of diagnostic categories. The association between PCOS and endometrial cancer is perhaps the most plausible, despite the paucity of epidemiological evidence to support it. In the interim, women with PCOS and oligo-/amenorrhea should therefore be screened by ultrasound for endometrial overgrowth and abnormal appearance, and they should be given therapy to promote regular endometrial shedding. Conservative treatment of endometrial hyperplasia may be appropriate in selected cases. There are published data on a few cases to indicate that patients with well-differentiated adenocarcinoma of the endometrium may also be treated conservatively with progestogens and ovulation induction, although only a few pregnancies are reported and the safest approach is probably still hysterectomy. However, it is important to note that the quality of the literature supporting this treatment is as poor as that linking PCOS with endometrial cancer. Let both the doctor and patient beware!

A link between PCOS and cancer of the breast appears probable on both theoretical grounds, although the epidemiological evidence is mixed.

An association between PCOS and ovarian cancer seems unlikely, leaving aside the putative association with ovulation-inducing drugs, which is an issue that should not apply to the modern approach to unifollicular ovulation induction in patients with PCOS and anovulatory infertility.

References

1. Gambrell RD, Jr, Bagnell CA, Greenblatt RB. Role of estrogens and progesterone in the etiology and prevention of endometrial cancer: review. Am J Obstet Gynecol 1983; 146:696–707.
2. Lobo RA, Granger L, Goebelsmann U, Mishell DR, Jr. Elevations in unbound serum estradiol as a possible mechanism for inappropriate gonadotropin secretion in women with PCO J Clin Endocrinol Metab 1981; 52:156–158.
3. Skov BG, Broholm H, Engel U, Franzmann MB et al. Comparison of the reproducibility of the who classifications of 1975 and 1994 of endometrial hyperplasia. Int J Gynecol Pathol 1997; 16:33–37.
4. Kurman RJ, Kaminski PF, Norris HJ. The behavior of endometrial hyperplasia. A long-term study of 'untreated' hyperplasia in 170 patients. Cancer 1985; 56:403–412.
5. Burke TW, Tortolero-Luna G, Malpica A, Baker VV et al. Endometrial hyperplasia and endometrial

cancer. Obst Gynecol Clin North Am 1996; 23:411–456.

6. Nagamani M, Hannigan EV, Dinh TV, Stuart CA. Hyperinsulinemia and stromal luteinization of the ovaries in postmenopausal women with endometrial cancer. J Clin Endocrinol Metab 1988; 67:144–148.

7. Rutanen EM, Stenman S, Blum W, Karkkainen T et al. Relationship between carbohydrate metabolism and serum insulin-like growth factor system in postmenopausal women: comparison of endometrial cancer patients with healthy controls. J Clin Endocrinol Metab 1993; 77:199–204.

8. Gamayunova VB, Bobrov YUF, Tsyrlina EV, Evtushenko TP, Berstein LM. Comparative study of blood insulin levels in breast and endometrial cancer patients. Neoplasma 1997; 44:123–126.

9. Straus DS. Growth-stimulatory actions of insulin in vitro and in vivo. Endocr Rev 1984; 5:356–369.

10. Nagamani M, Stuart CA. Specific binding and growth-promoting activity of insulin in endometrial cancer cells in culture. Am J Obstet Gynecol 1998; 179:6–12.

11. Kaaks R, Lukanova A, Kurzer MS. Obesity, endogenous hormones, and endometrial cancer risk: a synthetic review. Cancer Epidemiol Biomarkers Prev 2002; 11:1531–1543.

12. Colditz GA, Willett WC, Hunter DJ, Stampfer MJ et al. Family history, age, and risk of breast cancer. Prospective data from the Nurses' Health Study. JAMA 1993; 270:338–343.

13. Parslov M, Lidegaard O, Klintorp S, Pedersen B et al. Risk factors among young women with endometrial cancer: a danish case-control study. Ame J Obstet Gynecol 2000; 182:23–29.

14. Ibanez L, de Zegher F, Potau N. Premature pubarche, ovarian hyperandrogenism, hyperinsulinism and the polycystic ovary syndrome: from a complex constellation to a simple sequence of prenatal onset [review]. J Endocrinol Invest 1998; 21:558–566.

15. Nelson CL, Sellers TA, Rich SS, Potter JD et al. Familial clustering of colon, breast, uterine, and ovarian cancers as assessed by family history. Genet Epidemiol 1993; 10:235–244.

16. Huang Z, Hankinson SE, Colditz GA, Stampfer MJ et al. Dual effects of weight and weight gain on breast cancer risk. JAMA 1997; 278:1407–1411.

17. Key TJ, Allen NE, Spencer EA, Travis RC. The effect of diet on risk of cancer. Lancet 2002; 360:861–868.

18. Akhmedkhanov A, Zeleniuch-Jacquotte A, Toniolo P. Role of exogenous and endogenous hormones in endometrial cancer: review of the evidence and research perspectives. Ann NY Acad Sci 2001; 943:296–315.

19. Levi F, La Vecchia C, Negri E, Franceschi S. Selected physical activities and the risk of endometrial cancer. Br J Cancer 1993; 67:846–851.

20. McTiernan A, Kooperberg C, White E, Wilcox S et al. Recreational physical activity and the risk of breast cancer in postmenopausal women: the Women's Health Initiative Cohort Study. JAMA 2003; 290:1331–1336.

21. Fisher B, Costantino JP, Wickerham DL, Redmond CK et al. Tamoxifen for prevention of breast cancer: report of the National Surgical Adjuvant Breast and Bowel Project P-1 Study. J Natl Cancer Inst 1998; 90:1371–1388.

22. Sliwinska M, Wojtacki J, Sliwinski W. Endometrial cancer in patients with breast carcinoma treated with tamoxifen: report of two cases and the literature overview. Med Sci Monit 2000; 6:399–406.

23. Writing Group for the Women's Health Initiative Investigators. Risks and benefits of estrogen plus progestin in healthy postmenopausal women: principal results from the women's health initiative randomized controlled trial [see comments]. JAMA 2002; 288:321–333.

24. Anonymous. Effects of hormone replacement therapy on endometrial histology in postmenopausal women. The postmenopausal estrogen/progestin interventions (pepi) trial. The writing group for the PEPI trial [see comments]. JAMA 1996; 275:370–375.

25. Elwood JM, Cole P, Rothman KJ, Kaplan SD. Epidemiology of endometrial cancer. J Natl Cancer Inst 1977; 59:1055–1060.

26. Willett WC, Stampfer MJ, Colditz GA, Rosner BA, Hennekens CH, Speizer FE. Moderate alcohol consumption and the risk of breast cancer. N Engl J Med 1987; 316:1174–1180.

27. Swanson CA, Wilbanks GD, Twiggs LB, Mortel R et al. Moderate alcohol consumption and the risk of endometrial cancer. Epidemiology 1993; 4:530–536.

28. Landis SH, Murray T, Bolden S, Wingo PA. Cancer statistics. Cancer J Clinicians 1998; 48:6–29.

29. Jackson RL, Dockerty MB. The Stein–Leventhal syndrome. Analysis of 43 cases with special reference to endometrial cancer. Am J Obstet Gynecol 1957; 73:161–173.

30. Coulam CB, Annegers JF, Kranz JS. Chronic anovulation syndrome and associated neoplasia. Obstet Gynecol 1983; 61:403–407.

31. Smyczek-Gargya B, Geppert M. Endometrial cancer associated with polycystic ovaries in young women. Pathol Res Pract 1992; 188:946–948, discussion 948–950.

32. Ho SP, Tan KT, Pang MW, Ho TH. Endometrial hyperplasia and the risk of endometrial carcinoma. Singapore Med J 1997; 38:11–15.

33. Hardiman P, Pillay OS, Atiomo W. Polycystic ovary syndrome and endometrial carcinoma. Lancet 2003; 361:1810–1812.

34. Legro RS, Spielman R, Urbanek M, Driscoll D et al.

Phenotype and genotype in polycystic ovary syndrome. Recent Prog Horm Res 1998; 53: 217–256.

35. Dahlgren E, Friberg L-G, Johansson S, Lindstrom B et al. Endometrial carcinoma; ovarian dysfunction – a risk factor in young women. J Obstet Gynecol Reprod Biol 1991; 41:143–150.

36. Goldzieher JW, Axelrod LR. Clinical and biochemical features of polycystic ovarian disease. Fertil Steril 1963; 14:631–653.

37. Chamlian DL, Taylor HB. Endometrial hyperplasia in young women. Obstet Gynecol 1970; 36:659–666.

38. Aksel S, Wentz AC, Jones GS. Anovulatory infertility associated with adenocarcinoma and adenomatous hyperplasia of the endometrium. Obstet Gynecol 1974; 43:386–391.

39. Dahlgren E, Johansson S, Oden A, Lindstrom B, Janson PO. A model for prediction of endometrial cancer. Acta Obstet Gynecol Scand 1989; 68:507–510.

40. Henderson BE, Casagrande JT, Pike MC, Mack T et al. The epidemiology of endometrial cancer in young women. Br J Cancer 1983; 47:749–756.

41. Elwood JM, Cole P, Rothman KJ et al. Epidemiology of endometrial cancer. J Natl Cancer Inst 1977; 59:1055–1060.

42. MacMahon B. Risk factors for endometrial cancer. Gynecol Oncol 1974; 2:122–129.

43. Jackson RL, Dockerty MB. The Stein–Leventhal Syndrome: analysis of 43 cases with special reference to association with endometrial carcinoma. Am J Obstet Gynecol 1957; 73:161–173.

44. Coulam CB, Annegers JF, Kranz JS. Chronic anovulation syndrome and associated neoplasia. Obstet Gynecol 1983; 61:403–407.

45. Meirow D, Schenker JG. The link between female infertility and cancer: epidemiology and possible aetiologies. Hum Reprod Update 1996; 2:63–75.

46. Gibson M. Reproductive health and polycystic ovary syndrome. Am J Med 1995; 98:67S–75S.

47. Chamlian DL, Taylor HB. Endometrial hyperplasia in young women. Obstet Gynecol 1970; 36:659–666.

48. Potischman N, Hoover RN, Brinton LA, Siiteri P et al. Case-control study of endogenous steroid hormones and endometrial cancer. J Natl Cancer Inst 1996; 88:1127–1135.

49. Troisi R, Potischman N, Hoover RN, Siiteri P, Brinton LA. Insulin and endometrial cancer. Am J Epidemiol 1997; 146:476–482.

50. Speert H. Carcinoma of the endometrium in young women. Surg Gynecol Obstet 1949; 88:332–336.

51. Dockerty MB, Lovelady SB, Faust GT. Carcinoma of the corpus uteri in young women. Am J Obstet Gynecol 1951; 61:966–981.

52. Ramzy I, Nisker JA. Histologic study of ovaries from young women with endometrial adenocarcinoma. Am J Clin Pathol 1979; 71:253–256.

53. Gallup DG, Stock RJ. Adenocarcinoma of the endometrium in women 40 years of age or younger. Obstet Gynecol 1984; 64:417–420.

54. Murphy JE, Zhou S, Giese K, Williams LT et al. Long-term correction of obesity and diabetes in genetically obese mice by a single intramuscular injection of recombinant adeno-associated virus encoding mouse leptin. Proc Natl Acad Sci USA 1997; 94:13921–13926.

55. Escobedo LG, Lee NC, Peterson HB, Wingo PA. Infertility-associated endometrial cancer risk may be limited to specific subgroups of infertile women. Obstet Gynecol 1991; 77:124–128.

56. Dahlgren E, Friberg L-G, Johansson S, Lindstrom B et al. Endometrial carcinoma; ovarian dysfunction – a risk factor in young women. J Obstet Gynecol Reprod Biol 1991; 41:143–150.

57. Ho SP, Tan KT, Pang MW, Ho TH. Endometrial hyperplasia and the risk of endometrial carcinoma. Singapore Med J 1997; 38:11–15.

58. Pierpoint T, McKeigue PM, Isaacs AJ, Wild SH, Jacobs HS. Mortality of women with polycystic ovary syndrome at long-term follow-up. J Clin Epidemiol 1998; 51:581–586.

59. Wild S, Pierpoint T, McKeigue P, Jacobs H. Cardiovascular disease in women with polycystic ovary syndrome at long-term follow-up: a retrospective cohort study. Clin Endocrinol (Oxf) 2000; 52:595–600.

60. Chamlian DL, Taylor HB. Endometrial hyperplasia in young women. Obstet Gynecol 1970; 36:659–666.

61. Koss LG, Schreiber K, Oberlander SG, Moussouris HF, Lesser M. Detection of endometrial carcinoma and hyperplasia in asymptomatic women. Obstet Gynecol 1984; 64:1–11.

62. Briley M, Lindsell DR, The role of transvaginal ultrasound in the investigation of women with postmenopausal bleeding. Clin Radiol 1998; 53:502–505.

63. Fistonic I, Hodek B, Klaric P, Jokanovic L et al. Transvaginal sonographic assessment of premalignant and malignant changes in the endometrium in postmenopausal bleeding. J Clin Ultrasound 1997; 25:431–435.

64. Langer RD, Pierce JJ, O'Hanlan KA, Johnson SR et al. Transvaginal ultrasonography compared with endometrial biopsy for the detection of endometrial disease. Postmenopausal estrogen/progestin interventions trial [see comments]. N Engl J Med 1997; 337:1792–1798.

65. Cheung AP. Ultrasound and menstrual history in predicting endometrial hyperplasia in polycystic ovary syndrome. Obstet Gynecol 2001; 98:325–331.

66. Pike MC, Peters RK, Cozen W, Probst-Hensch NM et al. Estrogen-progestin replacement therapy and endometrial cancer [see comments]. J Natl Cancer Inst 1997; 89:1110–1116.

67. Hulka BS, Chambless LE, Kaufman DG, Fowler WC, Jr, Greenberg BG. Protection against endometrial carcinoma by combination-product oral contraceptives. JAMA 1982; 247:475–477.

68. Vessey MP, Painter R. Endometrial and ovarian cancer and oral contraceptives—findings in a large cohort study. Br J Cancer 1995; 71:1340–1342.

69. Weiderpass E, Adami HO, Baron JA, Magnusson C et al. Use of oral contraceptives and endometrial cancer risk (Sweden). Cancer Causes Control 1999; 10:277–284.

70. Voigt LF, Deng Q, Weiss NS. Recency, duration, and progestin content of oral contraceptives in relation to the incidence of endometrial cancer (Washington, USA). Cancer Causes Control 1994; 5:227–233.

71. McDonald TW, Malkasian GD, Gaffey TA. Endometrial cancer associated with feminizing ovarian tumor and polycystic ovarian disease. Obstet Gynecol 1977; 49:654–658.

72. Farhi DC, Nosanchuk J, Silverberg SG. Endometrial adenocarcinoma in women under 25 years of age. Obstet Gynecol 1986; 68:741–745.

73. Fechner RE, Kaufman RH. Endometrial adenocarcinoma in Stein–Leventhal syndrome. Cancer 1974; 34:444–452.

74. Muechler EK, Bonfiglio T, Choate J, Huang KE. Pregnancy induced with menotropins in a woman with polycystic ovaries, endometrial hyperplasia, and adenocarcinoma. Fertil Steril 1986; 46:973–975.

75. Kung FT, Chen WJ, Chou HH, Ko SF, Chang SY. Conservative management of early endometrial adenocarcinoma with repeat curettage and hormone therapy under assistance of hysteroscopy and laparoscopy. Hum Reprod 1997; 12:1649–1653.

76. Vinker S, Shani A, Open M, Fenig E, Dgani R. Conservative treatment of adenocarcinoma of the endometrium in young patients. Is it appropriate? Eur J Obstet Gynecol Reprod Biol 1999; 83:63–65.

77. Jafari K, Javaheri G, Ruiz G. Endometrial adenocarcinoma and the Stein–Leventhal syndrome. Obstet Gynecol 1978; 51:97–100.

78. Gammon MD, Thompson WD. Polycystic ovaries and the risk of breast cancer [see comments]. Am J Epidemiol 1991; 134:818–824.

79. Anderson KE, Sellers TA, Chen PL, Rich SS et al. Association of Stein–Leventhal syndrome with the incidence of postmenopausal breast carcinoma in a large prospective study of women in Iowa. Cancer 1997; 79:494–499.

80. Nugent D, Vandekerckhove P, Hughes E, Arnot M, Lilford R. Gonadotrophin therapy for ovulation induction in subfertility associated with polycystic ovary syndrome (Cochrane Review) In: The Cochrane Library, Issue 4. Oxford: Update Software, 2001:CD000410.

81. Balen A. Endocrine methods of ovulation induction [review]. Bailliere's Clin Obstet Gynaecol 1998; 12:521–539.

82. Risma KA, Clay CM, Nett TM, Wagner T et al. Targeted overexpression of luteinizing hormone in transgenic mice leads to infertility, polycystic ovaries, and ovarian tumors. Proc Natl Acad Sci USA 1995; 92:1322–1326.

83. Schildkraut JM, Schwingl PJ, Bastos E, Evanoff A, Hughes C. Epithelial ovarian cancer risk among women with polycystic ovary syndrome. Obstet Gynecol 1996; 88:554–559.

84. Solomon CG. The epidemiology of polycystic ovary syndrome- prevalence and associated disease risks. Endocrinol Metab Clin North Am 1999; 28:247–263.

Chapter 10

Disorders of the pilosebaceous unit: hirsutism and androgenic alopecia

Introduction

Women with polycystic ovary syndrome (PCOS) are plagued by a variety of peripheral androgen-excess disorders, including hirsutism, acne and androgenic alopecia. These all originate in the pilosebaceous unit (PSU), the common skin structure that gives rise to both hair follicles and sebaceous glands (Figure 10.1). Androgen excess most commonly leads to hirsutism, or what is referred to as androgen-dependent hirsutism. This concept may be too simplistic to explain pathological states of the PSU such as hirsutism, acne, and androgenic alopecia. Androgen can be viewed as a growth factor for stimulating development of the PSU, but it is just one among many factors that may contribute to its life cycle. Hyperinsulinemia, commonly found in women with PCOS may also contribute to the activation of the PSU.

Excess androgen-dependent hair growth present in women can result in clinically evident hirsutism. Paradoxically, androgens can exert opposite effects on the hair follicles of the scalp, causing conversion of terminal follicles to vellus-like follicles, a process termed miniaturization. This effect may lead to the development of androgenic alopecia in women or male pattern baldness characterized by frontal and sagittal scalp hair loss. Androgens can also cause increased sebum production and abnormal keratinization of the PSU, contributing to the development of seborrhea and acne evident at puberty and in women with androgen excess.

There are ethnic and genetic differences that can modify the effects of androgens on skin, as demonstrated by the lesser degree of hirsutism present in Eastern Asian women with PCOS.[1]

The prevalence of hyperandrogenism within different groups and ages of women with PCOS has not been determined. It appears that age has a major effect, with younger women more likely to experience acne and hirsutism, while older women experience hirsutism and androgenic alopecia. In a large multicenter trial of an insulin-sensitizing agent in PCOS, only 50% of the randomized subjects had evidence of hirsutism.[2] Thus hirsutism should not be viewed as essential to the diagnosis of PCOS.

This chapter will focus primarily on hirsutism, although androgenic alopecia will be discussed.

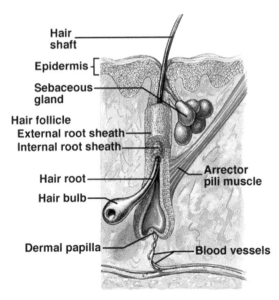

Figure 10.1

Diagram of a pilosebaceous unit.

Hair shaft
Epidermis
Sebaceous gland
Hair follicle
External root sheath
Internal root sheath
Hair root
Hair bulb
Dermal papilla
Arrector pili muscle
Blood vessels

The treatment of hirsutism is somewhat of a dismal science in that there have been few good large-scale randomized controlled trials. Female androgenic alopecia remains the poorer sister, with even less published in this area. Treatment for both of these conditions is still very much empirical.

The pilosebaceous unit

The PSU is the common skin structure that gives rise to both hair follicles and sebaceous glands (Figure 10.1), and which are found everywhere on the body except the palms, soles and lips. The density is greatest on the face and scalp (400–800 glands/cm²) and lowest on the extremities (50 glands/cm²). The number of PSUs does not increase after birth (about five million), but they can become more prominent through activation and differentiation. Generally, three phases of the hair growth cycle can be considered. The period of active growth is termed anagen, after which the hair follicle enters a resting or catagen phase, of varying length of time. During this transition the hair shaft separates from the dermal papillae at the base. The separated hair is then shed during the telogen phase. The period of anagen varies from three years on the scalp to four months on the face. For corresponding parts of the skin, men have longer anagen phases than women do, which may be partially due to their higher circulating androgen levels. Androgens stimulate the transformation of fine, unpigmented vellus hairs to coarse, pigmented, thickened terminal hairs, a process termed terminalization, in skin areas sensitive to the effects of androgens.

The peripheral effects of androgens are determined primarily by the intracellular actions of the enzymes 17β-ketosteroid reductase (converting androstenedione to testosterone) and 5α-reductase (converting testosterone to the more potent androgen dihydrotestosterone (DHT)), and the androgen receptor content. Before puberty, body hair is primarily composed of fine short unpigmented vellus hairs. The increase in androgen production observed with pubertal development transforms some of these, mainly in androgen-sensitive areas of skin such as the axilla and the genital triangle, into the coarser longer pigmented terminal hairs. It should be noted that not all skin areas are androgen sensitive. For example, the development of terminal hairs in body areas such as the eyebrows, eyelashes, and the temporal and occipital scalp is relatively androgen independent. Hirsutism is the presence of terminal (coarse) hairs in females in a male-like pattern. Excessive growth of coarse hairs of the lower forearms and lower legs alone does not constitute hirsutism, although women suffering from hirsutism may note an increase in the pigmentation and growth rate of hairs on these body areas.

Acne also has its origin in the PSU. This also contains a sebaceous gland that produces an oily protective secretion, sebum. The excessive production of sebum, in response to androgen action may lead to oily skin, clogged hair follicles, folliculitis, and the development of acne. Elevations in serum androgen levels have been noted in patients with acne,[3] particularly in those with concurrent hirsutism, although not all investigators agree.[4] Some investigators have observed that while serum androgen levels may be relatively normal in patients with acne, the conversion of androgens to DHT via 5α-reductase was increased in the affected skin.[5]

Assessment of hirsutism and balding

The methodology for the assessment of hirsutism, and response to treatment has been poorly validated.[6] Hirsutism scores are notoriously subjective,[27] and even the most frequently utilized standard of subjective hirsutism scores, the modified Ferriman–Gallwey score, utilizes non-midline, non-androgen-dependent body hair to make the diagnosis (Figure 10.2).[7] A subjective scale is important for discriminating unwanted excess hair with a diffuse distribution (hypertrichosis) from hirsutism. Other scales have focused on midline hair (Figure 10.3),[8,9] and the best discrimination between a control population and a hirsute population has been found using the sum of the scores for four regions: upper lip, chin, lower abdomen and thighs.[9] Interobserver coefficient of variation between two observers was good.[9]

Single-site assessments of the chin or lower abdomen have been found to be sensitive, but to have poor specificity in the larger population

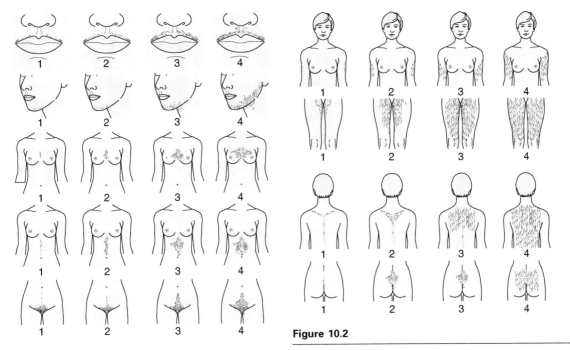

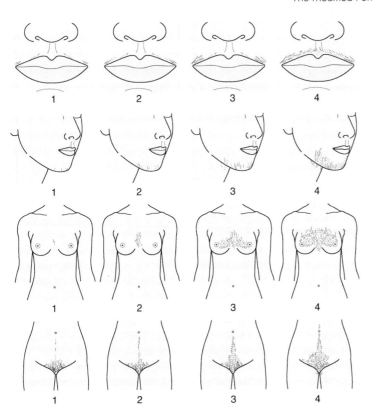

Figure 10.2

The modified Ferriman–Gallwey scale of hirsutism.

Figure 10.3

The Lorenzo scale of hirsutism.

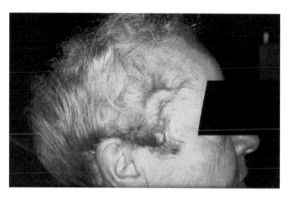

Figure 10.4

A post-menopausal woman with male pattern androgenic alopecia due to a virilizing Sertoli Leydig cell tumor of the ovary (courtesy of Edward Podczaski, MD).

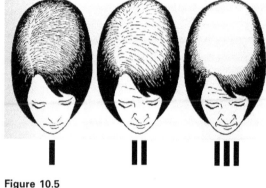

Figure 10.5

The Ludwig scale of female androgenic alopecia. Grade I mild to Grade III severe.

(positive predictive value in the general population of <60%).[10] The Food and Drug Administration's (FDA) approval of eflornithine hydrochloride cream for hirsutism was based on a Physician's Global Assessment (PGA) scale, evaluating facial hair 48 h after shaving on treatment compared to placebo (Vaniqa™ package insert). The methodology of this scale is not yet published.

A variety of objective measurements of hirsutism have been utilized including measuring hair shaft diameter,[11] weighing shaved hair from a specific area,[12] and computerized assessments of digitalized images of hirsute areas.[13] Another confounder of the assessment of hirsutism is the often robust mechanical means women utilize to remove hair, thus 'improving' the amount of hirsutism viewed by a subjective observer.[2]

Scalp hair loss as a consequence of androgen excess can take two forms. In severe cases, where massive androgen excess and virilization/masculinization is present, patients can demonstrate the typical pattern of balding found in men (i.e. premature male-pattern balding) (Figure 10.4). More common, however, is the so-called androgenic (also termed androgenetic as an inherited etiology is often suspected) alopecia of women (i.e. female-pattern balding). In female androgenic alopecia, a diffuse thinning of hair throughout the sagittal scalp is primarily noted. Most commonly the Ludwig scale is used to grade this type of female androgenic alopecia (Figure 10.5).

These grading schemes for hirstuism, and androgenic alopecia are primarily of interest for clinical trials, in clinical practice it is usually the patient's subjective assessment of efficacy that is important for the continuation or change in treatment (or the report of reduction in frequency of using physical methods of hair removal).

Treatment of hirsutism

Treatment options include cosmetic and medical therapies. As drug therapies may take six to nine months or longer before any improvement of hirsutism is perceived, physical treatments including electrolysis, waxing and bleaching may be helpful while waiting for medical treatments to work. For many years the most 'permanent' physical treatment for unwanted hair has been electrolysis. It is time-consuming, painful and expensive and should be performed by an expert practitioner. Regrowth is not uncommon and there is no really permanent cosmetic treatment, but the last few years have seen much development in the use of laser and photothermolysis techniques. There are many different types of laser in production and each requires evaluation of dose intensity, effectiveness and safety. The technique is promising, being faster and more effective than shaving, waxing or chemical depilation. Repeated treatments are required for a near-

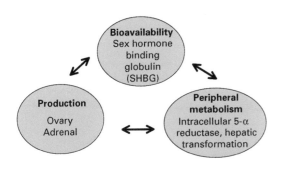

Figure 10.6

The triumvirate of androgen action and targets of therapy to improve hirustism.

permanent effect because only hair follicles in the growing phase are obliterated at each treatment. Hair growth occurs in three cycles, so six to nine months of regular treatments are typical. Patients should be appropriately selected (dark hair on fair skin is best), and warned that complete hair removal cannot be guaranteed and some scarring may occur. At present it is not widely available and is still an expensive option.

Medical regimens should stop further progression of hirsutism and decrease the rate of hair growth. Adequate contraception is important in women of reproductive age as transplacental passage of anti-androgens may disturb the genital development of a male fetus. Most medical methods, while improving hirsutism do not produce the dramatic results women desire, and treatment is often palliative rather than curative. Trials have been hampered by the methodology concerns discussed above, as well as by the small number of subjects. Some of the depilatory treatments utilized by patients are so effective that it is difficult to ever determine baseline hirsutism and response to treatment such that the patient's subjective assessment guides therapy. In general, combination therapies appear to produce better results than single-agent approaches,[14–16] however randomized trials have not established a primary treatment for hirsutism. The choice of combination therapies remains empirical, with variations on a theme as to the best combination.

There have been even fewer trials with androgenic alopecia, so in general, treatment for hirsutism is extrapolated to the treatment of other stigmata of hyperandrogenism at the PSU. In

terms of ameliorating the effects of androgen excess on the PSU, there are a triumvirate of targets to focus on: decreasing production of androgens, decreasing bioavailability of androgens and opposing the action of androgens (Figure 10.6). In terms of directly affecting the cell cycle in the PSU, there is a single agent available, eflornithine hydrochloride crème. It is ironic that this newer agent, which does not directly involve androgen metabolism at all (given the focus of this chapter and of much research in hirsutism) is the only FDA-approved pharmacological therapy of facial hirsutism in women in the US.

Anti-metabolite: eflornithine hydrochloride crème

Eflornithine hydrochoride crème is marketed under the brand name Vaniqa™. Eflornithine is a potent and irreversible inhibitor of the enzyme, ornithine decarboxylase (Figure 10.7). Ornithine decarboxylase is necessary for the production of polyamines, which are important for cell migration, proliferation, and differentiation. Inhibition of this enzyme limits cell division and function. This compound was originally used as a parenteral treatment for *Trypansomoa brucei gamiense*, which causes African sleeping sickness. One of the side-effects of this treatment was hair loss, and subsequently a topical preparation was developed and tested for this purpose.

It is given as a 13.9% crème of eflornithine hydrochloride, and applied to affected areas twice a day for a minimum of four hours each. Two randomized double-blind placebo-controlled trials involving 594 women (both pre- and postmenopausal) have been conducted. The publication of these studies in peer-reviewed journals

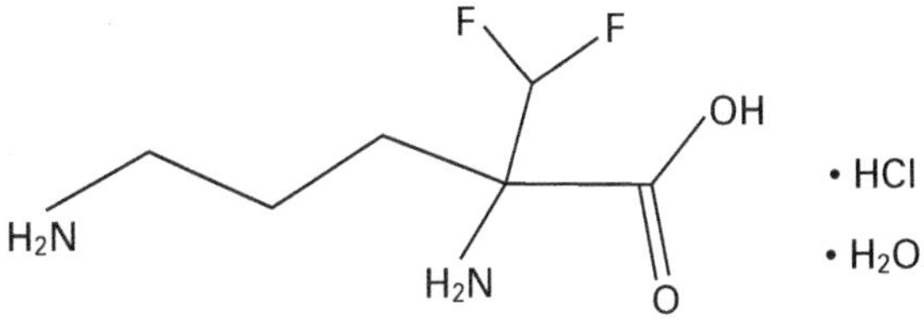

Figure 10.7

Chemical structure of eflornithine.

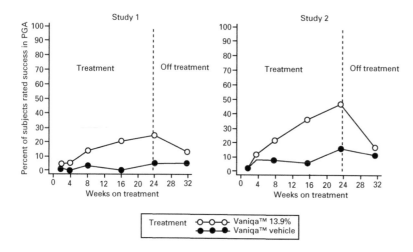

Figure 10.8

Improvement of the Physician's Global Assessment of hirsutism on treatment with eflornithine hydrochloride crème, and reversion to baseline after discontinuing therapy. Reproduced from the package insert.

should yield further information about their efficacy.[17] These studies lasted 24 weeks with an eight-week follow-up phase with no treatment. In these clinical trials, 32% of women showed marked improvement after 24 weeks compared with 8% of placebo-treated women and benefit was first noted at 8 weeks. A total of 58% of subjects experienced some overall improvement (Figure 10.8).

Improvement was assessed using a Physicans' Global Assessment, a four-point scale for evaluating response. Assessments (including the use of photographs) were made by the treating physician, 48 h after shaving, at several points during the study. Additionally, video analysis was performed, as well as patient self-assessment both of which supported the PGA. These trials involved both pre-menopausal and post-menopausal women with hirsutism, as well as an ethnically diverse patient population (60% Caucasian, 30% African American, and 7% Latino).

Eflornithine agent was generally well tolerated with the most common side-effects being stinging of the skin (8.5% of patients on eflornithine compared with 2.5% on placebo) and skin rash (2.8% in the eflornithine group compared with 1.5% of the placebo group). Eflornithine is pregnancy category C, with no known human or animal teratogenicity or toxicity – although theoretically an anti-mitotic, anti-proliferative, and anti-differentiation agent should be avoided during pregnancy and used cautiously in a

population of women seeking pregnancy. There appears to be minimal systemic absorption and circulation of the topical eflornithine when it is only applied to the face.[18] While it has not specifically been studied in other areas of the body, theoretically it would be effective for other midline areas of terminal hair.

Androgen-suppressive therapy

Women with documented hyperandrogenemia would theoretically benefit most from suppressive drugs, although in actual practice the clinical response to this type of therapy does not correlate with androgen levels. Suppression of ovarian androgen secretion has been achieved with oral contraceptives, progestins, or gonadotropin-releasing hormone (GnRH) analog treatment. Glucocorticoids have also been used to suppress adrenal hyperandrogenism, although they are not recommended because of their adverse effect on insulin resistance.

Combined oral contraceptive pills

No combined oral contraceptive pill (COCP) has an approved indication for the treatment of hirsutism in the US, although several forms have

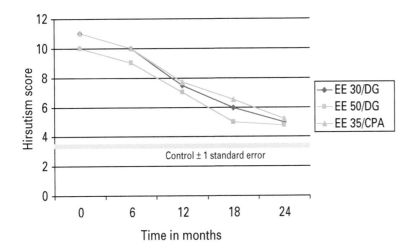

Figure 10.9

Improvement in hirsutism over two-year period. There are no differences according to pill type (EE = ethinyl estradiol, doses in µg, DG = desogestrel, CPA = cyproterone acetate). Adapted from Porcile and Gallardo, 1991.[23]

been approved to treat acne. There are unfortunately only small studies to confirm their benefit in improving hirsutism in PCOS, despite the theoretical appeal that they are the only treatment agent that can address all poles of the androgen action triumvirate (Figure 10.6). COCPs can lower ovarian androgen production by suppressing gonadotropins and indirectly suppressing ovarian androgen biosynthesis. They can markedly increase SHBG levels by the estrogen's effects on the liver. And, depending on the type of progestin chosen, they can also serve as androgen receptor antagonists. A number of observational or non-randomized studies have noted improvement in hirsutism in patients who take the oral contraceptive.[19-21] Few studies have compared varying types of oral contraceptives and no pill has been shown to be superior in treating hirsutism in PCOS.[22]

Onset of action may be prolonged, and is measured in months, if not years. One randomized study of different combination pills showed that hirsutism scores approached normal by two years (Figure 10.9).[23] One observational study of long-term effects noted that mild-to-moderate hirsutism took 36–60 cycles to resolve.[20] It was still present in about a third of women, though ameliorated in severe cases, after 60 cycles.[20] Acne may respond in a shorter time period (12–24 months) and there may be a greater remission rate.[20] A number of studies have found additive benefit when the oral contraceptive pill is combined with other treatment modalities, such as flutamide,[15] or with spironolactone.[24,25] It is noteworthy that both of these latter studies documenting a benefit with COCP and spironolactone, used Diane 35® (also known as Dianette®), which uses cyproterone acetate as its progestin.

The best oral contraceptive for women with PCOS is unknown, although arguably the pill containing a progestin that also functions as an anti-androgen, such as cyproterone acetate (never available in the US) is the best theoretical choice (i.e. Diane® or Dianette®).[26] A new COCP Yasmin® (Schering Healthcare Ltd) has recently been developed, containing ethinyl estradiol 30 µg and a new progestogen drospirenone (5 mg). Drospirenone is derived from 17α spironolactone, unlike most other current progestogens which are derived from 19-nortestosterone and therefore may have androgenic effects. Several studies have shown that drospirenone has a similar pharmacological profile to that of natural progesterone with clinically relevant anti-mineralocorticoid and anti-androgenic effects.[27] Drospirenone increases SHBG levels three- to four-fold. It also works as an antimineralocorticoid and its use may favor weight maintenance or even weight loss. These antimineralocorticoid effects preclude its use in women with renal disease or hyperkalemia. Additional benefit in terms of hirsutism is obtained by its antagonistic properties (much like spironolactone) at the level of the androgen receptor. Thus theoretically, this COCP would improve all three targets in the triumvirate of androgen action (Figure 10.6). There has also been published concern about a potential increased risk for thromboembolism in users, albeit concerning small numbers.[28] We have recently performed a pilot observational study to determine whether the clinical and biochemical features of PCOS are ameliorated by Yasmin®.[29] Seventeen women with PCOS aged 26.4 ± 5.3 years were recruited. Thirteen patients (76%) completed six months' therapy. Hirsutism scores did not change significantly in the women who were clinically hirsute (baseline Ferriman–Galleway score >10). There was, however, a significant improvement in the acne scores (ANOVA p <0.0001). Thus Yasmin® provides good cycle control and relief of acne without having a beneficial effect on hirsutism after 6 months' therapy. Larger randomized controlled trials are required.

Progestins alone

There are minimal data to guide the use of progestins alone in the treatment of hirsutism. A recent Cochrane Database systematic review of the use of progestins and estrogen/progestin combinations to control anovulatory bleeding found no randomized trials.[30] Both depot and intermittent oral medroxyprogesterone acetate (MPA 10 mg × 10 days) have been shown to suppress pituitary gonadotropins and circulating androgens in women with PCOS.[14,31] MPA may also directly inhibit some steroidogenic enzymes, including 3-beta hydroxysteroid dehydrogenase (3β-HSD).[33] However the use of medroxyprogesterone acetate has been associated with decreases in SHBG in PCOS.[34]

Cyproterone acetate alone has been used in many studies and has been found to be effective in treating hirsutism,[35,36] as well as alopecia.[37] This formulation was best for alopecia in obese hyperandrogenic women. The dose of cyproterone acetate when given as a progestin is usually markedly higher than the dose found in the COCP, and is usually 50 mg/day. This high dose is thought to have greater suppressive effects on the hypothalamic–pituitary axis. In at least one study of women with PCOS, this higher dose of progestin was more effective in treating hirsutism than spironolactone alone (Figure 10.10).

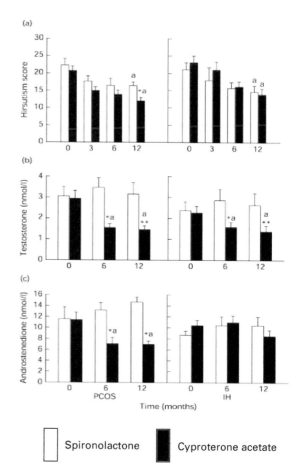

Figure 10.10

(a) Clinical scores for hirsutism with spironolactone and cyproterone acetate (CPA) in women with PCOS and idiopathic hirsutism. CPA. *p <0.05 vs spironolactone at 12 months; a: p <0.05 from baseline values. (b) Testosterone levels with spironolactone and CPA treatments. *p <0.005 vs spironolactone at 6 months; **p <0.05 vs spironolactone at 12 months; a: p <0.05 from baseline values. (c) Androstenedione levels with spironolactone and CPA treatments. *p <0.05 vs spironolactone at 6 and 12 months; a: p <0.05 from baseline values. From Spritzer et al, 2000.[36]

The best pharmacological treatment of proven effectiveness is a combination of the synthetic progestogen cyproterone acetate (CPA, 50–100 mg) which is anti-gonadotrophic and anti-androgenic with ethinyl estradiol (alone or as a COCP, as Dianette® in the UK). Estrogens lower circulating androgens by a combination of a slight inhibition of gonadotropin secretion and gonadotropin-sensitive ovarian steroid production, and by an increase in hepatic production of SHBG, resulting in lower free testosterone. The cyproterone is taken for the first 10 days of a cycle (the 'reversed sequential' method) and the estrogen for the first 21 days. After a gap of exactly 7 days, during which menstruation usually occurs, the regimen is repeated. As an easier and equally effective alternative, the preparation Dianette®, contains ethinylestradiol in combination with cyproterone, although at a lower dose (2 mg).[38] The effect on acne and seborrhea is usually evident within a couple of months. Cyproterone acetate can rarely cause liver damage, and liver function should be checked regularly (after 6 months and then annually). Serum levels of triglycerides, apolipoprotein A-1, A-2, and B may increase with Dianette®. Because of the relatively high dose of ethinyl-estradiol in Dianette® (35 µg) there is theoretically an increased risk of thromboembolism and so treatment should be switched to a lower dose COCP once symptom control has been achieved – usually after 6–9 months.

Gonadotropin-releasing hormone analogs

A GnRH agonist given alone may improve hirsutism, but results in unacceptable bone loss over time. When given in combination with add-back regimens, a GnRH agonist may cause greater lowering of circulating androgens, but little additive effect on improving hirsutism.[39,40] The expense is also prohibitive. Currently there appears to be a limited role for the use of GnRH agonists in the long-term management of hirsutism.

Glucocorticoids

Glucocorticoid suppression of the adrenal also offers theoretical benefits for hirsutism, but deterioration in glucose tolerance and induction of dyslipidemia is problematic for women with PCOS or other metabolic abnormalities, and long-term effects such as osteoporosis are a significant concern. Glucocorticoids may also lead to an iatrogenic exacerbation of a pre-existing Cushingoid habitus. Dexamethasone has been shown to slow hair growth rates in women

already on a GnRH agonist.[41] The use of glucocorticoids to treat hirsutism is rarely advised.

Anti-androgen therapy

None of the anti-androgen agents were developed or are FDA-approved to treat hyperandrogenism in women, and are used empirically in women with hirsutism. These compounds antagonize the binding of testosterone and other androgens to the androgen receptor. As a class therefore, they are teratogenic, and pose risk of feminization of the external genitalia in a male fetus should the patient conceive. This is one reason to use them in combination therapy with the oral contraceptive pill to prevent unexpected pregnancy. There may be additional benefits of this class of agents, including direct inhibition of steroidogenesis. Androgen antagonism may result in improvements in other metabolic variables such as insulin sensitivity and circulating lipids. All appear to offer some benefit, although the best choice for hirsutism is unknown. Randomized trials have found that spironolactone, flutamide and finasteride all have similar efficacy in improving hirsutism (Figure 10.11), although it should be noted that the sample sizes have been inadequate in many cases to detect true differences.[42–44]

Spironolactone

Although spironolactone has had a long and extensive use as an anti-androgen, and multiple clinical trials have been published showing a benefit, the overall quality of the trials and small numbers enrolled have limited the ability of a meta-analysis to document its benefit in the treatment of hirsutism.[45] Spironolactone, a diuretic and aldosterone antagonist, also binds to the androgen receptor with 67% of the affinity of DHT. It has other mechanisms of action, including inhibition of ovarian and adrenal steroidogenesis, competition for androgen receptors in hair follicles, and direct inhibition of 5α-reductase activity. The usual dose is 25–100 mg twice a day and the dose is titrated to balance efficacy with avoiding side-effects. There is a dose–response effect and a long period before benefit is observed – 6 months or more. About 20% of the women will experience increased menstrual

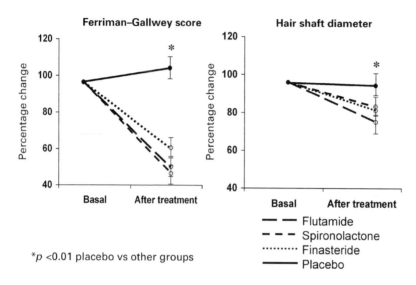

Figure 10.11

Results from a double-blind randomized trial. Changes after therapy (%) in modified Ferriman–Gallwey score and mean hair shaft diameter in the four treatment groups: spironolactone, flutamide, finasteride, and placebo. Error bars indicate standard error. From Moghetti et al, 2000.[44]

frequency and this is one reason for combining spironolactone therapy with a COCP. Because it can cause and exacerbate hyperkalemia, spironolactone should be used cautiously in women with renal impairment. The medication also has potential teratogenicity as an anti-androgen, although exposure has rarely resulted in ambiguous genitalia in male infants. Acne has also been successfully treated with spironolactone. Thus, despite extensive published experience with spironolactone, much of the treatment basis for hirsutism is empirical.

Flutamide

Flutamide is another non-steroidal anti-androgen which has been shown to be effective against hirsutism in observational trials.[46–48] The most common side-effect is dry skin but its use has rarely been associated with hepatitis and renal failure, and so is not recommended for young women with PCOS. A dose of 250 mg/day is given. There is greater risk of teratogenicity with this compound and contraception should be used. The mechanism, even with this agent can be debated as there is evidence to suggest that anti-androgens may also improve insulin sensitivity in hyperandrogenic women.[49]

Finasteride

There are two forms of the enzyme 5α-reductase, type 1 predominantly found in the skin and type 2,

predominantly found in the prostate and reproductive tissues. Finasteride inhibits both forms and is available as a 5 mg tablet for the treatment of prostate cancer and a 1 mg tablet for the treatment of male alopecia. It has been found to be effective for the treatment of hirsutism.[50,51] Finasteride is better tolerated than other anti-androgens with minimal hepatic and renal toxicity, but has the highest and clearest risk for teratogenicity in a male fetus, and adequate contraception must be used.

Increasing sex hormone binding globulin

Increasing SHBG is a legitimate treatment target for women with PCOS and hirsutism. SHBG is nature's androgen sponge. It soaks up circulating androgens (the preferred ligand, with much greater affinity than estrogens or progestins) and removes them from the bioavailable pool. The COCP is the classic drug for increasing SHBG as noted above. Since insulin also negatively regulates the hepatic production of SHBG, any improvement in insulin sensitivity should increase circulating levels of SHBG. The classic intervention to improve insulin sensitivity is weight loss, and this has been shown to increase SHBG levels in women with PCOS. This may not, however, translate into immediate improvements

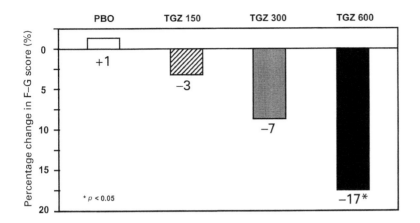

Figure 10.12

The percentage decrease in hirsutism, measured by a modified Ferriman–Gallwey (F–G) score, in patients treated with placebo (PBO) and three different doses (mg) of troglitazone (TGZ), TGZ 150, TGZ 300, and TGZ 600 mg. Note that the decrease in hirsutism score was significantly different from placebo with the use of TGZ 600. From Azziz et al and PCOS/Troglitazone Study Group, 2001.[2]

in hirsutism, which may require, as with the contraceptive pill, longer periods of treatment given the long latency of onset of medical treatments.[52] Pharmacological improvement of insulin sensitivity with biguanides and thiazolidinediones has also been used in women with PCOS.

Insulin-sensitizing agents

Insulin-sensitizing agents have been adapted from the treatment of type 2 diabetes and, by improving insulin sensitivity, improve ambient hyperinsulinemia. It is difficult to separate the effects of improving insulin sensitivity from that of lowering serum androgens, as any 'pure' improvement in insulin sensitivity can raise SHBG and thus lower bioavailable androgen. Given the long onset of action for improving hirsutism, longer periods of observation are needed. In the largest and longest randomized trial to date of these agents, troglitazone (TGZ) at the highest dose of 600 mg was found to significantly improve hirsutism in women with PCOS.[2] The mean percentage improvement was a modest 17% (Figure 10.12). This may have been mediated through a dose–response increase in SHBG, which saw a nearly 10-fold increase in the highest TGZ dose compared to placebo. There were also no differences in total testosterone or androstenedione between treatment groups, only a dose–response reduction in free testosterone, probably mediated through the increase in SHBG.

In small studies with metformin, hirsutism has been unchanged,[53,54] or has shown slight improvement with metformin treatment.[55,56] A recent Cochrane Database analysis of the efficacy of metformin in PCOS found only one study adequately designed to evaluate hirsutism, and this showed no treatment effect. There were no studies for androgenic alopecia.[57] However the meta-analysis did show a significant improvement in hyperinsulinemia and free androgen levels with the use of metformin in women with PCOS.[57] Further study is needed to detect differences between classes of insulin-sensitizing agents, and prolonged benefit over a longer duration of study.

Mechanical and chemical depilatory methods

Mechanical hair removal (shaving, plucking, waxing, depilatory creams, electrolysis, and laser vaporization) can control hirsutism, and often are the front-line treatment used by women. Shaving may be the most helpful and most frequently used temporary method. There is no evidence that shaving can increase hair follicle density or size of the hair shaft.[58] Judicious plucking can be helpful if tolerated, but care must be taken to avoid folliculitis, pigmentation, and scarring. Waxing and depilatories are used less commonly, and have potential adverse side-effects.[59] Depilating agents, while useful, can result in chronic skin irritation and worsening of hirsutism if used excessively or indiscriminately. The use of plucking and/or waxing in androgenized skin areas should be discouraged, since these

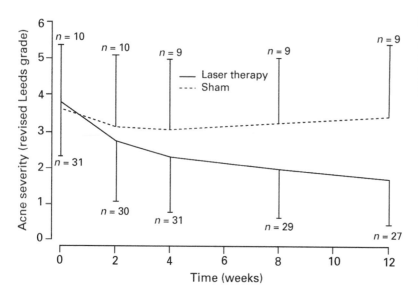

Figure 10.13

Change in acne severity over time with pulsed-dye laser therapy compared to sham treatment. Error bars indicate standard differences. From Seaton et al, 2003.[64]

techniques not only do not kill the hair follicles, but can also induce folliculitis and trauma to the hair shaft, with subsequent development of ingrown hairs and further skin damage.

Electrolysis

There are three electrolysis modalities.[60] With galvanic electrolysis, a direct current is passed down a needle inserted into the hair follicle, destroying the follicle. In thermolysis, a high-frequency alternating current is passed down the needle and produces destructive heat. The blend is the third modality, which combines galvanic electrolysis and thermolysis. Electrolysis satisfactorily removes hair from women and men with hypertrichosis, but women with hirsutism require concomitant hormonal management. Shaving one to five days before electrolysis greatly increases efficacy because it ensures that only growing anagen hairs are epilated. Electrolysis is tedious, highly operator dependent, and may be impractical for the treatment of large numbers of hairs. Electrologists are supervised to varying degrees in different states and countries.

Laser hair removal

The method for laser and light-assisted hair removal is based on the theory of selective photothermolysis.[61] The main objective of laser

therapy for hair removal is to selectively cause thermal damage of the hair follicle without destroying adjacent tissues, a process termed selective photothermolysis. Selective photothermolysis relies on the selective absorption of a brief radiation pulse to generate and confine heat at specific pigmented targets. Lasers useful in hair removal may be grouped into three categories based on the type of laser or light source each employs:

- red light systems (694 nm ruby)
- infrared light systems (755 nm alexandrite, 800 nm semiconductor diode, or 1064 nm neodymium:Yttrium-Aluminum-Garnet (Nd:YAG))
- intense pulsed light (IPL) sources (590–1200 nm).

After laser-assisted hair removal, most patients experience erythema and edema lasting no more than 48 h. Blistering or crusting may occur in 10–15% of patients. Temporary hyperpigmentation occurs in 14–25% of patients and hypopigmentation occurs in 10–17% of patients.

Dyspigmentation is less common with the use of longer wavelengths, as in the alexandrite or diode lasers, and longer pulse durations. Overall, laser hair removal is a promising technique for the treatment of the hirsute patient. Randomized studies have demonstrated a benefit over control areas,[62] but no specific laser type or method has been found to be superior for the treatment of hirsutism.[63] A recent well-designed trial for the treatment of inflammatory cystic acne found a significant treatment effect for a low irradiation density, pulsed-dye laser compared to a sham laser method (Figure 10.13).[64] Nonetheless, we should note that most studies have been uncontrolled and included fewer than 50 patients (and have not specifically focused on women with PCOS), none have been blinded, and all have used a variety of treatment protocols, equipment, skin types, and hair colors studied. Hair is damaged with wavelengths of light well absorbed by follicular melanin and pulse durations that selectively thermally damage the target without damaging surrounding tissue. Women with dark hair and light skin are ideal candidates, and it appears to be most effective during anagen. Due to the skew of hair follicles among varying segments of the hair growth cycle, multiple treatments may be necessary.

Summary

Androgen excess plays a pivotal role in the development of disorders of the PSU, but other factors also contribute. Hirsutism studies are difficult to perform due to the lack of a validated scale, as well as to the success of mechanical and depilatory agents in modifying the baseline and treated phenotype. There are a number of treatments available to treat hirsutism. Many of these are also applicable to the treatment of alopecia and acne. Most however are empirical and not FDA-approved. In general multi-agent treatment has been used to treat hirsutism through a variety of mechanisms. The oral contraceptive pill remains emblematic of this, as it offers benefits through a number of mechanisms. Avoiding unwanted pregnancy and potential unrecognized fetal exposure and teratogenicity is another benefit to contraceptive pill use, important considerations when anti-androgens are used. The combination of methods must be balanced not only against the benefit received, but also the costs of multiple agents, as well as potential side-effects and interactions with other medications.

Onset of action with medical treatments can last several months with years required to obtain the full benefit. Physical removal methods including electrolysis and laser are often used as adjuvant therapies after adequate medical suppression has been achieved. Further randomized trials of these mechanical methods are eagerly awaited. In the future we may see the continued development and utilization of agents that directly inhibit the cell cycle or cellular differentiation in the PSU such as is the case with eflornithine hydrochloride.

Key points

- There are a number of anti-androgens with differing degrees of efficacy:
  Eflornithine hydrochloride creme
  Combined oral contraceptive pill
  Cyproterone acetate (Dianette®)
  Drosperinone (Yasmin®)
  Spironolactone
  Anti-androgens (flutamide, finasteride)
  Progestogens
  GnRH agonists
  Insulin-lowering agents.
- Reliable contraception should be used.
- Physical methods include depilatory creams, electrolysis and laser therapy. These can be expensive but are a useful adjunct to medical treatment.
- Therapy for hirsutism may take at least 6 months before a benefit is observed.
- Androgen-dependent alopecia is very hard to treat, with therapies being palliative rather than curative.

References

1. Carmina E, Koyama T, Chang L, Stanczyk FZ, Lobo RA. Does ethnicity influence the prevalence of adrenal hyperandrogenism and insulin resistance in polycystic ovary syndrome? Am J Obstet Gynecol 1992; 167:1807–1812.
2. Azziz R, Ehrmann D, Legro RS, Whitcomb RW et al. and PCOS/Troglitazone Study Group. Troglitazone improves ovulation and hirsutism in the polycystic ovary syndrome: a multicenter, double blind, placebo-controlled trial. J Clin Endocrinol Metab 2001; 86:1626–1632.
3. Slayden SM, Moran C, Sams WM, Jr, Boots LR, Azziz R. Hyperandrogenemia in patients presenting with acne. Fertil Steril 2001; 75:889–892.
4. Cibula D, Hill M, Vohradnikova O, Kuzel D et al. The role of androgens in determining acne severity in adult women. Br J Dermatol 2000; 143:399–404.
5. Lookingbill DP, Horton R, Demers LM, Egan N et al. Tissue production of androgens in women with acne. J Am Acad Dermatol 1985; 12:481–487.
6. Barth JH. How robust is the methodology for trials of therapy in hirsute women? Clin Endocrinol (Oxf) 1996; 45:379–380.
7. Hatch R, Rosenfield RL, Kim MH, Tredway D. Hirsutism: implications, etiology, and management. Am J Obstet Gynecol 1981; 140:815–830.
8. Lorenzo EM. Familial study of hirsutism. J Clin Endocrinol Metab 1970; 31:556–564.
9. Derksen J, Moolenaar AJ, Van Seters AP, Kock DF. Semiquantitative assessment of hirsutism in dutch women. Br J Dermatol 1993; 128:259–263.
10. Knochenhauer ES, Hines G, Conway-Myers BA, Azziz R. Examination of the chin or lower abdomen only for the prediction of hirsutism. Fertil Steril 2000; 74:980–983.
11. Barth JH. Semi-quantitative measurements of body hair in hirsute women compare well with direct diameter measurements of hair shafts. Acta Derm Venereol 1997; 77:317–318.
12. Diani AR, Mulholland MJ, Shull KL, Kubicek MF et al. Hair growth effects of oral administration of finasteride, a steroid 5 alpha-reductase inhibitor, alone and in combination with topical minoxidil in the balding stumptail macaque. J Clin Endocrinol Metab 1992; 74:345–350.
13. Gruber DM, Berger UE, Sator MO, Horak F, Huber JC. Computerized assessment of facial hair growth. Fertil Steril 1999; 72:737–739.
14. Anttila L, Koskinen P, Erkkola R, Irjala K, Ruutiainen K. Serum testosterone, androstenedione and luteinizing hormone levels after short-term medroxyprogesterone acetate treatment in women with polycystic ovarian disease. Acta Obstet Gynecol Scand 1994; 73:634–636.
15. Ciotta L, Cianci A, Marletta E, Pisana L et al. Treatment of hirsutism with flutamide and a low-dosage oral contraceptive in polycystic ovarian disease patients. Fertil Steril 1994; 62:1129–1135.
16. De Leo V, Fulghesu AM, la Marca A, Morgante G et al. Hormonal and clinical effects of gnrh agonist alone, or in combination with a combined oral contraceptive or flutamide in women with severe hirsutism. Gynecol Endocrinol 2000; 14:411–416.
17. Balfour JA, McClellan K. Topical eflornithine [Review]. Am J Clin Dermatol 2001; 2:197–201.
18. Malhotra B, Noveck R, Behr D, Palmisano M. Percutaneous absorption and pharmacokinetics of eflornithine hcl 13.9% cream in women with unwanted facial hair. J Clin Pharmacol 2001; 41:972–978.
19. Sobbrio GA, Granata A, D'Arrigo F, Arena D et al. Short-term treatment of hirsutism related to micropolycystic ovary syndrome with a combination type oral contraceptive containing desogestrel. Acta Eur Fertil 1989; 20:35–37.
20. Falsetti L, Gambera A, Tisi G. Efficacy of the combination ethinyl oestradiol and cyproterone acetate on endocrine, clinical and ultrasonographic profile in polycystic ovarian syndrome. Hum Reprod 2001; 16:36–42.
21. Morin-Papunen LC, Vauhkonen I, Koivunen RM, Ruokonen A, Tapanainen JS. Insulin sensitivity, insulin secretion, and metabolic and hormonal parameters in healthy women and women with polycystic ovarian syndrome. Hum Reprod 2000; 15:1266–1274.
22. Sobbrio GA, Granata A, D'Arrigo F, Arena D et al. Treatment of hirsutism related to micropolycystic ovary syndrome (MPCO) with two low-dose oestrogen oral contraceptives: a comparative randomized evaluation. Acta Eur Fertil 1990; 21:139–141.
23. Porcile A, Gallardo E. Long-term treatment of hirsutism: desogestrel compared with cyproterone acetate in oral contraceptives. Fertil Steril 1991; 55:877–881.
24. Tartagni M, Schonauer LM, De Salvia MA, Cicinelli E et al. Comparison of Diane 35 and Diane 35 plus finasteride in the treatment of hirsutism. Fertil Steril 2000; 73:718–723.
25. Sahin Y, Dilber S, Kelestimur F. Comparison of Diane 35 and Diane 35 plus finasteride in the treatment of hirsutism. Fertil Steril 2001; 75:496–500.
26. Prelevic GM, Wurzburger MI, Balint-Peric L, Puzigaca Z. Effects of a low-dose estrogen-antiandrogen combination (Diane-35) on clinical signs of androgenization, hormone profile and ovarian size in patients with polycystic ovary syndrome. Gynecol Endocrinol 1989; 3:269–280.
27. Holdaway IM, Fraser A, Sheehan A, Croxson MS et al. Objective assessment of treatment response in hirsutism. Horm Res 1985; 22:253–259.

27. Krattenmacher R. Drospirenone: pharmacology and pharmacokinetics of a unique progestogen [review]. Contraception 2000; 62:29–38.
28. van Grootheest K, Vrieling T. Thromboembolism associated with the new contraceptive Yasmin. Br Med J 2003; 326:257.
29. Palep-Singh M, Barth JH, Mook K, Balen AH, An observational study of Yasmin in the management of polycystic ovary syndrome. J Fam Plann Reprod Health Care 2004; 30:163–165.
30. Hickey M, Higham J, Fraser IS. Progestogens versus oestrogens and progestogens for irregular uterine bleeding associated with anovulation (Cochrane Review). In: The Cochrane Library, Issue 2. Oxford Update Software, 2000:CD001895.
31. Petsos P, Ratcliffe WA, Anderson DC. Effects of medroxyprogesterone acetate in women with polycystic ovary syndrome. Clin Endocrinol (Oxf) 1986; 25:651–660.
33. Lee TC, Miller WL, Auchus RJ. Medroxy-progesterone acetate and dexamethasone are competitive inhibitors of different human steroido-genic enzymes. J Clin Endocrinol Metab 1999; 84:2104–2110.
34. Wortsman J, Khan MS, Rosner W. Suppression of testosterone-estradiol binding globulin by medroxy-progesterone acetate in polycystic ovary syndrome. Obstet Gynecol 1986; 67:705–709.
35. Carmina E, Lobo RA. Gonadotrophin-releasing hormone agonist therapy for hirsutism is as effec-tive as high dose cyproterone acetate but results in a longer remission. Hum Reprod 1997; 12:663–666.
36. Spritzer PM, Lisboa KO, Mattiello S, Lhullier F. Spironolactone as a single agent for long-term therapy of hirsute patients. Clin Endocrinol (Oxf) 2000; 52:587–594.
37. Vexiau P, Chaspoux C, Boudou P, Fiet J et al. Effects of minoxidil 2% vs. cyproterone acetate treatment on female androgenetic alopecia: a controlled, 12-month randomized trial. Br J Dermatol 2002; 146:992–999.
38. Barth JH, Cherry CA, Wojnarowska F, Dawber RPR. Cyproterone acetate for severe hirsutism: results of a double-blind dose-ranging study. Clin Endocrinol (Oxf) 1991; 35:5–10.
39. Carr BR, Breslau NA, Givens C, Byrd W et al. Oral contraceptive pills, gonadotropin-releasing hormone agonists, or use in combination for treat-ment of hirsutism: a clinical research center study. J Clin Endocrinol Metab 1995; 80:1169–1178.
40. Azziz R, Ochoa TM, Bradley EL, Jr, Potter HD, Boots LR. Leuprolide and estrogen versus oral contracep-tive pills for the treatment of hirsutism: a prospec-tive randomized study [see comments]. J Clin Endocrinol Metab 1995; 80:3406–3411 .
41. Rittmaster RS, Thompson DL. Effect of leuprolide and dexamethasone on hair growth and hormone

42. Wong IL, Morris RS, Chang L, Spahn MA et al. A prospective randomized trial comparing finasteride to spironolactone in the treatment of hirsute women. J Clin Endocrinol Metab 1995; 80:233–238.
43. Falsetti L, De Fusco D, Eleftheriou G, Rosina B. Treatment of hirsutism by finasteride and flutamide in women with polycystic ovary syndrome. Gynecol Endocrinol 1997; 11:251–257.
44. Moghetti P, Tosi F, Tosti A, Negri C et al. Comparison of spironolactone, flutamide, and finasteride efficacy in the treatment of hirsutism: a randomized, double blind, placebo-controlled trial. J Clin Endocrinol Metab 2000; 85:89–94.
45. Lee O, Farquhar C, Toomath R, Jepson R. Spironolactone versus placebo or in combination with steroids for hirsutism and/or acne (Cochrane Review). In: The Cochrane Library, Issue 4. Oxford: Update Software, 2000:CD000194.
46. Fruzzetti F, De Lorenzo D, Ricci C, Fioretti P. Clinical and endocrine effects of flutamide in hyperandro-genic women. Fertil Steril 1993; 60:806–813.
47. Cesur V, Kamel N, Uysal AR, Erdogan G, Baskal N. The use of antiandrogen flutamide in the treatment of hirsutism. Endocrinol J 1994; 41:573–577.
48. Pucci E, Genazzani AD, Monzani F, Lippi F et al. Prolonged treatment of hirsutism with flutamide alone in patients affected by polycystic ovary syndrome. Gynecol Endocrinol 1995; 9:221–228.
49. Moghetti P, Tosi F, Castello R, Magnani CM et al. The insulin resistance in women with hyperandro-genism is partially reversed by antiandrogen treat-ment - evidence that androgens impair insulin action in women. J Clin Endocrinol Metab 1996; 81:952–960.
50. Fruzzetti F, de Lorenzo D, Parrini D, Ricci C. Effects of finasteride, a 5 alpha-reductase inhibitor, on circulating androgens and gonadotropin secretion in hirsute women. J Clin Endocrinol Metab 1994; 79:831–835.
51. Moghetti P, Castello R, Magnani CM, Tosi F et al. Clinical and hormonal effects of the 5 alpha-reduc-tase inhibitor finasteride in idiopathic hirsutism. J Clin Endocrinol Metab 1994; 79:1115–1121.
52. Moran LJ, Noakes M, Clifton PM, Tomlinson L, Norman RJ. Dietary composition in restoring repro-ductive and metabolic physiology in overweight women with polycystic ovary syndrome. J Clin Endocrinol Metab 2003; 88:812–819.
53. Morin-Papunen LC, Koivunen RM, Ruokonen A, Martikainen HK. Metformin therapy improves the menstrual pattern with minimal endocrine and metabolic effects in women with polycystic ovary syndrome. Fertil Steril 1998; 69:691–696.

levels in hirsute women: the relative importance of the ovary and the adrenal in the pathogenesis of hirsutism. J Clin Endocrinol Metab 1990; 70:1096–1102.

54. Morin-Papunen LC, Vauhkonen I, Koivunen RM, Ruokonen A et al. Endocrine and metabolic effects of metformin versus ethinyl estradiol-cyproterone acetate in obese women with polycystic ovary syndrome: a randomized study. J Clin Endocrinol Metab 2000; 85:3161–3168.

55. Ibanez L, Valls C, Potau N, Marcos MV, de Zegher F. Sensitization to insulin in adolescent girls to normalize hirsutism, hyperandrogenism, oligo-menorrhea, dyslipidemia, and hyperinsulinism after precocious pubarche [see comments]. J Clin Endocrinol Metab 2000; 85:3526–3530.

56. Kolodziejczyk B, Duleba AJ, Spaczynski RZ, Pawelczyk L. Metformin therapy decreases hyper-androgenism and hyperinsulinemia in women with polycystic ovary syndrome. Fertil Steril 2000; 73:1149–1154.

57. Lord JM, Flight IHK, Norman RJ. Metformin in polycystic ovary syndrome: systematic review and meta-analysis. Br Med J 2003; 327:951–955.

58. Lord JM, Flight IH, Norman RJ. Metformin in polycystic ovary syndrome: systematic review and meta-analysis. Br Med J 2003; 327:951–953.

59. Inaba M, Anthony J, McKinstry C. Histologic study of the regeneration of axillary hair after removal with subcutaneous tissue shaver. J Invest Dermatol 1979; 72:224–231.

60. Richards RN, Uy M, Meharg G. Temporary hair removal in patients with hirsutism: a clinical study. Cutis 1990; 45:199–202.

61. Richards RN, Electrolysis for the treatment of hypertrichosis and hirsutism. Skin Therapy Lett 1999; 4:3–4.

62. Dierickx CC. Hair removal by lasers and intense pulsed light sources. Semin Cutan Med Surg 2000; 19:267–275.

63. Dierickx CC, Grossman MC, Farinelli WA, Anderson RR. Permanent hair removal by normal-mode ruby laser [see comments]. Arch Dermatol 1998; 134:837–842.

64. Handrick C, Alster TS. Comparison of long-pulsed diode and long-pulsed alexandrite lasers for hair removal: a long-term clinical and histologic study. Dermatol Surg 2001; 27:622–626.

65. Seaton ED, Charakida A, Mouser PE, Grace I et al. Pulsed-dye laser treatment for inflammatory acne vulgaris: randomised controlled trial. Lancet 2003; 362:1347–1352.

Chapter 11
Acne

Introduction

Acne vulgaris is a very common condition particularly in adolescents. It is basically caused by increased activity in sebaceous glands which is dependent on androgens. Acne in women may thus be considered as a manifestation of cutaneous androgenization. It often appears in the teenage years, induced by the burst of pubertal androgenic activity, but if persistent, particularly severe or of late onset, acne is commonly associated with polycystic ovary syndrome (PCOS).

Pathophysiology

Increased sebaceous gland function is of major importance in the etiology of acne. Fueled by overstimulation of the androgen receptors, an excess of sebum is produced. Without this overproduction of sebum, acne vulgaris would not occur. There then follow changes in the pattern of follicular keratinization, with cornification of the infrainfundibulum of the sebaceous gland. This results in impaired drainage, and consequently the formation of comedones. Abnormal microbial colonization of the pilosebaceous duct by *Proprionibacterium acnes* is the next step down the acne pathway which terminates with inflammation (Table 11.1).

When assessed histologically, the keratinous material in the comedone is very dense, has a high lipid content and the squames are coherent. The wall of the comedone, compared with the normal follicular wall, has an increased rate of cellular turnover which also contributes to the additional accumulation of keratinous material.[1]

The lipid content of the skin is also higher than in the normal population.

Hormonal associations

Androgens are known to play a central role in the etiology of acne and increased concentrations of testosterone, androstendione, dehydroepiandrosterone (DHEA) and its sulfate (DHEAS) from ovarian and/or adrenal origin have all been implicated. In addition, testosterone and its 5α-reduced metabolite, dihydrotestosterone (DHT), are androgens produced in the target-tissue.

Although acne and hirsutism are both androgen-driven conditions, both involving the single morphological entity of the pilosebaceous unit (PSU) and quite often presenting simultaneously, especially in PCOS, they do not always appear

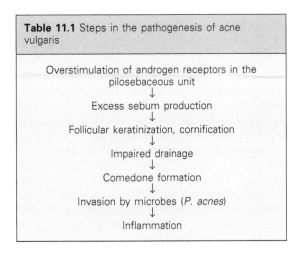

Table 11.1 Steps in the pathogenesis of acne vulgaris

Overstimulation of androgen receptors in the pilosebaceous unit
↓
Excess sebum production
↓
Follicular keratinization, cornification
↓
Impaired drainage
↓
Comedone formation
↓
Invasion by microbes (*P. acnes*)
↓
Inflammation

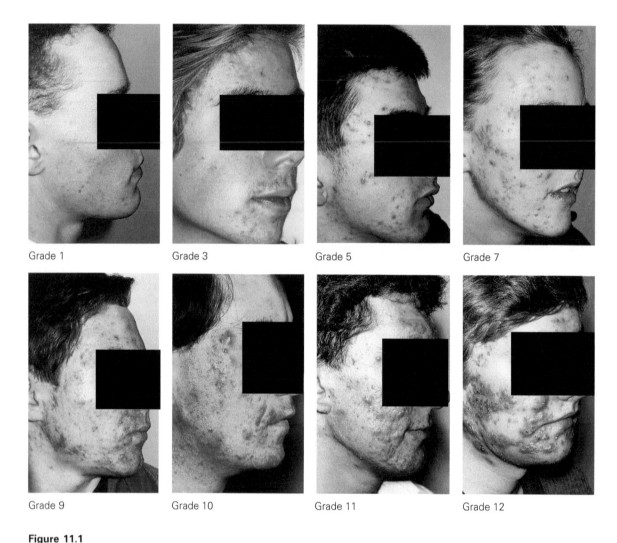

Grade 1   Grade 3   Grade 5   Grade 7

Grade 9   Grade 10   Grade 11   Grade 12

Figure 11.1

Grades of facial acne from 1–10. Cunliffe and Fernandez.[15]

concomitantly. It was hypothesized therefore that there may be some dichotomy in the final pathway of endocrine pathogenesis and, indeed it was found that dihydrotestosterone is further reduced to 3α-androstenediol and its glucuroneride only in hirsute patients but not in patients with acne.[2] These authors concluded that DHT may undergo different metabolic pathways at skin level, supporting the hypothesis that the two clinical entities may be expressions of the different metabolic fate of DHT itself.

The etiology of acne in early adolescence has been associated with increasing serum levels of DHEAS, whereas hirsutism has been more directly linked with high concentrations of free testosterone. The two structures comprising the PSU may have different degrees of sensitivity to similar androgenic stimulation.[2]

The hormonal profiles differ between women who have acne and ultrasonically demonstrated polycystic ovaries compared with women who have acne but morphologically normal ovaries.[3]

Those with polycystic ovaries had raised concentrations of androstendione, DHEA, DHEAS, and luteinizing hormone:follicle-stimulating hormone (LH:FSH) ratio compared with those with normal ovaries. However, within the group of women with polycystic ovaries, hormonal levels differ. Bunker et al, examined a large group of women with polycystic ovaries; those with acne alone were much less likely to have the biochemical features of PCOS (e.g. raised LH and testosterone concentrations), compared with those who had hirsutism and other non-dermatological manifestations of PCOS. This suggested to the authors that those with polycystic ovaries and acne without other clinical characteristics of PCOS may be a distinct subpopulation of women with PCOS.[4]

Grading

Although the clinical severity of acne may be appraised by evaluating the consecutive phases of development (Figure 11.1) (comedo, papules or pustules, nodular or scarring lesions), most physicians (and certainly gynaecologists) use a simpler grading system:

- *mild:* fewer than 10 papules on one side of the face
- *moderate:* more than 10 papules and pustules on one side of the face *or* spread to the shoulders and neck
- *severe:* the above plus deep infiltrates.

Prevalence of polycystic ovary syndrome in women with acne

The majority of women who have acne will have PCOS. The most informative large study examined the ultrasound appearance of the ovaries in 82 females referred to a dermatology clinic with acne vulgaris as the presenting symptom.[5] Of these, 68 (83%) had polycystic ovaries. This staggering figure compares with 19% of women in a control group with no acne who had polycystic ovaries on ultrasound examination. Smaller studies have found a prevalence of ultrasound-diagnosed polycystic ovaries in 52–80% of women with persistent, moderate to severe acne.[3,6] In our view, these types of study have revolutionized much of the treatment of acne, by informing and emphasizing for dermatologists and gynecologists alike, the role of PCOS in its etiology, and applying anti-androgenic therapeutic principles accordingly.

The prevalence of acne in women with PCOS has been less clearly documented, probably due to the fact that it is usually accompanied by more dominant hyperandrogenic symptoms such as hirsutism. However, more than 50% of adolescents who had PCOS were found to have moderate to severe acne.[7]

Treatment of acne

In view of the role that androgens play in the development of acne and seborrhea, anti-androgens are today the cornerstone of the treatment for acne. However, more traditional dermatological treatment is still being used, either alone or combined with anti-androgen therapy. These include antibiotics, administered either topically for mild cases, or systemically for more severe acne. When small nodules are present in more severe types, systemic tetracyclines in combination with topical benzoyl peroxide 5% or tretinoin have been widely applied by dermatologists. Other antibiotics that are prescribed include erythromycin and minocycline. In cases of severe scarring from the acne, tretinoin is often used.

As the acne associated with PCOS undoubtedly arises from over-stimulation of the PSU by androgens, then anti-androgens are the most effective long-term treatment option.

Anti-androgens

There are a number of effective options for anti-androgen therapy, each having its particular site of action to block the synthesis or action of androgens: cyproterone acetate (CPA), spironolactone, flutamide and finasteride (Figure 11.2) (see also Chapter 10).

Excluding North America, a combination of CPA, an orally active progestogen, and ethinyl estradiol (EE) is probably the most widely used anti-androgen (Dianette®, Schering Healthcare

Insulin ← (weight loss, insulin sensitizers)

5α-Reductase (finasteride, CPA)

P450c17α → Androstendione → Testosterone → Dihydrotestosterone

(Receptor blockers – Flutamide, spironolactone, CPA)

LH ← (CPA+EE)

Figure 11.2

Sites of action of anti-androgen agents. Possible treatments are in parentheses. CPA = cyproterone acetate, EE = ethinyl estradiol.

Ltd). CPA has an anti-androgen action at several sites:[8]

1. in combination with EE, suppression of LH release by the anterior pituitary
2. it competes for the androgen receptor which it blocks
3. as a progestogen in suppressing the action of 5α-reductase
4. with EE, it increases SHBG concentrations.

Adrenal steroidogenesis is reduced by CPA, which acts by decreasing the metabolic clearance of cortisol, and is more effective and less appetite inducing than glucocorticoid therapy (taken before sleep) in lowering androgen levels. The combination of CPA (2 mg/day) and EE (35 µg/day) given cyclically has proved very effective in the treatment of acne as well as serving as an excellent contraceptive. Acne has been successfully treated in almost 100% of cases using this minimal dose.[9] The addition of CPA in a dose of 10–100 mg/day on the first 10 days of the combined medication has proved effective for more severe cases. Success rates in reversing or severely diminishing symptoms, and maintaining improvement with minimal side-effects are high, but patients need to be informed that this treatment is not 'instant' and that at least 3–5 months of treatment are needed to see an improvement of the acne. Acne will be cleared in 60% of patients in 6 months and after 12 months, 95% should be free of acne. Side-effects of CPA in combination with EE are similar to those of oral contraceptives, are usually mild and transient, and include mastodinia, increased appetite, change of libido, and headaches. The effects on the lipid profile are usually slight and probably

clinically irrelevant, and include an increase in triglycerides and a small increase in cholesterol, mainly due to an increase in the high-density lipoprotein (HDL) fraction. No significant hepatotoxicity has been reported in a woman using CPA cyclically. Once symptom control has been achieved, standard practice is to switch to a lower dose combined oral contraceptive pill (e.g. one containing 20 µg of EE).

Spironolactone is an aldosterone antagonist but its anti-androgen action is exerted by competitive inhibition of testosterone and DHT binding to the androgen receptor. In the usual dose of 100 mg/day, spironolactone does not seem to suppress either androgen or LH levels. When spironolactone is given to previously cycling women, some menstrual disturbances, particularly polymenorrhea, may occur which are often transient and resolve within a few months. Mild breast tenderness occurs frequently.

A new combined oral contraceptive pill, Yasmin® (Schering Healthcare Ltd) contains drosperinone a derivative of spironolactone, and is currently being evaluated for use in women with PCOS. We have recently observed a significant improvement in acne scores after 6 months of use.[10]

Flutamide is a non-steroidal anti-androgen which has primarily been used in advanced prostatic carcinoma in that it inhibits DHT binding to the androgen receptors. Flutamide has also proved effective in the treatment of hirsutism and acne in women.[11] The efficacy, non-interference with ovulation and generally good tolerance of flutamide, have been tempered by rare reports of hepatotoxicity which may be severe, and the incidence of which seems to increase with higher doses. Careful monitoring of liver function is therefore advised if flutamide is to be used for the treatment of acne and for this reason is seldom advised.

Finasteride has quite a different site of action. It acts by inhibiting the activity of 5α-reductase, the enzyme responsible for the conversion of testosterone to DHT, which is particularly potent at hair follicle level. This treatment is taken orally in a dose of 1–5 mg/day and is effective without any appreciable side-effects although it may need more prolonged treatment to achieve the goal. As with spironolactone and flutamide, contraceptive use is recommended with finasteride in order to avoid the potential risk of feminization of a male fetus.

In patients who have PCOS, these medications have mostly been studied using hirsutism as the end-point, so it is a little difficult to compare their efficacy for the treatment of acne (see Chapter 10). From our personal experience, the combination of CPA and EE has proved effective, simple to use and has had minimal side-effects and good compliance.

However effective these anti-androgen medicines may be, they ameliorate symptoms while they are being taken but fail to 'cure' the cause. After the withdrawal of treatment with spironolactone, flutamide or CPA, acne may relapse, regardless of which anti-androgen therapy is used. What is now becoming clear is that the longer the duration of treatment (at least with CPA/EE) the less the chance of relapse within a given period of time.

An essential element in the successful compliance of the patient on anti-androgen treatment is the accuracy and fullness of information given to her by the physician. First and foremost, it is important to convey the fact that a good clinical response to treatment takes time. Second, it is important to explain the need for long-term maintenance treatment, even when obvious clinical improvement has been achieved. Third, there is the possibility of relapse some time after treatment is terminated.

Weight loss

About 40% of women who have PCOS are obese, and it is well documented that obesity, by exacerbating insulin resistance, increases the severity of the clinical manifestations of PCOS. Acne is no exception. Failure to respond to anti-androgen therapy is much more common in the obese, so

changes in diet and lifestyle for these patients must be recommended in order to achieve full therapeutic success.

Insulin sensitizers

The use of metformin as treatment when acne is the sole symptom is not justified as there is not yet enough supporting evidence. The one (uncontrolled) study using acne as a specific end-point found a significant decrease in the severity of acne when metformin was given in a dose of 500 mg three times a day for 12 weeks.[12] Pioglitazone also significantly improved acne when given to a small group of obese patients with PCOS.[13]

Laparoscopic ovarian drilling (LOD)

While obviously not in contention as treatment for acne, it is interesting to note that long-term follow-up after laparoscopic ovarian drilling (LOD) revealed that 10 of 25 patients who had acne experienced long-term improvement.[14]

Summary

There is little that can be more devastating to a young healthy woman than the stigma of acne which is there for everyone to see. It is a frequent presenting symptom of PCOS, caused by stimulation of the PSU by androgens. The most logical and successful treatment is therefore with anti-androgens. In our experience, the combination of CPA and EE fulfils this role best and has the added advantage of improving hirsutism and regulating menstrual cyclicity.

Key points
• The presence of acne in women with PCOS is androgen dependent.
• Anti-androgens are the mainstay of treatment (e.g. combined oral contraceptive pill, CPA and spironolactone).

References

1. Dramusic V. Hyperandrogenism. In: Dramusic V, Ratnam SS, eds. Clinical approach to paediatric and adolescent gynaecology. Singapore: Oxford University Press 1998:176–179.

2. Toscano V, Balducci R, Bianchi P et al. Two different pathogenic mechanisms may play a role in acne and in hirsutism. Clin Endocrinol (Oxf) 1993; 39:551–556.

3. Betti R, Bencini PL, Lodi A et al. Incidence of polycystic ovaries in patients with late onset or persistent acne: hormonal reports. Dermatologica 1990; 181:109–111.

4. Bunker CB, Newton JA, Conway GS et al. The hormonal profile of women with acne and polycystic ovaries. Clin Exp Dermatol 1991; 16:420–423.

5. Bunker CB, Newton J, Kilborn J et al. Most women with acne have polycystic ovaries. Br J Dermatol 1989; 121:675–680.

6. Jebraili R, Kaur S, Kanwar AJ et al. Hormone profile and polycystic ovaries in acne vulgaris. Ind J Med Res 1994; 100:73–76.

7. Dramusic V, Rajan U, Wong YC et al. Adolescent polycystic ovary syndrome. Ann NY Acad Sci 1997; 816:194–208.

8. Diamanti-Kandarakis E, Tolis G, Duleba A. Androgens and therapeutic aspects of anti-androgens in women. 1995; 2:577–592.

9. van Waygen RG, van den Ende A. Experience in the long term treatment of hisutism and/or acne with cyproterone acetate-containing preparations. Efficacy, metabolic and endocrine effects. Expl Clin Endocrinol Diabetes 1995; 103:241–251.

10. Palep-Singh M, Barth JH, Mook K, Balen AH. An observational study of Yasmin in the management of polycystic ovary syndrome. Br J Fam Plann 2004; 30:163–165.

11. Moghetti P, Castello R, Negri C et al. Flutamide in the treatment hirsutism: long term clinical effects, endocrine changes and androgen receptor behaviour. Fertil Steril 1995; 64:511–517.

12. Kolodziejczyk B, Duleba AJ, Spaczynski RZ, Pawelczyk L. Metformin therapy decreases hyperandrogenism and hyperinsulinemia in women with polycystic ovary syndrome. Fertil Steril 2000; 73:1149–1154.

13. Romualdi D, Guido M, Ciampelli M et al. Selective effects of pioglitazone on insulin and androgen abnormalities in normo-and hyperinsulinaemic obese patients with polycystic ovary syndrome. Hum Reprod 2003; 18:1210–1218.

14. Amer SA, Gopalan V, Li TC et al. Long term follow-up of patients with polycystic ovary syndrome after laparoscopic ovarian drilling: clinical outcome. Hum Reprod 2002; 17:2035–2042.

15. Cunliffe JW, Fernandez C. The Leeds acne grading system. J Dermatol Treat 1998; 9:215–220.

Chapter 12
Menstrual disturbances

Introduction

Menstrual disturbance, particularly oligo- and amenorrhea, is one of the cardinal signs and symptoms of polycystic ovary syndrome (PCOS). This symptom, when associated with polycystic ovaries and/or signs of hyperandrogenism, usually infers absent or irregular ovulation which is mostly implicated as the source of infertility in these patients.

Definitions

- *Oligomenorrhea:* occurrence of menstrual bleeding at an interval of 35 days to 6 months.
- *Amenorrhea:* no menstrual bleeding for 6 months or more.
- *Polymenorrhea:* menstrual bleeding at a frequency of more than once in 21 days. This type of bleeding is usually associated with anovulation.
- *Regular cycles:* menstrual bleeding occurring at intervals of between 22 and 35 days and not varying in length by more than 2 to 3 days each month.

Incidence

Because of different definitions that have been used, it is difficult to estimate the prevalence of menstrual disturbances in PCOS. However, in the largest series published using ultrasonically diagnosed polycystic ovaries as the marker,[1] 29.7% had normal cycles, 47% oligomenorrhea, 19.2% amenorrhea, 2.7% polymenorrhea, and 1.4% menorrhagia. These figures are remarkably consistent with those of a smaller study from a different center that examined the prevalence of menstrual disturbance in women who had both ultrasound features of polycystic ovaries and clinical and/or biochemical evidence of hyperandrogenism, i.e. PCOS.[2] In this study, 73.6% had oligo-/amenorrhea and 26.4% had regular menses.

Looking from another angle, 87% of women with oligomenorrhea and 26% of those with amenorrhea presenting at a gynecological endocrine clinic were found to have polycystic ovaries on ultrasound examination.[3] Clearly, menstrual disturbance is a very prevalent feature of PCOS, and polycystic ovaries are found in the vast majority of women with oligomenorrhea.

Associations

The presence and severity of menstrual disturbances have variously been associated with a number of factors. These include obesity, insulin resistance, serum androgen and luteinizing hormone (LH) concentrations, and the size of the follicle cohort.

Regular menstrual cycles were present in 32% of women with polycystic ovaries and a body mass index (BMI) <30 kg/m^2 in contrast to 22% of those with a BMI of >30.[1] The intimate association of obesity and its exacerbating effect on insulin resistance in women with PCOS has prompted a number of studies to investigate whether insulin insensitivity influences menstrual regularity. Groups of women with polycystic ovaries, hyperandrogenism and oligomenorrhea, and those with polycystic ovaries, hyperandrogenism, and regular periods were examined for insulin resistance.[2] Insulin sensitivity was significantly decreased in those with oligomenorrhea compared with women with PCOS but regular cycles, and compared with controls with normal ovaries. The combination of insulin insensitivity and polycystic ovaries is thus associated with anovulation and irregular cycles.

Menstrual irregularity may be related to the magnitude of insulin sensitivity or insulin secretion.[4]

High LH concentrations have also been associated with menstrual irregularity. In a series of 1741 women with ultrasonically detected polycystic ovaries, those with LH concentrations >10 IU/l had a very significantly increased incidence of cycle disturbance compared with those who had an LH concentration <10 IU/l.[1] In adolescents, hypersecretion of LH is the most common abnormality in those with oligomenorrhea with or without hyperandrogenism.

The possible association of the size of the antral follicle cohort with menstrual regularity is fascinating. Polycystic ovaries contain approximately double the number of antral follicles compared with normal ovaries.[5] It has been long established that wedge resection of polycystic ovaries involving a reduction in the number of follicles, is capable of restoring normal menstrual regularity in a large proportion of patients. This leads to the postulate that an enlarged antral follicle cohort is an etiological factor in the irregularity of cycles prevalent in PCOS. Elting et al[6] therefore examined whether a reduction in the antral follicle cohort due to aging would lead to regular menstrual cycles in women with PCOS.[6] On questioning more than 200 patients, they found a highly significant linear trend for a shorter menstrual cycle length with increasing age in these patients, and a lack of influence of any other factors. They concluded that the development of a new balance in the polycystic ovary, caused solely by follicle loss due to aging, explained the restoration of menstrual regularity.

It is interesting to note that laparoscopic ovarian drilling significantly improves menstrual regularity. Following the operation, 67% had regular menstrual cycles compared with 8% before the drilling.[7] Whether the mechanism causing this improvement is the same as that following wedge resection of the ovaries is still a matter for conjecture.

Treatment

The aim of treatment for the menstrual disturbances associated with PCOS is to provide a regular menstrual cycle. This can be achieved using measures that will also relieve symptoms associated with hyperandrogenism, particularly hirsutism and acne, will prevent endometrial hyperplasia, and may help prevent long-term health consequences (see also Chapter 9).

As with the treatment of all other symptoms associated with PCOS in obese patients, weight loss should be the first line of treatment. This alone has an excellent chance of restoring normal menstrual regularity in patients who succeed in losing >5% of their body weight.[8] This improvement is associated with a reduction in circulating insulin and androgen levels, which can also be achieved by using insulin-sensitizing drugs. Although evidence is still flimsy, metformin does appear to improve cyclicity in about 50% of patients with oligo-/amenorrhea. In a compilation of data from controlled trials, Harborne et al found that women on metformin had 41 cycles per 100 patient-months compared with 21 cycles per patient-month in those receiving placebo.[9] They concluded that these improvements were variable and modest. It seems therefore that insulin sensitizers cannot yet be recommended as treatment when menstrual irregularity is the primary complaint.

For those who have symptoms of hyperandrogenism associated with their menstrual irregularity, the cyclical administration of the combination of ethinyl estradiol (EE) and the anti-androgen cyproterone acetate (CPA) would seem to be the optimal treatment. This has also been described at length in other chapters but, briefly, this combined pill containing 35 µg of EE and 2 mg of CPA has the advantage of not only ensuring a regular cycle but also of successfully decreasing symptoms of hyperandrogenism such as hirsutism and acne, preventing endometrial hyperplasia, and providing contraception. As untreated PCOS may be regarded as a progressive syndrome, at least up to the age of 40, it is reasonable to assume that treatment with this combination of EE and CPA, which markedly reduces androgen concentrations and their untoward effects, will put the syndrome 'on hold', so improving the prospects of success of fertility treatment when it is discontinued. All other cyclically administered contraceptive pills will of course regularize the cycle, and should be substituted after 6 months with the higher dose EE/CPA combination – because of the putative increased risk of thromboembolism. Cyclical progestogen therapy (using the less androgenic progestogens such as medroxyprogesterone acetate and dydrogesterone) may also be used to induce regular mestruation. A progesterone releasing IUCD (Mirena® system) may also be used to provide endometrial protection (see Chapter 9).

Mainly due to the lack of availability of CPA in the US, other anti-androgenic drugs have been employed for the treatment of PCOS. These include spironolactone, flutamide and finestride but, again, these are not usually utilized as first-line treatment when menstrual irregularity is the primary complaint, especially for adolescents.

Women undergoing ovulation induction and who have amenorrhea are less likely to ovulate on clomifene treatment compared with those who have oligomenorrhea.[10] This hints that amenorrhea may reflect a more 'severe' degree or progression of the syndrome than oligomenorrhea.

Summary

Menstrual irregularity, particularly oligo- or amenorrhea, is one of the most common symptoms of PCOS. It is frequently associated with hyperinsulinemia and obesity, but also with hyperandrogenemia, high LH concentrations and a large antral follicle cohort. A combination of CPA and EE is the most popular form of treatment for those not wishing to conceive.

References

1. Balen AH, Conway GS, Kaltsas G et al. Polycystic ovary syndrome: the spectrum of the disorder in 1741 patients. Hum Reprod 1975; 10:2705–2712.

2. Robinson S, Kiddy D, Gelding SV et al. The relationship of insulin insensitivity to menstrual pattern in women with hyperandrogenism and polycystic ovaries. Clin Endocrinol (Oxf) 1993; 39:351–355.

3. Adams J, Polson DW, Franks S. Prevalence of polycystic ovaries in women with anovulation and idiopathic hirsutism. Br Med J 1986; 293:355–359.

4. Legro RS, Bentley-Lewis R, Driscoll D, Wang SC, Dunaif A. Insulin resistance in the sisters of women with polycystic ovary syndrome: Association with hyperandrogenemia rather than menstrual irregularity. J Clin Endocrinol Metab 2002; 87:2128–2133.

5. Hughesdon PE. Morphology and morphogenesis of the Stein–Leventhal ovary and of so-called 'hyperthecosis'. Obstet Gynec Survey 1982; 37:59–77.

6. Elting MW, Korsen TJM, Rekers-Mombarg LTM, Schoemaker J. Women with polycystic ovary syndrome gain regular menstrual cycles when ageing. Hum Reprod 2000; 15:24–28.

7. Amer SA, Goplaan V, Li TC, Ledger WL, Cooke ID. Long term follow-up of patients with polycystic ovarian syndrome after laparoscopic ovarian drilling: clinical outcome. Hum Reprod 2002; 17:2035–2042.

8. Kiddy DS, Hamilton-Fairley D, Bush A et al. Improvement in endocrine and ovarian function during dietary treatment of obese women with polycystic ovary syndrome. Clin Endocrinol (Oxf) 1992; 36:105–111.

9. Harborne L, Fleming R, Lyall H, Norman J, Sattar N. Descriptive review of the evidence for the use of metformin in polycystic ovary syndrome. Lancet 2003; 361:1894–1900.

10. Imani B, Eijkemans MJC, Te Velde ER et al. A nomogram to predict the probability of live birth after clomiphene citrate induction of ovulation in normogonadotrophic oligoamenorrheic infertility. Fertil Steril 2002; 77:91–97.

Chapter 13

The management of infertility associated with polycystic ovary syndrome

Introduction

Polycystic ovary syndrome (PCOS) is the most common cause of anovulatory infertility. Treatment modes available are numerous, mainly relying on ovarian stimulation with follicle-stimulating hormone (FSH), a reduction in circulating insulin concentrations and a decrease in luteinizing hormone (LH) levels as the basis of the therapeutic principles. Clomifene citrate is still the first-line treatment, and if unsuccessful is usually followed by stimulation with exogenous FSH. This should be given in a low-dose protocol, essential to avoid the otherwise prevalent complications of ovarian hyperstimulation syndrome and multiple pregnancies. The addition of a gonadotropin-releasing hormone (GnRH) analog, while very useful during in vitro fertilization/embryo transfer (IVF/ET), adds little to ovulation induction success, whereas the position of GnRH antagonists is not yet clear. Hyperinsulinemia is the commonest contributor to the state of anovulation and its reduction, by weight loss or insulin-sensitizing agents such as metformin, will alone often restore ovulation or will improve results when used in combination with other agents. Laparoscopic ovarian diathermy is proving equally as successful as FSH for the induction of ovulation, particularly in thin patients with high LH concentrations. Aromatase inhibitors are presently being examined and may replace clomifene in the future. When all else has failed, IVF/ET produces excellent results. The aim of ovulation induction therapy should be to correct the underlying disturbance and achieve safe, repeated unifollicular ovulation in order to achieve the livebirth of singleton babies. There are today very few women suffering from anovulatory infertility associated with PCOS who cannot be successfully treated.

Polycystic ovary syndrome and anovulatory infertility

PCOS is associated with approximately 80–90% of women who suffer from infertility due to anovulation.[1,2] PCOS is a very heterogeneous syndrome both in its clinical presentation and laboratory manifestations. The majority of women with anovulation due to PCOS have menstrual irregularities, usually oligomenorrhea or amenorrhea, associated with clinical and/or biochemical evidence of hyperandrogenism. The main disturbances in this syndrome are:

- abnormal morphology of the ovary, detected by a characteristic hyperechogenic enlarged central stroma and >9 small follicles of 2–9 mm diameter on transvaginal ultrasound examination of the ovaries[3]
- abnormal steroidogenesis, mainly increased ovarian production of androgens but also increased progesterone and estradiol production
- hyperinsulinemia, present in about 80% of obese women and 30–40% of women of normal weight with PCOS,[4] and more strongly associated with anovulation than any other feature of the syndrome
- abnormal gonadotropin secretion, most commonly manifested as increased serum LH

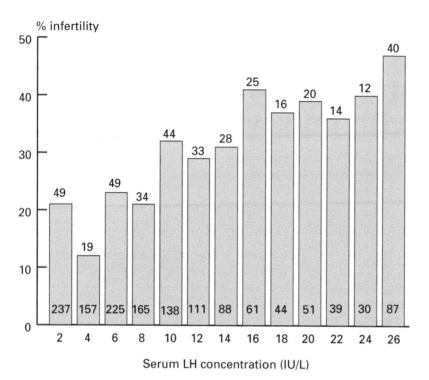

% infertility

Serum LH concentration (IU/L)

Figure 13.1

A rising serum LH concentration associated with an increased risk of infertility, taken from a series of 1741 women with PCOS.[5] The number at the top of each column represents the number of women with infertility with a given LH concentration and the number at the bottom of the column the total numbers with that LH level.

concentrations in 40% of women with ultra-sonically detected PCO (Figure 13.1).[5] A functional deficiency of the endogenous action of FSH also seems to be present in women with anovulatory PCOS.

Several modes of inducing ovulation for these patients will now be described. It will be seen that they basically depend on either a reduction of insulin concentrations, FSH stimulation or a reduction of LH concentrations – or a combination of these.

Weight loss

Excess body weight is a common problem of modern society, reaching epidemic proportions in some countries. For women with PCOS, an excess of body fat accentuates insulin resistance and its associated clinical sequelae. Central obesity and BMI are major determinants of insulin resistance, hyperinsulinemia and hyperandrogenemia. The rate of insulin resistance in women with PCOS is

50–80% and a large majority of these women are obese.[6,7] They almost inevitably have the stigmata of hyperandrogenism and irregular or absent ovulation. Insulin stimulates pituitary LH and ovarian androgen secretion, and decreases sex hormone binding globulin (SHBG) concentrations.[8]

The successful treatment of obesity and hyperinsulinemia is capable of reversing their deleterious effects, of which there are several, on the outcome of treatment. More gonadotropins are required to achieve ovulation in insulin-resistant women.[9,10] Obese women being treated with low-dose therapy have inferior pregnancy and miscarriage rates.[11] Both obese and insulin-resistant women with PCOS, even on low-dose FSH stimulation, have a much greater tendency to a multifollicular response and thus a relatively high cycle cancellation rate in order to avoid hyperstimulation.[10,12]

Just as obesity expresses and exaggerates the signs and symptoms of insulin resistance, then loss of weight can reverse this process by improving ovarian function and the associated hormonal abnormalities.[13–15] Loss of weight induces a reduction of insulin and androgen concentrations and an increase in SHBG concentrations. Curiously, in obese women with PCOS, a loss of just 5–10% of body weight is enough to restore reproductive function in 55–100% within 6 months of weight reduction.[13–15] Weight loss has the undoubted advantages of being effective and cheap with no side-effects, and should be the first line of treatment in obese women with anovulatory infertility associated with PCOS.

Even moderate obesity – BMI >27 kg/m² – is associated with a reduced chance of ovulation,[16] and a visceral body fat distribution leading to an increased waist:hip ratio appears to have a more important effect than body weight alone.[17,18] Obese women (BMI >30 kg/m²) should be encouraged to lose weight. A study by Clark et al looked at the effect of a weight loss and exercise program on women with anovulatory infertility, clomifene resistance and a BMI >30 kg/m².[19] The emphasis of the study was a realistic exercise schedule combined with positive reinforcement of a suitable eating program over a six-month period of time. Thirteen out of the 18 women enrolled completed the study. Weight loss had a significant effect on endocrine function, ovulation and subsequent pregnancy. Fasting insulin and serum testosterone concentrations fell and 12 of the 13 subjects resumed ovulation, 11 becoming pregnant (five naturally and the remainder now becoming sensitive to clomifene). Thus, with appropriate support, patients may ovulate spontaneously without medical therapy. An extension of this study, in women with a variety of diagnoses, demonstrated that in 60 out of 67 subjects, weight loss resulted in spontaneous ovulation with lower than anticipated rates of miscarriage and a significant saving in the cost of treatment.[20]

A reduction in body weight of 5–10% will cause a 30% reduction in visceral fat, which is often sufficient to restore ovulation and reduce markers for metabolic disease.[21] Weight loss should also be encouraged prior to ovulation induction treatments, as they appear to be less effective when the BMI is greater than 28–30 kg/m².[22] Much has been written about diets that are said to be particularly helpful for women with PCOS. In reality, however, there is no evidence that women with PCOS require anything different in their diet than overweight women with normal ovaries.[18] The aim is to eat foods that produce a 'low glycemic response' – such as vegetables, fruit, fiber, protein and fat. Refined foods, high in carbohy-drate, cause an increased glycemic response and also reduce satiety, which results in overeating.

Exercise is important in helping to achieve weight loss and improve insulin sensitivity and reproductive function. Visceral fat is affected more than subcutaneous fat and as little as two hours of exercise a week may be sufficient. A study of 970 female twins reported that physical activity was the strongest independent predictor of central abdominal fat and total fat mass.[23] A difference of one hour's exercise between twins was found to account for a 1 kg difference in body fat. Regular aerobic exercise is most beneficial, and a strategy should be developed to maintain exercise activity.

Clomifene citrate

The introduction of even small amounts of FSH into the circulation either directly with FSH injections or indirectly with pulsatile GnRH or clomifene citrate, is capable of inducing ovulation and pregnancy in a large number of anovulatory women with PCOS. Antiestrogen therapy with clomifene citrate or tamoxifen has traditionally been used as first-line therapy for anovulatory PCOS. Clomifene citrate (CC) has been available for many years and its use has tended not to have been closely monitored. There have been no prospective, randomized studies comparing the efficacy of CC with other therapies,[24] and it may be time to rethink our approach to the initial management of anovulation. Furthermore, the original published studies were not in patients with clearly defined PCOS, as we now know it.

Clomifene citrate is given in a dose of 50–250 mg per day for 5 days starting from day 2–5 of spontaneous or induced bleeding, starting with the lowest dose and raising the dose in increments of 50 mg/day each cycle until an ovulatory cycle is achieved. In practice there is rarely any advantage in using a dose of greater than 100 mg per day as 150 mg seems to significantly increase neither the ovulation rate nor follicular recruitment. Careful monitoring of ovarian response with serial ultrasound scans is essential and in those who respond sensitively to 50 mg, a lower dose of 25 mg may be used. A course of three to six ovulatory cycles is usually sufficient to know whether pregnancy will be achieved using clomifene citrate, before moving on to more complex treatment, as approximately 75% of the pregnancies achieved with clomifene occur within the first three cycles of treatment.[25] If the patient is ovulating, it is not necessary to increase the dose if conception does not occur, and conception is expected to occur at a rate determined by factors such as the patient's age. All women who are prescribed clomifene should be carefully monitored with a combination of endocrine and ultrasonographic assessment of follicular growth and ovulation, because of the risk of multiple pregnancy (reported to be 7–11%).[26] Clomifene therapy should therefore be prescribed and managed by specialists in reproductive medicine.

Ovulation is restored in approximately 80% but will result in pregnancy in only about 35–40% of patients who are given clomifene.[25-27] Additionally, around 20–25% of anovulatory women with PCOS will not respond at all to CC and are considered to be 'clomifene resistant'.[28,29] Patients who do not respond to clomifene are likely to be more obese, insulin resistant and hyperandrogenic than those who do respond.[29] As CC induces a discharge of LH as well as FSH, and elevated LH concentrations are believed to impede conception, those with high basal LH levels are also less likely to respond to clomifene treatment.[30] The most probable factor involved in this large discrepancy between ovulation and pregnancy rates in patients treated with clomifene is the anti-estrogenic effects of clomifene at the level of the endometrium and cervical mucus. While the depression of the cervical mucus, occurring in about 15% of patients, may be overcome by performing intra-uterine insemination (IUI), suppression of endometrial proliferation, unrelated to dose or duration of treatment but apparently idiosyncratic, indicates a poor prognosis for conception in my experience, when endometrial thickness never reaches 8 mm. Monitoring of the clomifene-treated cycle by ultrasound evaluation of follicular growth, endometrial thickness and even estradiol and progesterone concentrations on day 12–14 of the cycle is justified by the identification of those who are not responding or have depressed endometrial thickness, and is helpful in the timing of natural intercourse or IUI. Although this monitoring implies added expense, this is neutralized by the prevention of protracted periods of possibly

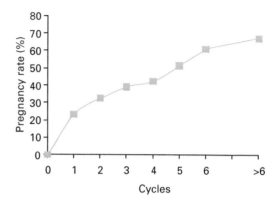

Figure 13.2

The modern use of clomifene citrate.[31]

inappropriate therapy and delay in the inception of more efficient treatment (Figure 13.2).

Kousta et al reported treatment with CC of 167 patients in whom there was a cumulative conception rate of 67.3% over 6 months in those who had no other subfertility factors, which continued to rise up to 12 cycles of therapy.[31] They reported a multiple pregnancy rate of 11%, similar to that described in other series, and a miscarriage rate of 23.6%, with those who miscarried tending to have a higher serum LH concentration immediately after clomifene administration. Recent reviews about the safety of CC with respect to congenital anomalies indicate that there is no increased risk.[32]

Shoham and colleagues studied the hormonal profiles in a series of 41 women treated with CC, of whom 28 ovulated.[33] In those who ovulated, 17 exhibited normal patterns of hormone secretion and five conceived, while 11 exhibited an abnormal response, characterized by significantly elevated serum concentrations of LH from day 9 until the LH surge, together with premature luteinization and higher estradiol levels throughout the cycle – none of the patients with this abnormal response conceived. This strengthens the argument for careful monitoring of therapy and discontinuation if the response is abnormal. A useful approach for clomifene-resistant patients is the administration of progesterone prior to CC treatment,[34] which, at an intramuscular dose of

50 mg over 5 days, caused a suppression of FSH and LH secretion. LH levels fell in seven out of ten women treated with progesterone; all became responsive to clomifene (those whose LH levels were not suppressed remained unresponsive) and three conceived in the first cycle of treatment. Such pre-treatment with progesterone has therefore been shown to improve ovarian response and the endocrine profile and is a seldom used, yet most useful adjunct, to CC therapy.

Clomifene is currently licensed for only six months' use in the UK as the initial application for the license was only made for six months. It has been suggested that there is an association between clomifene and ovarian cancer with more than 12 months' therapy, although in most cases of prolonged use the indication was unexplained infertility rather than anovulation.[35] It would seem reasonable that patients should be counseled about the possible risks if treatment is to continue beyond six months. If pregnancy has not occurred after 10–12 normal ovulatory cycles it is then appropriate to offer the couple assisted conception.

The results of clomifene treatment may be improved by cotreatment with several proposed adjuvants. The addition of an ovulatory dose of human chorionic gonadotropin (hCG), 5,000–10,000 IU is only theoretically warranted when the reason for a non-ovulatory response is that the LH surge is delayed or absent despite the presence of a well-developed follicle. Although the routine addition of hCG at mid-cycle seems to add little to the improvement of conception rates it may be useful if given when an ultrasonically demonstrated leading follicle attains a diameter of 18–24 mm, for the timing of intercourse or IUI.[36]

Daily doses of dexamethasone, 0.5 mg at bedtime, as an adjunct to clomifene therapy, suppress the adrenal androgen secretion and may induce responsiveness to clomifene in previous non-responders, mostly hyperandrogenic women with PCOS with elevated concentrations of dehydroepiandrosterone sulfate (DHEAS).[37,38] Although this method meets with some success, glucocorticoid steroid therapy often induces side-effects including increased appetite, weight gain and insulin resistance, which is not an appealing proposition for women with PCOS.

The term 'clomifene resistance' should be applied to mean failure to ovulate (i.e. no response) rather than failure to conceive despite ovulation, which should be termed 'clomifene failure'. The therapeutic options for patients with anovulatory infertility who are resistant to anti-estrogens are either parenteral gonadotropin therapy or laparoscopic ovarian diathermy.

The combined treatment of clomifene with metformin is dealt with in the section on metformin.

Aromatase inhibitors

Aromatase inhibitors have been suggested as an alternative treatment to clomifene as the discrepancy between ovulation and pregnancy rates with CC has been attributed to its anti-estrogenic action and estrogen receptor depletion. The aromatase inhibitors do not possess the adverse anti-estrogenic effects of clomifene but, by suppressing estrogen production, mimic the central reduction of negative feedback through which clomifene works. Letrozole, the most widely used anti-aromatase for this indication, has been shown to be effective, in early trials, in inducing ovulation and pregnancy in women with anovulatory PCOS and inadequate clomifene response,[39] and improving ovarian response to FSH in poor responders.[40] Evidence from larger trials is still awaited but some encouragement may be taken from the solidity of the working hypothesis and the success of the preliminary results. Possible teratogenicity of letrozole has to be fully elucidated and anastrozole is being examined as a possible alternative.

Gonadotropin therapy

Gonadotropin (FSH or human menopausal gonadotropin (hMG)) therapy is the usual next step following failure with clomifene. Gonadotropin therapy is indicated for women with anovulatory PCOS who have been treated with anti-estrogens, if they have either failed to ovulate or if they have a response to clomifene that is likely to reduce their chance of conception (e.g. persistent hypersecretion of LH, or anti-estrogenic effect on cervical mucus). The literature on gonadotropin therapy contains many articles with different starting points and different definitions of clomifene resistance – including those who ovulate in response to CC but fail to conceive. The main complications of gonadotropin therapy, ovarian hyperstimulation syndrome (OHSS) and multiple pregnancies, are the result of multiple follicular development – to which anovulatory women with PCOS are particularly prone.

Acceptable cumulative conception rates have been achieved using conventional step-up treatment with gonadotropins for women with PCOS (Figures 13.3 and 13.4). However, because of the peculiarly high sensitivity of polycystic ovaries to gonadotropin stimulation, this form of treatment, employing incremental dose rises of 75 IU every 5–7 days, characteristically induces multiple follicular development, resulting in a high frequency of multiple pregnancies and OHSS. A review by Hamilton-Fairley and Franks reported a mean multiple pregnancy rate of 34% and severe OHSS rate of 4.6%.[41] In a further study, although this traditional protocol produced a cumulative conception rate of 82% after six cycles, it was plagued by an unacceptable rate of multiple pregnancies and OHSS.[42] The supraphysiological doses of FSH used in the conventional protocol provoke an initial development of a large cohort, stimulate additional follicles, and even rescue those follicles destined for atresia.[43] Levels of FSH well above the threshold induce a multiple follicular development. While this can be utilized for the induction of superovulation for in vitro fertilization (IVF) and embryo transfer, for the induction of ovulation in women with PCOS the problem of achieving the desired monofollicular ovulation is particularly difficult due to the extreme sensitivity of the polycystic ovary to gonadotropic stimulation. This is not due to a difference of FSH threshold levels of the polycystic ovaries, but probably to the fact that they contain twice the number of available FSH-sensitive antral follicles in their cohort compared with the normal ovary.[44] Any dose of FSH overstepping the threshold of the polycystic ovary will, therefore, produce multifollicular development and impending danger of multiple pregnancy and OHSS. Polycystic ovaries have twice the number of FSH-sensitive follicles as normal ovaries and so great care is required with the use of stimulation regimens.[44]

The chronic low-dose regimen of FSH was designed to reduce the rate of complications due to multiple follicular development,[45] the reason-

- Step up
- Low-dose step up
- Step down

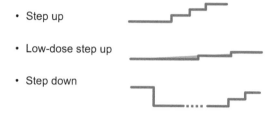

Figure 13.3

Gonadotropin regimens

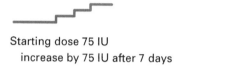

Starting dose 75 IU
  increase by 75 IU after 7 days
  and then every 3–5 days until response

(a) **Conventional step up**

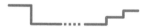

Start with 37.5–75 IU
Do not increase for 14 days (1st cycle)
or 7 days (subsequent cycles)
Increments of 25–37.5 IU every 7 days until threshold

(b) **low-dose step up**

Dominant follicle becomes more sensitive to lower concentration of FSH

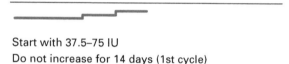

Decrease when follicle is recruited
may decrease again 3 days later until day of hCG, sometimes requires an increase to maintain response

(c) **step down**

Figure 13.4

Gonadotropin regimens. (a) Step up; (b) low-dose step up; (c) step down

ing being that the 'threshold theory', demanding the attainment and maintenance of follicular development with exogenous FSH, without exceeding the threshold requirement of the ovary, should be employed. The principle of the classic chronic low-dose regimen is to employ a

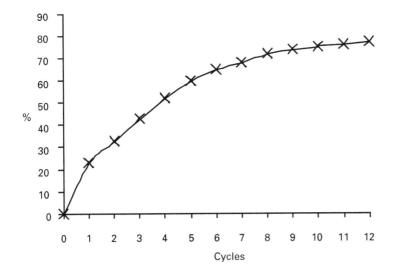

Figure 13.5

Cumulative conception rates with gonadotrophin therapy in 103 patients with clomiphene citrate resistant PCOS.[118]

low starting dose for 14 days and then use small incremental dose rises when necessary, at intervals of not less than 7 days, until follicular development is initiated.[46,47] The dose that initiates follicular development is continued until the criteria for giving hCG are attained. This form of therapy aims to achieve the development of a single dominant follicle rather than the development of many large follicles and thereby avoid the complications of OHSS and multiple pregnancies.

A comparative prospective study of the conventional regimen with chronic low-dose administration of FSH for anovulation associated with PCOS,[42] involved 50 participants treated with FSH, half of them using a conventional stepwise protocol (incremental dose rises of 75 IU every 5–7 days when necessary) and half with a regimen of chronic low dose as described above. Both methods of treatment had an initial dose of 75 IU FSH. Compared with the conventional dose protocol, the chronic low-dose regimen yielded slightly improved pregnancy rates (40% versus 24%) while completely avoiding OHSS and multiple pregnancies, which were prevalent (11% OHSS and 33% multiple pregnancies) with conventional therapy. Uniovulation was induced in 74% versus 27% of cycles, and the total number of follicles >16 mm and estradiol concentrations were half those observed on conventional therapy. A large French multicenter study with an identical objective and protocol design compared conventional and chronic low-dose regimens in 103 anovula-

tory World Health Organization (WHO) Group II (that is essentially polycystic ovary syndrome) women.[48] The comparison of low with conventional dose revealed pregnancy rates of 33.3% versus 20%, and a multiple/twins pregnancy rate of 14% and 22%, respectively. The total number of follicles >10 mm and estradiol concentrations on the day of hCG in the low-dose group were half those seen on conventional therapy. Additionally, the low-dose regimen tended to produce a higher rate of mono- or bifollicular development in this study.

Reported results using a chronic low-dose protocol identical to that described above, show a remarkably consistent rate of uniovulatory cycles of around 70% and an acceptable pregnancy rate of 40% of the patients and 20% per cycle (Figure 13.5).[45,49,118] However, the justification for the adoption of the chronic low-dose protocol may be seen in the almost complete elimination of OHSS and a multiple pregnancy rate of <6% (Figure 13.6).

In the normal ovulatory cycle, decreasing FSH concentrations are seen throughout the follicular phase. Experimental studies have indicated that initiation of follicular growth requires a 10–30% increment in the dose of exogenous FSH, and the threshold changes with follicular growth, due to an increased number of FSH receptors, so that the concentration of FSH required to maintain growth is less than that required to initiate it.[50] In order to mimic more closely the events of the normal ovulatory cycle, the Rotterdam group examined a

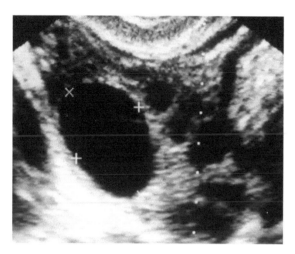

Figure 13.6

A transvaginal ultrasound scan of a single preovulatory folli-cle in a polycystic ovary. Multiple pregnancy rates can be minimized by strict criteria for the administration of hCG (e.g. no more than a total of two follicles ≥14 mm including a lead follicle of ≥17 mm), careful monitoring with serial ultrasound scans and low-dose stimulation regimens.

step-down dose regimen with a starting dose of 150 IU and decreasing the dose by 0.5 ampoules when a follicle of 10 mm ensued and by the same amount every 3 days if follicular growth contin-ued.[51] A comparison of this regimen with the classic step-up regimen from the same group demonstrated a monofollicular growth rate of 88% of cycles in the step-down regimen compared with 56% with the step-up protocol.[52] In the step-down group, duration of treatment and gonadotropin requirement were significantly reduced. However, a recently concluded random-ized, French multicenter study comparing the step-up versus the step-down protocol demon-strated superiority of the step-up regimen in relation to the rates of monofollicular develop-ment, overstimulation and ovulation.[53]

Assuming that the step-up protocol is superior to the step-down version, do the initial dose, the duration of its administration and the incremental dose rise influence results? From the largest published series of chronic low-dose FSH therapy it was possible to compare the results of a starting dose of 75 IU with that of 52.5 IU for an initial 14-day period with an incremental dose rise of 37.5 IU or 22.5 IU respectively.[12] There were no significant differences between the two groups,

but pregnancy rate/patient, uni-ovulatory cycle rate and miscarriage rate were all in favor of the smaller starting dose.

Although the majority of patients with PCOS will reach criteria for hCG administration within 14 days using 75 IU/day of urinary FSH or 50 IU/day of recombinant FSH, some have attempted to cut down the initial period of 14 days without changing the dose to 7 days.[12] A compar-ison of 14-day versus 7-day starters in 50 patients showed no significant differences other than a slightly higher rate of multiple pregnancies in the 7-day group.[45] As we regarded a multiple pregnancy as a 'failure' of treatment, we reverted back to the 14-day initial period without any change of dose.

A recently completed multicenter study employing a step-up protocol starting with doses of 50 IU/day of Puregon® for a minimum of 7 days, compared two randomized groups using incre-mental dose rises of 25 IU or 50 IU when needed (HJ Out, personal communication). The use of the smaller incremental dose rises was significantly more beneficial in terms of monofollicular devel-opment, ovulation rates and cancellation rates.

It can be extremely difficult to predict the response to stimulation of a women with polycys-tic ovaries. In order to prevent OHSS and multiple pregnancy, however, the strategy of cancelling cycles on day 8 of stimulation if there are more than seven follicles (≥8 mm) seems to be reason-able.[54] The chance of multiple pregnancy can be minimized if strict criteria are used for the admin-istration of hCG. We suggest that there should be no more than a total of two follicles greater than 14 mm in diameter with the largest being at least 17 mm.

The different gonadotropin preparations appear to work equally well. A meta-analysis of urinary FSH (uFSH) compared with hMG found no difference in pregnancy or miscarriage rates.[55] Interestingly there was an apparent reduction in the incidence of OHSS with FSH compared with hMG in stimulation cycles without the concomi-tant use of a GnRH agonist (odds ratio (OR) = 0.20; 95% confidence interval (CI) = 0.08–0.46) and a higher rate of overstimulation when a GnRH agonist was used with gonadotropin therapy (OR = 3.15; 95% CI = 1.48–6.70).[55] Also in the Cochrane review of recombinant FSH (rFSH) versus uFSH there were no significant differences demon-strated for the relevant outcomes.[56] The review identified four trials of which three compared rFSH with uFSH,[57–59] and one compared two different treatment regimens using rFSH.[60] A total of 451 women were included in the trials comparing rFSH with uFSH and in the study of Hedon et al 103 women were included.[60] The OR for ovulation rate was 1.19 (95% CI = 0.78–1.80), for pregnancy rate 0.95 (95% CI = 0.64–1.41), for miscarriage rate 1.26 (95% CI = 0.59–2.70), for multiple pregnancy rate 0.44 (95% CI = 0.16–1.21) and for OHSS 1.55 (95% CI = 0.50–4.84).

To summarize, low-dose, step-up gonadotropin therapy should be preferred to the now outdated conventional therapy for patients with PCOS. Small starting doses in the first cycle for a 14-day initial period without a dose change, and then a small incremental dose rise if required, seem, on present evidence, to give the best results.

Gonadotropin-releasing hormone agonists

The ability of GnRH agonists to suppress LH concentrations before and during ovarian stimulation has earned them an undisputed place in IVF treatment protocols. They confer the advantage of eliminating, almost completely, the annoying occurrence of premature luteinization. In addition, some investigators have reported more pregnancies, possibly better quality eggs and fewer miscarriages.[61] Their possible application during ovulation induction should therefore be particularly relevant in the presence of the chronic, tonic, high serum concentrations of LH observed in a high proportion of women with PCOS. Theoretically, by suppressing LH concentrations, GnRH agonists should eliminate premature luteinization and alleviate the relatively low pregnancy rates and high miscarriage rates witnessed in this group of patients.[9] In a large study, 239 women with PCOS received hMG with or without GnRH agonist for ovulation induction or superovulation for IVF/embryo transfer.[62] Of pregnancies achieved with GnRH agonist, 17.6% miscarried compared with 39% of those achieved with gonadotropins alone. Cumulative live-birth rates after four cycles for GnRH agonist were 64% compared with 26% for gonadotropins only.[62]

The GnRH agonist has not become standard treatment for ovulation induction in PCOS despite the fact that our experience and that of others has shown an increased pregnancy rate and lower miscarriage rate in women receiving combination treatment of agonist and gonadotropins, when tonic LH concentrations are high.[63] There are several reasons for this apparent anachronism. Cotreatment with GnRH agonist and low-dose gonadotropin therapy is more cumbersome, longer, requires more gonadotropins to achieve ovulation, and has a greater prevalence of multiple follicle development and consequently more OHSS and multiple pregnancies. This combination therapy should be reserved for women with high serum concentrations of LH who have repeated premature luteinization, persistently do not conceive on gonadotropin therapy alone, or who have conceived and had early miscarriages on more than one occasion.

There is no doubt that GnRH agonists cannot help to reduce the incidence of OHSS and multiple pregnancies in PCOS ovulation induction. If anything, combining GnRH agonist with gonadotropin stimulation will exacerbate the problem of multiple follicular development and therefore increase rates of cycle cancellation, OHSS and multiple pregnancy.[63–65] This may be due to several factors: loss of the endogenous feedback mechanism when using GnRH agonist, reduction of intrafollicular androgen levels following pituitary downregulation and consequently postponed atresia and, most probably, greater stimulation of follicles by the larger amounts of gonadotropins needed when using GnRH agonist. A GnRH agonist is not the solution to the problem of multiple follicular development.

The two main complications of ovulation induction for PCOS are multifollicular development and the possible deleterious effects of high LH levels, low conception rates and high miscarriage rates. A combination of chronic low-dose FSH stimulation with GnRH agonist therapy should theoretically therefore yield the best results. Scheele et al studied women with PCOS undergoing ovulation induction with chronic low-dose FSH therapy, one group with and one without adjuvant GnRH agonist therapy.[66] A very low rate of monofollicular ovulation was achieved (14%) in the agonist cycles compared with 44% of those treated with low-dose FSH alone. Treatment with GnRH agonist abolished neither the inter- nor intra-individual variability of the FSH dose required to induce ongoing follicular growth but also seemed to induce an even further increase in the sensitivity of the polycystic ovary follicles to gonadotropin stimulation once the threshold FSH dose had been reached.

Gonadotropin-releasing hormone antagonists

The GnRH antagonists have some advantages over the agonists and may well become utilized in the treatment of anovulatory PCOS. First, antagonists act by the mechanism of competitive binding, and this allows a modulation of the degree of hormonal suppression by adjustment of the dose. Further, antagonists suppress gonadotropin release within a few hours, have no flare-up effect, and gonadal function resumes without a lag effect following their discontinuation. If we apply these advantages to an ovulation-induction protocol for PCOS, one can visualize that, used in combination with low-dose FSH administration, the antagonist could be given in single or repeated doses when a leading follicle of 13–14 mm is produced. This would theoretically prevent premature luteinization, protect the oocyte from the deleterious effects of high LH concentrations and still allow the follicle to grow unhindered to ovulatory size. Compared with agonist-treated cycles this would confer the, again, theoretical advantages of a much shorter cycle of treatment, promise more conceptions and fewer miscarriages, reduce the amount of gonadotropin required, and increase the incidence of monofollicular ovulation, with a consequent reduction in the prevalence of OHSS and multiple pregnancies. Only one trial employing a GnRH antagonist with recombinant FSH, specifically for women with PCOS, has been published to date.[67] Following pretreatment with oral contraceptives, a treatment with GnRH antagonist was started in 20 patients on day 2 of the cycle. When LH concentrations were found to be suppressed, concurrent antagonist and recombinant FSH therapy was started and continued until the day of hCG treatment. LH was effectively suppressed by one dose of antagonist, and all patients ovulated. Overall clinical pregnancy rates were 44% and ongoing pregnancy rates 28%. This is a preliminary trial and large randomized controlled trials (RCTs) are needed to confirm these results.

Metformin

This strong association between hyperinsulinemia and anovulation would suggest that a reduction of insulin concentrations could be of great importance.[68,69] Weight loss for the obese can reverse this situation as mentioned above, but for those who fail to lose weight or are of normal weight but hyperinsulinemic, an insulin-sensitizing agent such as metformin is indicated. However, the indications for the administration of metformin to anovulatory women with PCOS in an ovulation induction program have widened, as it seems to be difficult to predict which individuals will respond well with this medication.[69]

Metformin is an oral biguanide, well established for the treatment of hyperglycemia, that does not cause hypoglycemia in normoglycemic patients. The sum total of its actions is a decrease in insulin levels and, as a consequence, a lowering of circulating total and free androgen levels with a resulting improvement of the clinical sequelae of hyperandrogenism. It is metformin that has been extensively used in the management of insulin-resistant states and that has been most thoroughly investigated for the management of PCOS.

Metformin, a biguanide, is a non-steroidal compound that appears both indirectly and directly to influence ovarian function. Metformin is claimed to have a multifactorial action with primary effects on insulin sensitivity. It lowers blood glucose mainly by enhancing peripheral glucose uptake and inhibiting hepatic glucose production. Metformin also enhances insulin sensitivity at post-receptor levels and stimulates insulin-mediated glucose disposal without affecting pancreatic insulin secretion. There is evidence that metformin also has a direct effect on androstenedione and testosterone production by theca cells *in vitro* by inhibiting the expression of steroidogenic acute regulatory (StAR) protein and 17-alpha-hydroxylase (CYP17).[70]

The major concern with biguanides has been the risk of lactic acidosis. This is a very rare and serious metabolic complication of metformin therapy, occurring mainly in women with renal impairment, and does not appear to be a problem for otherwise fit women with PCOS who are not frankly diabetic and who have normal renal and liver function. The most commonly reported minor side-effects of metformin include bloating, nausea, vomiting, flatulence, and diarrhea. These symptoms appear to be dose dependent and may be substantially minimized by taking the tablet with meals. It is likely that an incremental dosage protocol (500 mg up to 850 mg initially once and then twice daily) will be helpful to acclimatize patients and minimize undesirable gastrointestinal complaints.

In the last few years a number of mostly uncontrolled short-term studies have assessed the effects of metformin on insulin sensitivity and endocrine profile in women with PCOS. Velazquez et al demonstrated that an improvement in insulin sensitivity induced by 1500 g of metformin a day for 8 weeks, leads to a favorable change in serum concentrations of androgens, SHBG and gonadotropins.[71] Metformin resulted in a rapid fall in insulin and the insulin to glucose ratio, with a concurrent significant decrease in serum concentrations of testosterone (T), free T, DHEAS and androstenedione.[71] A significant increase in the concentration of SHBG was also noted. As far as gonadotropin concentrations were concerned, there was a significant decrease in LH concentrations, an increase in FSH and a normalization of the LH:FSH ratio.

Not all the data, however, have been so encouraging. Two trials with essentially identical recruitment criteria and using slightly higher doses of metformin (850 mg twice and three times a day) over similar lengths of time, showed little or no benefit with respect to insulin metabolism, hormone concentrations or lipid variables.[72,73] In one of these, Ehrmann et al, in a study that was designed to balance dietary intake and sustain body weight, found that hyperinsulinemia and androgen excess in obese non-diabetic women with PCOS were not improved by the administration of high-dose metformin.[73] The reasons for these disagreements are unclear but could be due to different methods used to assess insulin action and large BMI differences (29 versus 39 kg/m^2) between the study groups. In fact, it has been claimed that the ability of metformin to alter insulin sensitivity in individuals with major obesity (BMI of 40 kg/m^2 and above) is limited.[74]

Metformin, by reducing fasting insulin and insulin response to glucose in hyperinsulinemic PCOS patients, reduces the hyperinsulinemia-driven hyperandrogenism and can reverse the endocrinopathy, often enough to allow regular menstrual cycles, reversal of infertility, and spontaneous pregnancy. The achievement of normal menstrual cycles may also reduce the risk of endometrial hyperplasia and adenocarcinoma associated with PCOS.

Evidence supporting ovarian responsiveness to metformin has accumulated from several institutions through small studies published during the past decade. For example, among 22 PCOS patients receiving metformin for 6 months, Velazquez et al demonstrated a restoration of menstrual cyclicity in 96% of oligo-/amenorrhoeic women.[75] This menstrual regularization was accompanied by an ovulatory response in 87% of patients with regular menses, and pregnancy rates of 19%. All patients who had normalization of menstrual irregularities showed a metformin-induced reduction in insulin levels at baseline, and after a glucose load that was associated with a substantial decrease in serum-free T concentrations and the LH/FSH ratio.

Similarly, an extensive two-year investigation of 43 amenorrheic, hyperinsulinemic PCOS patients treated with metformin demonstrated return of normal menses in more than 90% of women.[76] Many other studies have shown, to varying degrees, improvements in both spontaneous and drug-induced ovulatory function, development of normal menses and restoration of fertility, independent of changes in body weight. Indeed a significant decline in serum concentrations of testosterone and LH occurred within one week in a small group of patients, indicating a rapid effect of metformin on ovarian function.[77] The reasons for the striking differences in clinical response to metformin might reflect the heterogeneity in the pathogenesis of the syndrome and different patient populations.

There are now a large number of studies published on the effect of metformin in a dose of 1500–2550 mg/day in women with PCOS. The vast majority of these studies have demonstrated a significant improvement in insulin concentrations, insulin sensitivity, and serum androgen concentrations accompanied by decreased LH and increased SHBG concentrations.[78] The restoration of regular menstrual cycles by metformin has been reported in the large majority of published series, and the reinstatement of ovulation occurred in 78–96% of patients.[68,69,78–81] Fleming et al, in a large RCT, demonstrated a significantly increased frequency of ovulation with metformin compared with placebo in a

Review: Insulin-sensitizing drugs (metformin, troglitazone, rosiglitazone, pioglitazone, D-*chiro*-inositol) for polycystic ovary syndrome
Comparison: 01 Metformin versus placebo or no treatment (clinical outcomes)
Outcome: 03 Ovulation rate

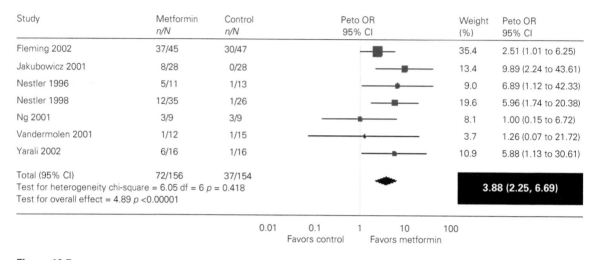

Study	Metformin n/N	Control n/N	Peto OR 95% CI	Weight (%)	Peto OR 95% CI
Fleming 2002	37/45	30/47		35.4	2.51 (1.01 to 6.25)
Jakubowicz 2001	8/28	0/28		13.4	9.89 (2.24 to 43.61)
Nestler 1996	5/11	1/13		9.0	6.89 (1.12 to 42.33)
Nestler 1998	12/35	1/26		19.6	5.96 (1.74 to 20.38)
Ng 2001	3/9	3/9		8.1	1.00 (0.15 to 6.72)
Vandermolen 2001	1/12	1/15		3.7	1.26 (0.07 to 21.72)
Yarali 2002	6/16	1/16		10.9	5.88 (1.13 to 30.61)
Total (95% CI)	72/156	37/154			**3.88 (2.25, 6.69)**

Test for heterogeneity chi-square = 6.05 df = 6 p = 0.418
Test for overall effect = 4.89 p <0.00001

```
       0.01      0.1        1        10       100
              Favors control  Favors metformin
```

Figure 13.7

Cochrane meta-analysis of metformin versus placebo with respect to ovulation rate.[87]

group of 92 oligomenorrheic women with PCOS.[77] This was achieved without any significant changes in the insulin response to glucose challenge after 14 weeks of metformin treatment in a dose of 850 mg, twice a day. Interestingly, significantly more patients withdrew in the metformin arm due to side-effects (15 vs 5, p <0.05). The patients treated with metformin were found to have an increased rate of ovulation (23% vs 13%, p <0.01) and a quicker first time to ovulation (24 vs 42 days, p <0.05). Significant weight loss was reported in the treated group, while the placebo group gained weight (p <0.05) over the 14 weeks of therapy, although glucose tolerance was not improved in either group. The study also reported an inverse relationship between body mass and efficacy of metformin. The largest prospective placebo-controlled double-blind study to date recruited 143 women with anovulatory PCOS and a BMI of >30 kg/m².[82] The mean BMI was approximately 37 kg/m² in each arm of the study, and while significant weight loss improved menstrual cyclicity there was no difference either in the degree of weight loss or the degree of improvement between those treated

with metformin or placebo. It is likely that a higher dose of metformin is required for very obese women with PCOS, although data are lacking on predictive factors for response and appropriate dosages.

In an RCT performed on clomifene-resistant infertile patients with PCOS, compared with placebo, metformin markedly improved ovulation and pregnancy rates with clomifene treatment.[83] In a large study, 46 anovulatory obese women with PCOS who did not ovulate on metformin or placebo for 35 days, were given 50 mg of clomifene daily for five days while continuing metformin or placebo. Of those on metformin, 19 of 21 ovulated compared with 2 of 25 on placebo.[79]

When women with clomifene-resistant PCOS were administered FSH with or without pre-treatment with metformin for one month in an RCT, those receiving metformin developed significantly fewer large follicles, produced less estradiol and had fewer cycles cancelled due to excessive follicular development. The reduction of insulin concentrations induced by metformin seemed to favor a more orderly follicular growth in response

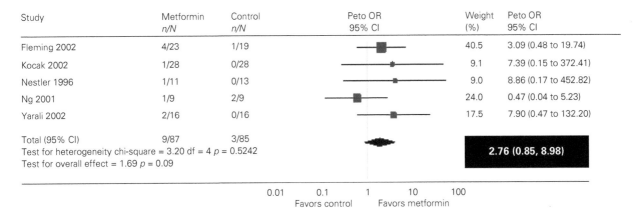

Review: Insulin-sensitizing drugs (metformin, troglitazone, rosiglitazone, pioglitazone, D-chiro-inositol) for polycystic ovary syndrome
Comparison: 01 Metformin versus placebo or no treatment (clinical outcomes)
Outcome: 02 Pregnancy rate

Study	Metformin n/N	Control n/N	Peto OR 95% CI	Weight (%)	Peto OR 95% CI
Fleming 2002	4/23	1/19		40.5	3.09 (0.48 to 19.74)
Kocak 2002	1/28	0/28		9.1	7.39 (0.15 to 372.41)
Nestler 1996	1/11	0/13		9.0	8.86 (0.17 to 452.82)
Ng 2001	1/9	2/9		24.0	0.47 (0.04 to 5.23)
Yarali 2002	2/16	0/16		17.5	7.90 (0.47 to 132.20)
Total (95% CI)	9/87	3/85			2.76 (0.85, 8.98)

Test for heterogeneity chi-square = 3.20 df = 4 p = 0.5242
Test for overall effect = 1.69 p = 0.09

0.01   0.1   1   10   100
Favors control   Favors metformin

Figure 13.8

Cochrane meta-analysis of metformin versus placebo with respect to clinical pregnancy rate.[87]

to exogenous gonadotropins for ovulation induction.[84] In the one published study on the effects of metformin on clomifene resistant patients undergoing IVF/ICSI (intracytoplasmic sperm injection), the results of cycles preceded by treatment with metformin were compared retrospectively to those in which metformin was not given. Those receiving metformin had a decreased total number of follicles but no difference in the mean number of oocytes retrieved. There were more mature oocytes, embryos cleaved, increased fertilization and clinical pregnancy rates (70% vs 30%) in the metformin group.[85] These latter two studies would seem to confirm that both obese,[12] and insulin-resistant women,[10] with PCOS have a much greater tendency to a multi-follicular response and thus a relatively high cycle cancellation rate on low-dose FSH stimulation.

The evidence so far is encouraging concerning the efficiency and safety of metformin as a single agent or in combination with clomifene citrate or gonadotropins for induction of ovulation in women with hyperinsulinemic PCOS.[86] A recent Cochrane review has confirmed a beneficial effect of metformin in improving rates of ovulation when compared with placebo (Figures 13.7 and 13.8), and also in improving both rates of ovulation and pregnancy when used with clomifene citrate compared with clomifene citrate alone (Figures 13.9 and 13.10).[87] The data indicate that serum concentrations of insulin and androgens improve although, contrary to popular belief, body weight does not fall (Figure 13.11).

It remains to be seen whether metformin, which probably also has a direct androgen-lowering action on the ovary, will be of help to all women with PCOS wishing to conceive. Not only does metformin seem to be safe when continued throughout pregnancy, but preliminary data suggest that this strategy may decrease the high miscarriage rate usually associated with PCOS[88,89] (see also Chapter 14). It is hoped that the apparent lack of teratogenicity and beneficial effect of metformin on miscarriage rates will be confirmed by future studies.

The use of troglitazone, the first oral thiazolidinedione approved for the treatment of type 2 diabetes, has a beneficial effect upon insulin resistance in PCOS.[90] In some studies it was found that administration at a dose of 400 mg daily

Review: Insulin-sensitizing drugs (metformin, troglitazone, rosiglitazone, pioglitazone, D-chiro-inositol) for polycystic ovary syndrome
Comparison: 01 Metformin versus placebo or no treatment (clinical outcomes)
Outcome: 03 Ovulation rate

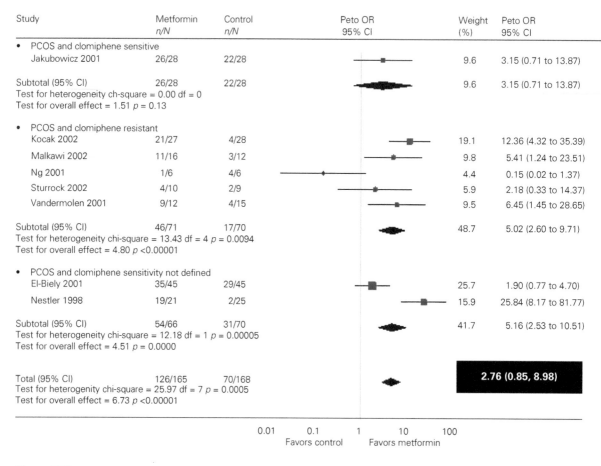

Figure 13.9

Cochrane meta-analysis of insulin sensitizers with ovulation induction versus ovulation induction alone with respect to ovulation rate.[87]

improved total body insulin sensitivity, lowered circulating insulin levels and ameliorated the metabolic and hormonal derangements in obese PCOS women.[91,92] Unfortunately troglitazone has been removed from clinical practice because of its hepatotoxicity. Later generations of thiazolidinediones, such as rosiglitazone and pyoglitazone, may have a role in the future, although there is natural reluctance to introduce them for the treatment of women of reproductive years because of the uncertainty regarding long-term side-effects and teratogenicity.

Laparoscopic ovarian diathermy

For many years, from the 1930s to the early 1960s, wedge resection of the ovary was the only treatment for PCOS. Wedge resection required a laparotomy, removal of up to 75% of each ovary and often resulted in extensive pelvic adhesions. In the modern day, the minimal access alternative to gonadotropin therapy for clomifene-resistant PCOS is laparoscopic ovarian surgery. Laparoscopic ovarian surgery is free of the risks of multiple pregnancy and

Review: Insulin-sensitizing drugs (metformin, troglitazone, rosiglitazone, pioglitazone, D-*chiro*-inositol) for polycystic ovary syndrome
Comparison: 03 Metformin combined with ovulation induction agent versus ovulation induction agent alone (clinical outcomes)
Outcome: 02 Clinical pregnancy rate

Study	Treatment n/N	Control n/N	Peto OR 95% CI	Weight (%)	Peto OR 95% CI
El-Biely 2001	13/45	4/45		42.5	3.64 (1.27 to 10.39)
Kocak 2002	3/27	0/28		8.8	8.29 (0.83 to 83.27)
Malkawi 2002	9/16	2/12		20.7	4.95 (1.10 to 22.31)
Sturrock 2002	4/10	1/9		11.8	4.10 (0.56 to 30.02)
Vandermolen 2001	6/12	1/15		16.2	8.78 (1.60 to 48.07)
Total (95% CI)	35/110	8/109			**4.88 (2.46, 9.67)**

Test for heterogeneity chi-square = 0.99 df = 4 p = 0.9108
Test for overall effect = 4.54 p = 0.0000

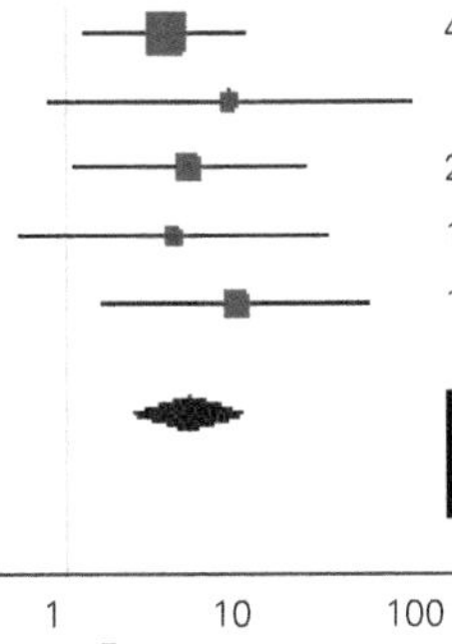

0.01   0.1   1   10   100
Favors control   Favors treatment

Figure 13.10

Cochrane meta-analysis of insulin sensitizers with ovulation induction versus ovulation induction alone with respect to clinical pregnancy rate.[87]

Review: Insulin-sensitizing drugs (metformin, troglitazone, rosiglitazone, pioglitazone, D-*chiro*-inositol) for polycystic ovary syndrome
Comparison: 01 Metformin versus placebo or no treatment (clinical outcomes)
Outcome: 06 Body mass index (kg/m^2)

Study	Metformin n	Mean (SD)	Control n	Mean (SD)	Weighted mean difference (fixed) 95% CI	Weight (%)	Weighted mean difference (fixed) 95% CI
Fleming 2002	25	35.20 (8.90)	39	35.30 (8.60)		2.7	−0.10 (−4.51 to 4.31)
Jakubowicz 2001	26	31.80 (1.52)	22	31.70 (1.52)		69.6	0.10 (−0.76 to 0.96)
Kocak 2002	27	30.47 (5.25)	28	31.10 (3.50)		9.3	−0.63 (−3.00 to 1.74)
Moghetti 2000	11	26.00 (4.64)	12	31.90 (3.81)		4.3	−5.90 (−9.39 to −2.41)
Nestler 1996	11	34.10 (4.31)	13	35.20 (6.85)		2.5	−1.10 (−5.61 to 3.41)
Ng 2001	8	24.40 (4.30)	7	22.70 (3.50)		3.3	1.70 (−2.25 to 5.65)
Pasquali 2000	10	36.40 (7.40)	8	38.00 (6.20)		1.3	−1.60 (−7.88 to 4.68)
Vandermolen 2001	11	35.40 (10.28)	14	38.40 (7.43)		1.0	−3.00 (−10.21 to 4.21)
Yarali 2002	16	29.80 (3.40)	16	29.80 (4.90)		6.1	0.00 (−2.92 to 2.92)
Total (95% CI)	145		159				**−0.27 (−0.98, 0.45)**

Test for heterogeneity chi-square = 12.65 df = 8 p = 0.1245
Test for overall effect = 0.72 p = 0.5

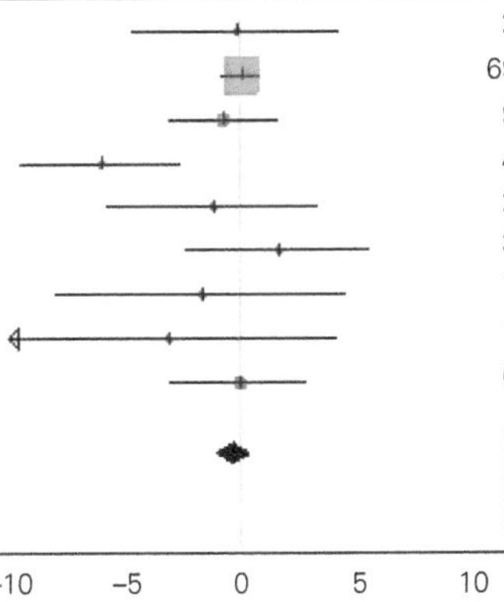

−10   −5   0   5   10

Figure 13.11

Cochrane meta-analysis of metformin versus placebo with respect to weight change.[87]

ovarian hyperstimulation, and does not require intensive ultrasound monitoring. Furthermore, a number of authors have suggested that ovarian diathermy is as effective as routine gonadotropin therapy in the treatment of clomifene-insensitive PCOS.[93–95] The most recent Cochrane review, however, is more cautious in its conclusions.[96]

Laparoscopic ovarian surgery is a useful therapy for anovulatory women with PCOS who fail to respond to clomifene and who either persistently hypersecrete LH, need a laparoscopic assessment of their pelvis, or who live too far away from the hospital to be able to attend for the intensive monitoring required of gonadotropin therapy. Surgery, does of course carry its own risks and must be performed only by fully trained laparoscopic surgeons.

After laparoscopic ovarian surgery, with restoration of ovarian activity serum concentrations of LH and testosterone fall.[97] A fall in serum LH concentrations both increases the chance of conception and reduces the risk of miscarriage, as demonstrated by Armar and Lachelin,[98] who observed a miscarriage rate of 14% in 58 pregnancies compared with the expected miscarriage rate of 30–40% seen in reports of hormonal induction of ovulation in women with PCOS.[99] Whether patients respond to laparoscopic ovarian diathermy (LOD) appears to depend on their pre-treatment characteristics, with patients with high basal LH concentrations having a better clinical and endocrine response.[100] In that study it was found that neither the pre-treatment testosterone level, BMI or ovarian volume could be used to predict outcome. A small prospective study randomized women to receiving either unilateral or bilateral LOD.[101] It was found that unilateral diathermy restored bilateral ovarian activity, with the contralateral, untreated ovary often being the first to ovulate after the diathermy treatment. In that study, the only significant difference between the responders and non-responders was a post-diathermy fall in serum LH concentration.

Commonly employed methods for laparoscopic surgery include monopolar electrocautery (diathermy),[102] and laser,[103] while multiple biopsy alone is less commonly used. In the first reported series, ovarian diathermy resulted in ovulation in 90% and conception in 70% of the 62 women treated.[102] A number of subsequent studies have produced similarly encouraging results, although the techniques used and degree of ovarian damage vary considerably. Gjonnaess cauterized each ovary at five to eight points, for 5–6 s at each point with 300–400 W.[102] Naether et al treated 5–20 points per ovary, with 400 W for approximately 1 s.[104] They found that the rate of adhesions was 19.3% and 16.6% when peritoneal lavage with saline was used.[105] In an earlier study,

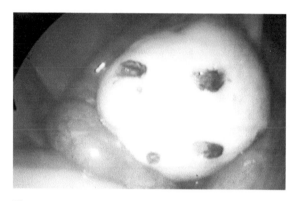

Figure 13.12

Photograph taken at laparoscopy after 4-point monopolar ovarian diathermy.

Naether et al found that the post-diathermy fall in serum testosterone concentration was proportional to the degree of ovarian damage, with up to 40 cauterization sites being used in some patients.[106] The greater the amount of damage to the surface of the ovary, the greater the risk of peri-ovarian adhesion formation. This led Armar to develop a strategy of minimizing the number of diathermy points to four per ovary for 4 s at 40 W – it is this technique that we favor.[107] The high pregnancy rate (86% of those with no other pelvic abnormality) reported by Armar and Lachelin,[98] indicates that the small number of diathermy points used leads to a low rate of significant adhesion formation (Figure 13.12).

Wedge resection of the ovaries resulted in significant adhesions – in 100% of cases in some published series. The risk of adhesion formation is far less after laparoscopic ovarian diathermy (10–20% of cases), and the adhesions that do form are usually fine and of limited clinical significance. Our technique involves instilling 200 ml Hartmann's solution or Adept® into the pouch of Douglas, which by cooling the ovaries prevents heat injury to adjacent tissues and reduces adhesion formation. The risk of peri-ovarian adhesion formation may be further reduced by abdominal lavage and early second-look laparoscopy, with adhesiolysis if necessary.[108] We have also used liberal peritoneal lavage to good effect.[101,107] In another study, 40 women undergoing laser photocoagulation of the ovaries using an Nd-YAG laser set at 50 W at 20–25 points per ovary, were randomized to a second-look laparoscopy and adhesiolysis.[109] Of those who underwent a second-look laparoscopy, adhesions that were described as minimal or mild were found in 68%, yet adhesiolysis did not appear to be necessary, as the cumulative conception rate after 6 months was 47% compared with 55% in the expectantly managed group (not a statistically significant difference).

An additional concern is the possibility of ovarian destruction leading to ovarian failure, an obvious disaster in a women wishing to conceive. Cases of ovarian failure have been reported after both wedge resection and laparoscopic surgery,[110] but this event is, fortunately, very uncommon. For those in whom LOD is successful, the duration of effect is variable. A recently reported large series of 116 patients found that the beneficial effects could be sustained for up to 9 years in the majority.[111]

It is therefore important that a minimum amount of ovarian destruction should be employed. Furthermore, a combined approach may be suitable for some women whereby low-dose diathermy is followed by low-dose ovarian stimulation. Ostrzenski, for example, commenced all his patients on either clomifene or FSH therapy, immediately after laser wedge resection,[112] and Farhi et al also demonstrated an increased ovarian sensitivity to gonadotropin therapy after LOD.[113] Now that we recognize the importance of insulin resistance in the pathophysiology of anovulation in PCOS, studies are needed of the use of metformin in patients who do not ovulate after LOD.

Laser treatment seems to be as efficacious as diathermy, and it has been suggested that it may result in less adhesion formation,[103,114] although the only study to compare the two techniques was non-randomized, reported similar ovulation and pregnancy rates, and did not examine adhesion formation.[115] Various types of laser have been used from the CO_2 laser, to the Nd:YAG and KTP lasers. As with the use of laser in other spheres of laparoscopic surgery, whether laser or diathermy is employed appears to depend upon the preference of the surgeon and the availability of the equipment.

It has been suggested that to demonstrate a 20% increase in pregnancy rate over 6 months from 50% to 70%, with an 80% power, at least 235 patients would be required in each arm of a study to compare LOD with gonadotropin therapy.[96] The current meta-analysis in the Cochrane Database includes a total of only 303 women.[96] The first prospective study to suggest that LOD appeared to be as effective as gonadotropin therapy in the treatment of clomifene-insensitive PCOS, prospectively randomized 88 patients,[93] who had failed to conceive after six CC cycles, to receiving either hMG, FSH or LOD. There were no differences in the rates of ovulation or pregnancy between the groups, although those treated with LOD had fewer cycles with multiple follicular growth, and a lower rate of miscarriage.[93] There have been few other prospective randomized studies since, that have attempted to compare LOD with gonadotropin therapy. Farquhar et al randomized 50 patients and reported similar and somewhat disappointing cumulative pregnancy rates of 28% at 6 months for LOD and 33% after three cycles of gonadotropin therapy.[95]

The ongoing pregnancy rate following ovarian drilling compared with gonadotropins differed according to the length of follow up. Overall, the pooled OR for all studies was not statistically significant (OR = 1.27; 95% CI = 0.77–1.98). Multiple pregnancy rates were reduced in the ovarian drilling arms of the four trials where there was a direct comparison with gonadotropin therapy (OR = 0.16; 95% CI = 0.03–0.98). There was no difference in miscarriage rates in the drilling group when compared with gonadotropin in these trials (OR = 0.61; 95% CI = 0.17–2.16).

The duration of follow up varied among the studies that were included in the meta-analysis. Furthermore it is difficult to produce a temporal comparison, as not all women receiving gonadotropin therapy are treated in consecutive months, and so it is therefore necessary to compare treatment cycles. The meta-analysis found that when comparing 6 months after ovarian drilling with six cycles of gonadotropin therapy, the ongoing cumulative pregnancy rate was higher among women who received gonadotropins (OR = 0.48; 95% CI = 0.28–0.81). One large study (n =168) involved the administration of CC and then rFSH to those who were anovulatory after LOD.[116] They reported an improved cumulative ongoing pregnancy rate with six cycles of recombinant FSH (67%), compared with LOD 6 months after surgery (37%) (OR = 0.28; 95% CI = 0.15–0.52), and after 12 months the OR was 1.37 (95% CI = 0.70–2.69) for ovarian drilling (with the addition of rFSH for women who were anovulatory) compared with rFSH.

Thus it was concluded that there is insufficient evidence of a difference in cumulative ongoing pregnancy rates between laparoscopic ovarian drilling after 6–12 months follow up and 3–6 cycles of ovulation induction with gonadotropins as a primary treatment for subfertile patients with anovulatory PCOS. The greatest advantage is that multiple pregnancy rates are considerably reduced.

In vitro fertilization/embryo transfer

If all else fails for the infertile PCOS patient then IVF is a last resort providing excellent results. Although a smaller percentage of recovered oocytes are fertilized, the larger number of oocytes recovered from PCOS patients balances out the pregnancy rate in comparison with, for example, women with a mechanical factor.[61] In vitro maturation (IVM) of oocytes from women with PCOS may become a possible option.[117] However, it is proving technically difficult at present and concerns over the wellbeing of pregnancies achieved from IVM have not yet been fully answered.

Future developments

There is interest in the development of genetically modified gonadotropin compounds which may have a longer half-life than the more 'natural' recombinantly derived products. These may be able to be administered less frequently than the current requirement for daily injections – possibly even on a weekly basis. Synthetic gonadotropin analogs – for both parenteral and oral administration – are also being explored as possibilities for the future.

Conclusions

Following weight loss if warranted, CC is the usual first-line treatment. If clomifene fails to induce ovulation and pregnancy, several therapeutic paths are open, depending on the individual case: low-dose FSH therapy, addition of metformin to clomifene or gonadotropin treatment, LOD and finally, IVF. Alternative possibilities for treatment in the near future include aromatase inhibitors and IVM of oocytes. Whatever the treatment option used, there are very few women today who suffer from pure anovulatory infertility due to PCOS who will remain involuntarily childless.

Key points

- PCOS is the most common cause of anovulatory infertility.
- Strategies to achieve weight loss and improve insulin sensitivity, including the use of drugs such as metformin, enhance reproductive function. Therapies to induce ovulation involve first the use of the anti-estrogen clomifene citrate, then, for those who fail to ovulate in response to clomifene citrate, the principal options include parenteral gonadotropin therapy or laparoscopic ovarian diathermy.
- First-line therapy should include lifestyle modification and weight loss.
- Clomifene citrate therapy requires careful monitoring with serial ultrasound scans.
- Clomifene resistance is defined as the failure to ovulate in response to doses of usually up to 100 mg.
- Aromatase inhibitors are showing early promise and have the advantage of not having an anti-estrogenic effect on the endometrium.
- Gonadotropin therapy is best administered in a low-dose step-up regimen, with a starting dose of 37.5–50 units of FSH or hMG. Ultrasound monitoring is obligatory.
- The chance of multiple pregnancy can be minimized if strict criteria are used for the administration of hCG: no more than a total of two follicles greater than 14 mm in diameter with the largest at least 17 mm.
- Laparoscopic ovarian diathermy is successful in inducing ovulation and is associated with lower rates of multiple pregnancy than gonadotropin therapy. Cumulative conception rates are lower than with gonadotropins at 6 months but similar by 12 months.
- Insulin-lowering agents, such as metformin, ameliorate the endocrine and metabolic consequences of PCOS and may enhance both spontaneous reproductive function and the response of the polycystic ovary to ovulation induction agents such as clomifene citrate.

References

1. Adams J, Polson DW, Franks S. Prevalence of polycystic ovaries in women with anovulation and idiopathic hirsutism. Br Med J 1986; 293:355–359.

2. Hull, MG. Epidemiology of infertility and polycystic ovarian disease: endocrinological and demographic studies. Gynaecol Endocrinol 1987; 1:235–245.

3. Adams J, Franks S, Polson DW, Mason HD et al. Multifollicular ovaries: clinical and endocrine features and response to pulsatile gonadotrophin releasing hormone. Lancet 1985; ii:1375–1378.

4. Dunaif A, Segal K, Futterweit W, Dobrjansky A. Profound peripheral resistance independent of obesity in polycystic ovary syndrome. Diabetes 1989; 38:1165–1174.

5. Balen AH, Conway GS, Kaltsas G, Techatrasak K et al. Polycystic ovary syndrome: the spectrum of the disorder in 1741 patients. Hum Reprod 1995; 10:2107–2111.

6. Legro RS, Finegood D, Dunaif A. A fasting glucose to insulin ratio is a useful measure of insulin sensitivity in women with polycystic ovary syndrome. J Clin Endocrinol Metab 1998; 83:2694–2698.

7. Carmina E, Lobo RA. Polycystic ovary syndrome: arguably the most common endocrinopathy is associated with significant morbidity in women. J Clin Endocrinol Metab 1999; 84:1897–1899.

8. Poretsky L, Cataldo NA, Rosenwaks, Z Giudice LA. The insulin-related ovarian regulatory system in health and disease. Endocrinol Rev 1999; 20:535–582.

9. Homburg R. Adverse effect of luteinizing hormone on fertility: fact or fantasy. Bailliere's Clin Obstet Gynaecol 1996; 12:555.

10. Dale O, Tanbo T, Haug E, Abyholm T. The impact of insulin resistance on the outcome of ovulation induction with low-dose FSH in women with polycystic ovary syndrome. Hum Reprod 1998; 13:567–570.

11. Hamilton-Fairley D, Kiddy D, Watson H, Paterson C, Franks S. Association of moderate obesity with a poor pregnancy outcome in women with polycystic ovary treated with low dose gonadotrophin. Br J Obstet Gynaecol 1992; 99:128–131.

12. White DM, Polson DW, Kiddy D, Sagle P et al. Induction of ovulation with low-dose gonadotrophins in polycystic ovary syndrome: an analysis of 109 pregnancies in 225 women. J Clin Endocrinol Metab 1996; 81:3821–3824.

13. Kiddy DS, Hamilton-Fairley D, Bush A, Anyaoku V et al. Improvement in endocrine and ovarian function during dietary treatment of obese women with polycystic ovary syndrome. Clin Endocrinol (Oxf) 1992; 36:1105–1111.

14. Pasquali R, Antenucci D, Casmirri F, Venturoli S et al. Clinical and hormonal characteristics of obese amenorrheic hyperandrogenic women before and after weight loss. J Clin Endocrinol Metab 1989; 68:173–179.

15. Clark AM, Ledger W, Galletly C, Tomlinson L et al. Weight loss results in significant improvement in pregnancy and ovulation rates in anovulatory obese women. Hum Reprod 1995; 10: 2705–2712.

16. Grodstein F, Goldman MB, Cramer DW. Body mass index and ovulatory infertility. Epidemiology 1994; 5:247–250.

17. Zaazdstra BM, Seidell JC, Van Noord PA et al. Fat and female fecundity: prospective study of effect of body fat distribution on conception rates. Br Med J 1993; 306:484–487.

18. Lord J, Wilkin T. Polycystic ovary syndrome and fat distribution: the central issue? Hum Fertil 2002; 5:67–71.

19. Clarke AM, Ledger W, Galletly C, Tomlinson L et al. Weight loss results in significant improvement in pregnancy and ovulation rates in anovulatory obese women. Hum Reprod 1995; 10:2705–2712.

20. Clark AM, Thornley B, Tomlinson L, Galletley C, Norman RJ. Weight loss in obese infertile women results in improvement in reproductive outcome for all forms of fertility treatment. Hum Reprod 1998; 13:1502–1505.

21. Despres JP, Lemieux I, Prud'homme D. Treatment of obesity: need to focus on high risk, abdominally obese patients. Br Med J 2001; 322:716–720.

22. Hamilton-Fairley D, Kiddy DS, Watson H, Sagle M, Franks S. Low-dose gonadotrophin therapy for induction of ovulation in 100 women with polycystic ovary syndrome. Hum Reprod 1991; 6:1095–1099.

23. Samaras K, Kelly PJ, Chiano MN et al. Genetic and environmental influences on total body and central abdominal fat: the effect of physical activity in female twins. Ann Int Med 1999; 130:873–882.

24. Hughes E, Collins J, Vandekerckhove P. Clomifene citrate for ovulation induction in women with oligo-amenorrhoea (Cochrane Review). In: The Cochrane Library, Issue 2. Oxford: Update Software, 2000:CD000056.

25. Gysler M, March CM, Mishell DR, Bailey EJ. A decade's experience with an individualized clomifene treatment regimen including its effects on the postcoital test. Fertil Steril 1982; 37:161–167.

26. MacGregor AH, Johnson JE, Bunde CA: Further clinical experience with clomifene citrate. Fertil Steril 1968; 19:616–622.

27. Imani B, Eijkemans MJ, te Velde ER. A nomogram to predict the probability of live birth after clomifene citrate induction of ovulation in normogonadotropic oligomenorrheic infertility. Fertil Steril 2002; 77:91–97.

28. Franks S, Hamilton Fairley D. Ovulation induction: gonadotrophins. In: Adashi EY, Rock JA, Rosenwacks Z, eds. Reproductive endocrinology, surgery and technology. Philadelphia: Lipincott-Raven, 1996.

29. Imani B, Eijkemans MJ, te Velde ER, Habbema JD, Fauser BC. Predictors of patients remaining anovulatory during clomifene citrate induction of ovulation in normogonadotropic oligomenorrheic infertility. J Clin Endocrinol Metab1998; 83:2361–2365.

30. Homburg R, Armar NA, Eshel A, Adams J, Jacobs HS. Influence of serum luteinising hormone concentrations on ovulation, conception and early pregnancy loss in polycystic ovary syndrome. Br Med J 1988; 297:1024–1026.

31. Kousta E, White DM, Franks S. Modern use of clomifene citrate in induction of ovulation. Hum Reprod Update 1997; 3:359–365.

32. Venn A, Lumley J. Clomifene citrate and pregnancy outcome. Aust NZ J Obstet Gynaecol 1994; 34:56–66.

33. Shoham Z, Borenstein R, Lunenfeld B, Pariente C. Hormonal profiles following clomifene citrate therapy in conception and nonconception cycles. Clin Endocrinol (Oxf) 1990; 33:271–278.

34. Homburg R, Weissglass L, Goldman J. Improved treatment for anovulation in polycystic ovarian disease utilizing the effect of progesterone on the inappropriate gonadotrophin release and clomifene citrate response. Hum Reprod 1988; 3:285–288.

35. Rossing MA, Dalling JR, Weiss NS et al. Ovarian tumours in a cohort of infertile women. N Engl J Med 1994; 331:335–339.

36. Agrawal SK, Buyalos RP. Corpus luteum function and pregnancy rates with clomifene citrate therapy: comparison of human chorionic gonadotrophin-induced versus spontaneous ovulation. Hum Reprod 1995; 10:328–331.

37. Diamant YZ, Evron, S. Induction of ovulation by combined clomifene citrate and dexamethasone treatment in clomifene citrate non-responders. Eur J Obstet Gynecol Biol 1981; 11:335–340.

38. Daly DC, Walters CA, Soto-Albors CE, Tohan N, Riddick DH. A randomized study of dexamethasone in ovulation induction with clomifene citrate. Fertil Steril 1984; 41:844–848.

39. Mitwally MF, Casper RF. Use of aromatase inhibitor for induction of ovulation in patients with an inadequate response to clomifene citrate. Fertil Steril 2001; 75:305–309.

40. Mitwally MF, Casper RF. Aromatase inhibition improves ovarian response to FSH: a potential option for low responders during ovarian stimulation. Fertil Steril 2001; 75:88–89.

41. Hamilton-Fairley D, Franks S. Common problems in induction of ovulation. Balliere Clin Obstet Gynaecol 1990; 4:609–625.

42. Homburg R, Levy T, Ben-Rafael Z. A comparative prospective study of conventional regimen with chronic low-dose administration of follicule-stimulating hornone for anovulation associated with polycystic ovary syndrome. Fertil Steril 1995; 63:729–733.

43. Insler V. Gonadotrophin therapy: new trends and insights. Int J Fertil 1988; 33:85–91.

44. Van der Meer M, Hompes P, de Boer J, Schats R, Schoemaker J. Cohort size rather than follicle-stimulating hormone threshold levels determines ovarian sensitivity in polycystic ovary syndrome. J Clin Endocrinol Metab 1988; 83:423–426.

45. Homburg R, Howles CM. Low dose FSH therapy for anovulatory infertility associated with polycystic ovary syndrome: rationale, reflections and refinements. Hum Reprod Update 1999; 5:493–499.

46. Seibel MM, Kamrava MM, McArdle C, Taymor ML. Treatment of polycystic ovarian disease with chronic low dose follicle stimulating hormone: biochemical changes and ultrasound correlation. Int J Fertil 1984; 29:39–43.

47. Polson DW, Mason HD, Saldahna MBY, Franks S. Ovulation of a single dominant follicle during treatment with low-dose pulsatile FSH in women with PCOS. Clin Endocrinol (Oxf) 1987; 26:205–212.

48. Hedon B, Hugues JN, Emperaire JC, Chabaud JJ et al. A comparative prospective study of a chronic low dose versus a conventional ovulation stimulation regimen using recombinant human follicle-stimulating hormone in anovulatory infertile women. Hum Reprod 1998; 13:2688–2692.

49. Ben Rafael Z, Levy T, Schoemaker J. Pharmacokinetics of follicle-stimulating hormone: clinical significance. Fertil Steril 1995; 63:689–700.

50. Schoot BC, Hop WC, de Jong FH, van Dessel TJ, Fauser BC. Initial oestradiol response predicts outcome of exogenous gonadotrophins using a step-down regimen for induction of ovulation in PCOS. Fertil Steril 1995; 64:1081–1087.

51. Van Dessel HJHM, Schoot BC, Schipper I, Dahl KD, Fauser BC. Circulating immunoreactive and bioactive follicle-stimulating hormone concentrations in anovulatory infertile women during gonadotrophin induction of ovulation using a decremental dose regimen. Hum Reprod 1995; 11:101–108.

52. Van Santbrink, EJP, Fauser, BCJM. Urinary follicle-stimulating hormone for normogonadotrophic clomifene resistant anovulatory infertility: prospective, randomized comparison between low dose step-up and step-down dose regimens. J Clin Endocrinol Metab 1997; 82:3597–3602.

53. Christin-Maitre S, Hugues JN. A comparative randomized multicentric study comparing the step-up versus the step-down protocol in polycystic ovary syndrome. Hum Reprod 2003; 18:1626–1631.

54. Farhi J, Jacobs HS. Early prediction of ovarian

multifollicular response during ovulation induction in patients with polycystic ovary syndrome. Fertil Steril 1997; 67:459–462.

55. Nugent D, Vandekerckhove P, Hughes E, Arnot M, Lilford R. Gonadotrophin therapy for ovulation induction in subfertility associated with polycystic ovary syndrome (Cochrane Review). In: The Cochrane Library, Issue 4. Oxford: Update Software, 2000:CD000410.

56. Bayram N, van Wely M, van der Veen F. Recombinant FSH versus urinary gonadotrophins or recombinant FSH for ovulation induction in subfertility associated with polycystic ovary syndrome (Cochrane Review). In: The Cochrane Library, Issue 2, Oxford: Update Software, 2001:CD002121.

57. Loumaye E, Martineau I, Piazzi A, O'Dea L et al. Clinical assessment of human gonadotrophins produced by recombinant DNA technology. Hum Reprod 1996; 11(suppl 1):95–107.

58. Coelingh Bennink HJT, Fauser BCJM, Out HJ. Recombinant follicle-stimulating hormone (FSH; Puregon) is more efficient than urinary FSH (Metrodin) in women with clomifene citrate-resistant, normogonadotropic, chronic anovulation: a prospective, multicenter, assessor-blind, randomized, clinical trial. Fertil Steril 1998; 69:19–25.

59. Yarali H, Bukulmez O, Gurgan T. Urinary follicle-stimulating hormone (FSH) versus recombinant FSH in clomifene citrate-resistant, normogonadotropic, chronic anovulation: a prospective randomized study. Fertil Steril 1999; 72:276–281.

60. Hedon B, Hugues JN, Emperaire JC, Chabaud JJ et al. A comparative prospective study of a chronic low dose versus a conventional ovulation stimulation regimen using recombinant human follicle stimulating hormone in anovulatory infertile women. Hum Reprod 1998; 13:2688–2692.

61. Homburg R, Berkovitz D, Levy T, Feldberg D et al. In-vitro fertilization and embryo transfer for the treatment of infertility associated with polycystic ovary syndrome. Fertil Steril 1993; 60:858–863.

63. Homburg R, Levy T, Berkovitz D. GnRH agonist reduces the miscarriage rate for pregnancies conceived in women with polycystic ovary syndrome. Fertil Steril 1993; 59:527–531.

64. Homburg R, Eshel A, Kilborn J, Adams J, Jacobs HS. Combined luteinizing hormone releasing hormone analogue and exogenous gonadotrophins for the treatment of infertility associated with polycystic ovaries. Hum Reprod 1990; 5:32–37.

65. Van der Meer M, Hompes, PGA, Scheele F. The importance of endogenous feedback for monofollicular growth in low-dose step-up ovulation induction with FSH in PCOS, a randomized study. Fertil Steril 1996; 66:571.

66. Scheele F, Hompes, PGA, van der Meer M, Schoute E, Schoemaker J. The effects of a gonadotrophin-releasing hormone agonist on treatment with low dose luteinizing hormone in polycystic ovary syndrome. Hum Reprod 1993; 8:699–704.

67. Elkind-Hirsch KE, Webster BW, Brown CP, Vernon, MW. Concurrent ganirelix and follitropin-beta therapy is an effective and safe regimen for ovulation induction in women with polycystic ovary syndrome. Fertil Steril 2003; 79:603–607.

68. Velazquez EM, Acosta A, Mendoza SG. Menstrual cyclicity after metformin therapy in polycystic ovary syndrome. Obstet Gynecol 1997; 90:392–395.

69. Fleming R, Hopkinson ZE, Wallace AM, Greer IA, Sattar N. Ovarian function and metabolic factors in women with oligomenorrhea treated with metformin in a randomized double blind placebo-controlled trial. J Clin Endocrinol Metab 2002; 87:569–574.

70. Attia GR, Rainey WE, Carr BR. Metformin directly inhibits adrogen production in human theca cells. Fertil Steril 2001; 76:517–524.

71. Velazquez EM, Mendoza S, Hamer T, Sosa F, Glueck CJ. Metformin therapy in polycystic ovaries reduces hyperinsulinaemia, insulin resistance, hyperandrogenaemia and systolic blood pressure, while facilitating normal menses and pregnancy. Metabolism 1994; 43:647–654.

72. Acbay O, Gundogdu S. Can metformin reduce insulin resistance in polycystic ovary syndrome? Fertil Steril 1996; 65:946–949.

73. Ehrmann DA, Cavaghan MK, Imperial J, Sturis J et al. Effects of metformin on insulin secretion, insulin action and ovarian steroidogenesis in women with polycystic ovary syndrome. J Clin Endocrinol Metab 1997; 82:1241–1247.

74. Kahn SE, Prigeon RL, Mcculloch DK, Bayco EJ et al. Quantification of the relationship between insulin sensivity and b cell function in human subjects. Diabetes 1993; 42:1663–1672.

75. Velazquez EM, Mendoza SG, Wang P, Glueck CJ. Metformin therapy is associated with a decrease in plasminogen activator inhibitor-1, lipoprotein(a) and immunoreactive insulin levels in patients with PCOS. J Clin Endocrinol Metab 1997; 82:524–530.

76. Glueck CJ, Wang P, Fontaine R, Tracy T, Sieve-Smith L. Metformin-induced resumption of normal menses in 39 of 43 (91%) previously amenorrheic women with the polycystic ovary syndrome. Metabolism 1999; 48:511–519.

77. Pirwany IR, Yates RWS, Cameron IT, Fleming R. Effects of the insulin sensitizing drug metformin on ovarian function, follicular growth and ovulation rate in obese women with oligomenorrhoea. Hum Reprod 1999; 14:2963–2968.

78. Nestler JE, Stovall D, Akhter N, Iuorno MJ, Jacubwicz DJ. Strategies for the use of insulin-sensitizing drugs to treat infertility in women with

polycystic ovary syndrome. Fertil Steril 2002; 77:209–215.

79. Nestler JE, Jakubowicz DJ, Evans WS, Pasquali R. Effects of metformin on spontaneous and clomifene-induced ovulation in the polycystic ovary syndrome. N Engl J Med 1998: 338:1876–1880.

80. Moghetti P, Castello R, Negri C, Tosi F et al. Metformin effects on clinical features, endocrine and metabolic profiles, and insulin sensitivity in polycystic ovary syndrome: a randomized, double blind, placebo-controlled 6-month trial, followed by open, long-term clinical evaluation. J Clin Endocrinol Metab 2000; 85:139–146.

81. Ibanez L, Valls C, Ferrer A et al. Sensitization to insulin induces ovulation in non-obese adolescents with anovulatory hyperandrogenism. J Clin Endocrinol Metab 2001; 16:3595–3598.

82. Tang T, Hayden C, Glanville J, Balen AH. A prospect randomised placebo controlled study of metformin in anovulatory PCOS (submitted for publication).

83. Vandermolen DT, Ratts VS, Evans WS, et al. Metformin increases the ovulatory rate and pregnancy rate with clomifene citrate in patients with polycystic ovary syndrome who are resistant to clomifene citrate alone. Fertil Steril 2001; 75:310–315.

84. De Leo V, la Marca A, Ditto A et al. Effects of metformin on gonadotropin-induced ovulation women with polycystic ovary syndrome. Fertil Steril 1999; 72:282–285.

85. Stadtmauer LA, Toma SK, Riehl RM, Talbert LM. Metformin treatment of patients with polycystic ovary syndrome undergoing in vitro fertilization improves outcomes and is associated with modulation of the insulin-like growth factors. Fertil Steril 2001; 75:505–509.

86. Homburg R. Should patients with polycystic ovary syndrome be treated with metformin? Hum Reprod 2002; 17:853–856.

87. Lord JM, Flight IHK, Norman RJ. Metformin in polycystic ovary syndrome: systematic review and meta-analysis. Br Med J 2003; 327:951–955.

88. Glueck CJ, Wang P, Goldenberg N, Sieve-Smith L. Pregnancy outcomes among women with polycystic ovary syndrome treated with metformin. Hum Reprod 2002; 17:2858–2864.

89. Jakubowicz DJ, Iuorno MJ, Jakubowicz S, Roberts KA, Nestler JE. Effects of metformin on early pregnancy loss in the polycystic ovary syndrome. J Clin Endocrinol Metab 2002; 87:524–529.

90. Diamanti-Kandarakis E, Zapanti E. Insulin sensitizers and antiandrogens in treatment of polycystic ovary syndrome. Ann NY Acad Sci 2000; 900:203–212.

91. Dunaif A, Scott D, Finegood D, Quintana B,

Whitcomb R. The insulin-sensitizing agent, troglitazone, improves metabolic and reproductive abnormalities in the polycystic ovary syndrome. J Clin Endocrinol Metab 1996; 81:3299–3306.

92. Ehrmann DA, Schneider DJ, Sobel BE, Cavaghan MK et al. Troglitazone improves defects in insulin action, insulin secretion ovarian steroidogenesis and fibrinolysis in women with polycystic ovary syndrome. J Clin Endocrinol Metab 1997; 82:2108–2116.

93. Abdel Gadir A, Mowafi RS, Alnaser HMI, Alrashid AH et al. Ovarian electrocautery versus human menopausal gonadotrophins and pure follicle stimulating hormone therapy in the treatment of patients with polycystic ovarian disease. Clin Endocrinol (Oxf) 1990; 33:585–592.

94. Donesky BW, Adashi EY. Surgically induced ovulation in the polycystic ovary syndrome: wedge resection revisited in the age of laparoscopy. Fertil Steril 1995; 63:439–463.

95. Farquhar CM, Williamson K, Gudex G, Johnson NP et al. A randomised controlled trial of laparoscopic ovarian diathermy versus gonadotrophin therapy for women with clomifene citrate-resistant polycystic ovary syndrome. Fertil Steril 2002; 78:404–411.

96. Farquhar C, Vandekerckhove P, Lilford R. Laparoscopic 'diathermy' by diathermy or laser for ovulation induction in anovulatory polycystic ovary syndrome (Cochrane Review). In: The Cochrane Library, Issue 4. Oxford: Update Software, 2001:CD001122.

97. Balen AH. PCOS – Medical or surgical treatment? In: Templeton A, Cooke I, O'Brien PMS, eds. Evidence-based fertility treatment, RCOG Study Group. London: RCOG Press, 1998:157–177.

98. Armar NA, Lachelin GCL. Laparoscopic ovarian diathermy: an effective treatment for anti-oestrogen resistant anovulatory infertility in women with polycystic ovaries. Br J Obstet Gynaecol 1993; 100:161–164.

99. Homburg R, Armar NA, Eshel A, Adams J, Jacobs HS. Influence of serum luteinising hormone concentrations on ovulation, conception and early pregnancy loss in polycystic ovary syndrome. Br Med J 1988; 297:1024–1026.

100. Abdel Gadir A, Alnaser HMI, Mowafi RS, Shaw RW. The response of patients with polycystic ovarian disease to human menopausal gonadotrophin therapy after ovarian electrocautery or a luteinizing hormone-releasing hormone agonist. Fertil Steril 1992; 57:309–313.

101. Balen AH, Jacobs HS. A prospective study comparing unilateral and bilateral laparoscopic ovarian diathermy in women with the polycystic ovary syndrome. Fertil Steril 1994; 62:921–925.

102. Gjoannaess H. Polycystic ovarian syndrome treated by ovarian electrocautery through the laparoscope. Fertil Steril 1984; 41:20–25.

103. Daniell JF, Miller N. Polycystic ovaries treated by laparoscopic laser vaporization. Fertil Steril 1989; 51:232–236.

104. Naether OGJ, Fischer R, Weise HC, Geiger-Kotzler L et al. Laparoscopic electrocoagulation of the ovarian surface in infertile patients with polycystic ovarian disease. Fertil Steril 1993; 60:88–94.

105. Naether OGJ, Fischer R. Adhesion formation after laparoscopic electrocoagulation of the ovarian surface in polycystic ovary patients. Fertil Steril 1993; 60:95–99.

106. Naether O, Weise HC, Fischer R. Treatment with electrocautery in sterility patients with polycystic ovarian disease. Geburtsh Frauenheilk 1991; 51:920–924.

107. Armar NA, McGarrigle HHG, Honour JW, Holownia P et al. Laparoscopic ovarian diathermy in the management of anovulatory infertility in women with polycystic ovaries: endocrine changes and clinical outcome. Fertil Steril 1990; 53:45–49.

108. Naether OGJ. Significant reduction in of adnexal adhesions following laparoscopic electrocautery of the ovarian surface by lavage and artificial ascites. Gynaecol Endosc 1995; 4:17–19.

109. Gurgan T, Urman B et al. The effect of short internal laparoscopic lysis of adhesions in pregnancy rates following ND:YAG laser photocoagulation of PCO. Obstet Gynaecol 1992; 80:45–47.

110. Cohen BM. Laser laparoscopy for polycystic ovaries. Fertil Steril 1989; 52:167–168.

111. Amer SAKS, Banu Z, Li TC, Cooke ID. Long-term follow-up of patients with polycystic ovary syndrome after laparoscopic ovarian diathermy: endocrine and ultrasonographic outcomes. Human Reprod 2002; 11:2851–2857.

112. Ostrzenski A. Endoscopic carbon dioxide laser ovarian wedge resection in resistant polycystic ovarian disease. Int J Fertil 1992; 37:295–299.

113. Farhi J, Soule S, Jacobs H. Effect of laparoscopic ovarian electrocautery on ovarian response and outcome of treatment with gonadotrophins in clomifene citrate resistant patients with PCOS. Fertil Steril 1995; 64:930–935.

114. Keckstein G, Rossmanith W, Spatzier K, Schneider V et al. The effect of laparoscopic treatment of polycystic ovarian disease by CO_2-laser or Nd:YAG laser. Surg Endosc 1990; 4:103–107.

115. Heylen SM, Puttemans PJ and Brosens LH. Polycystic ovarian disease treated by laparoscopic argon laser capsule diathermy: comparison of vaporization versus perforation technique. Hum Reprod 1994; 9:1038–1042.

116. Bayram N, van Wely M, Kaajik EM, Bossuyt PMM, van der Veen. Using an electrocautery strategy or recombinant follicle stimulating hormone to induce ovulatioin in polycystic ovary syndrome: randomized controlled trial. Br Med J 2004; 328:192–195.

117. Child TJ, Phillips SJ, Abdul-Jalil AK, Gulekli B, Tan SL. A comparison of in-vitro maturation and in-vitro fertilization for women with polycystic ovary syndrome. Obstet Gynecol 2002; 100:665.

118. Balen AH, Braat DD, West C, Patel A, Jacobs HS. Cumulative conception and live birth rates after the treatment of anovulatory infertility: safety and efficacy of ovulation induction in 200 patients. Hum Reprod 1994; 9:1563–1570.

Chapter 14

Polycystic ovary syndrome, pregnancy and miscarriage

Introduction

Whether pregnancy is achieved spontaneously or with assistance, women with polycystic ovary syndrome (PCOS) face an increased risk of pregnancy complications and the potential for a poor outcome. Several pregnancy-related issues have been reported to have a particular association with PCOS, although the strength of the evidence in this field is often weak. In this chapter we review the links between PCOS and miscarriage, gestational diabetes and pregnancy-related hypertension. Much of the data have been obtained by retrospective audit and are prone to ascertainment and publication bias. The reader will note a practically uniform trend for major risk associations in early papers to diminish over time with later, often more rigorous, publications.

Miscarriage and polycystic ovary syndrome

The evidence that miscarriage might be more common in women with PCOS compared to average started to appear in the 1980s soon after the application of high-resolution ultrasound. In reviewing this literature we need to consider the strategies that can be used to explore the association. The studies differ in their starting clinical source. One experiment would be to identify a large group of women planning to conceive and to classify them according to PCOS status, and then to compare this diagnosis with the miscarriage rate. This type of design was used in an early paper using serum luteinizing hormone (LH) rather than PCOS as a clinical marker.[1] Of course, large numbers of women would be required if we

estimate that 5% have PCOS (as opposed to the percentage who show polycystic ovaries on ultrasound), of whom 20% may miscarry. Thus a study group of 20 women with PCOS *and* miscarriage would require a starting population of 2000 women.

A second strategy would be to identify women presenting with PCOS, whether it be with hirsutism, oligomenorrhea or infertility, and then to track their pregnancy experience with comparison population data on miscarriage. This type of study provides an outcome that is more relevant to women receiving the diagnosis of PCOS for the first time, and wanting to know the implications for pregnancy. In practice however, the study groups in these papers have used fertility clinics as the starting clinical material because the imminent pregnancy data can be audited over a short time. That is, only the infertile subgroup (perhaps a minority) of women with PCOS has been studied, so the relevance of such data for women with mainly androgenic symptoms remains obscure.

A third strategy is to use data from a recurrent miscarriage clinic, in order to find whether the prevalence of polycystic ovaries is more common than expected. Once again, there is then some confusion as to how many would be considered to have PCOS and we do not find out how close the link between the two conditions is for women recently diagnosed with PCOS.

Lastly, we have to consider confounding factors common to PCOS and miscarriage risk which might link the two conditions. The main risk factors for miscarriage – thrombophilias and certain uterine anomalies – are not thought to be more common than expected in PCOS. Additional risk factors such as maternal age, obesity and diabetes may well become important when comparing women with PCOS to controls.

Gestational diabetes, in particular, has to be taken into account together with related obesity as either of these might contribute to an apparent link between PCOS and miscarriage, which may not be direct.[2,3]

Prevalence of miscarriage in polycystic ovary syndrome

There is no good prospective study that quantifies the risk of miscarriage for the broad spectrum of women presenting with PCOS. For the subgroup of women with PCOS who proceed to fertility treatments, miscarriage may be more common. In an IVF setting, women with polycystic ovaries on ultrasound were reported to have a miscarriage rate of 36% compared with 24% for women with normal ovaries,[4] although it must be accepted that a group identified in this way is highly selected and the comparison group had a mix of pathologies that led to the need for in vitro fertilization (IVF). A similar smaller study failed to find an excess of miscarriage in women with polycystic ovaries on ultrasound.[5] Wang et al carried out a similar analysis, this time separating an IVF population into those with PCOS and those without.[6] Simple univariate analysis showed a significantly greater spontaneous abortion rate of 25% in PCOS compared with 18% in controls – a significance which was eliminated on multiple regression analysis controlling for obesity and treatment type.

An analysis of 62,228 pregnancies achieved with assisted reproduction technologies found an overall spontaneous abortion rate of 14.7%, which was considered no different from the population average.[7] Assuming that in many of these women the underlying diagnosis was PCOS, and that a major increase in miscarriage risk would therefore have been manifest in the whole population, we can conclude that any association between PCOS and miscarriage must be slight. In a smaller study of 1196 pregnancy cycles in an IVF clinic, the risk of early pregnancy loss in the PCOS group (120 cycles) was 26% compared with 15% in the non-PCOS group (1076) cycles, which was marginally significant only on univariate analysis but not when confounders were controlled for.[8]

We can conclude from these few papers that the evidence for an excess risk of miscarriage in women with PCOS is weak. There is a real need for a prospective series spanning the full spectrum of women with PCOS in order to clarify this link. Polycystic ovaries on ultrasound may segregate with miscarriage in women undergoing IVF, but the two may be epiphenomena rather than causally related.

Polycystic ovary syndrome and recurrent miscarriage

Several papers have explored the prevalence of polycystic ovaries on ultrasound in women presenting with recurrent miscarriage, usually defined as three or more consecutive spontaneous abortions, within the same relationship, before 12 weeks gestation.[9–13] These papers agree that polycystic ovary morphology is more common than expected in women with recurrent miscarriage, with rates varying between 36 and 56% compared with 20–23% in reference populations.[14–16] The polycystic ovary morphology and markers of the syndrome such as serum LH or testosterone concentrations, however, do not influence the risk of subsequent miscarriage.[13,17] In addition, thrombophilias, the most widely recognized risk for recurrent miscarriage, are not more prevalent in women with PCOS.[18]

Despite the fact that hyperinsulinemia and obesity have not been shown to be closely related to miscarriage risk,[8,13,19] several reports have focused on the possible effect of metformin in the recurrent miscarriage setting. As is often the case, early papers demonstrated a dramatic effect of metformin in reducing miscarriage risk, however, the retrospective/prospective design of such studies make interpretation difficult and tends to lead to an over-estimation of effect – in these studies patients were used as their own retrospective controls. Nevertheless, Glueck et al quote a fall in miscarriage rate from 62% to 26% after the introduction of metformin to the clinic.[19] Of course, it may be that instruction in diet and exercise also changed over this time, so the direct effect of metformin is unclear. A second retrospective study also reports a miscarriage rate of 41.9% in women with PCOS receiving metformin, and 8.8% in those not so treated.[20] Clearly, this reduced miscarriage risk is enticing, but the magnitude of the benefit will only emerge when prospective randomized trials are completed.

Luteinizing hormone and miscarriage in polycystic ovary syndrome

Early retrospective or observational studies showed a relationship between LH hypersecretion and reduced conception rate or miscarriage in women with PCOS undergoing fertility treatment.[21–23] In addition, Regan et al, studying a normal population intending spontaneous pregnancy, reported an association between raised serum LH concentrations and miscarriage, without reference to PCOS status.[1] These studies led to the notion that LH might have a deleterious effect at several stages of fertility, including propensity to miscarriage. While two retrospective studies suggested that suppression of LH with gonadotropin-releasing hormone (GnRH) analogs was associated with a reduced miscarriage rate,[4,24] a prospective study in recurrent miscarriage failed to show a benefit from this strategy.[25] An appropriately timed pre-ovulatory surge of LH both initiates the cascade of local events that result in follicular rupture, as well as initiating the resumption of meiosis within the oocyte. It has been hypothesized that chronic hypersecretion of LH might disrupt normal oocyte maturation, although this has yet to be proven.[26] The influence of LH on fertility outcome remains elusive, with little strong evidence for an association through miscarriage rates having emerged over recent years.

Gestational diabetes mellitus

With the clear evidence that type II diabetes occurs more frequently than expected in young women with PCOS and that polycystic ovaries are over-represented in an older age group with type II diabetes, it comes as no surprise that in intermediate years, gestational diabetes (GDM) should be associated with PCOS. Nearly all studies agree on this raised risk of diabetes in pregnancy (Table 14.1) with the relative risk varying from double to 13-fold. It must be remembered, however, that these figures relate to women in fertility clinics and not to women with PCOS who conceive spontaneously.

Some of the studies that fail to find any association may have been underpowered.[27] On the

Table 14.1 Papers showing an increased prevalence of gestational diabetes mellitus in women with polycystic ovary syndrome

	Women wit PCOS (n)	% GDM in next pregnancy	
		PCOS	Controls
Radon 1999	22	40	3
Mikola 2001	99	20	8.9
Bjerke et al 2002	52	7	0.6

other hand, several larger studies using careful case matching have also failed to show an association between PCOS and GDM, suggesting that it is not PCO per se but obesity that mediates the risk of diabetes.[28–30] Using similar case matching, however, Urman et al still found a significant excess of GDM in PCOS women.[31] Some of the discrepancies between the positive and negative papers in this field may be explained by the fact that the criteria for allocation to a 'GDM group' are always arbitrary. For instance, Turhan et al failed to find a difference in the prevalence of GDM in PCOS, but found that obesity was the strongest predictor of GDM status.[32] By analyzing glucose concentrations during an oral glucose tolerance test, however, they found that impaired glucose tolerance was related to PCOS pregnancies.

Using the opposite strategy, several groups have determined the prevalence of polycystic ovaries in women identified by virtue of their GDM status (Table 14.2). The results from these studies are remarkably consistent with the prevalence of polycystic ovary morphology being found twice to ten times greater in women with GDM.

Accepting the risk of GDM is raised in women with PCOS undergoing fertility treatment, there is a real preventative health opportunity to limit this process with some intervention. This may become an ever more pressing need as the population grows more obese and with the use of metformin in ovulation induction enabling women at high risk of GDM to conceive. The most sensible program would be to introduce a careful diet and exercise program as part of pre-pregnancy education. Inevitably, however, some

Table 14.2 Prevalence of polycystic ovary morphology on ultrasound in women presenting with gestational diabetes mellitus

	Women with GDM (n)	% with polycystic ovary morphology	
		GDM	Controls
Antilla 1998	31	44	7
Holte 1998	34	41	3
Kousta 2000	91	52	27
Koivunen 2001	33	39	16.7

will question whether a less arduous pharmaceutical route may be an acceptable alternative, and the world's eyes are on metformin. Glueck et al report GDM in 22 of 72 pregnancies in women with PCOS who took metformin before and throughout pregnancy compared with 1 of 33 women with PCOS who did not take metformin.[19] Once again, this is not a scientific trial, but a retrospective/prospective audit, and so the magnitude of benefit may by over-estimated and changes in management other than metformin therapy may account for the effect. Also, we are a long way from being able to provide valid safety data for the use of metformin in pregnancy, and we know that it does cross the placenta.[33,34] At the time of writing therefore, the use of metformin in pregnancy remains a research topic and, other than in the context of clinical trials, we currently recommend that it is discontinued as soon as pregnancy is confirmed (see Chapter 13).

Pregnancy-related hypertension

The background of obesity, insulin resistance and GDM in women with PCOS would suggest that hypertension might be a greater risk than expected in this group when pregnant, particularly as hypertension is an integral feature of the metabolic syndrome X. Several reports have suggested that a higher than expected risk of pre-eclampsia exists in women with PCOS.[35–38] Kashyap et al quote the excess risk of pregnancy-induced hypertension to be 31.8% in 22 women with PCOS, compared with 3.7% in their control group of 27 women.[38] A similar excess risk was

reported by Radon et al who included weight matching in their study.[37]

Once again we see that later, larger studies try to refine this observation by controlling more precisely for confounding factors using regression analysis. Mikola et al studied 99 pregnancies in women with PCOS, compared them with a control population, and found that pre-eclampsia was related only to nulliparous status and was not influenced by PCOS status.[39] Haakova et al also reported a negative case-control study in 66 women with PCOS who were carefully controlled for age and weight.[30] The discrepancies in these papers are likely to be the results of differing definitions of pre-eclampsia, and variations in the category of PCOS women under investigation and in the nature of the control group.

Fridstrom et al used a different strategy by comparing blood pressure measurements throughout pregnancy in 33 women with PCOS, compared with 66 controls.[27] Blood pressure showed no difference in the first two trimesters, but in the third trimester the PCOS group had significantly higher readings.

Summary

There is a good deal of disagreement about the risk of pregnancy complications in women with PCOS. The best consensus relates to an excess risk of GDM, although this risk association may have been over-estimated in papers which fail to control for obesity. Even on current evidence it seems sensible to advise a diabetes prevention plan before and during pregnancy in women with PCOS. In the absence of a good trial showing the benefit of metformin in pregnancy, such a program should be based primarily on lifestyle changes. Weight reduction prior to pregnancy is likely to be associated with better antenatal and postnatal health, and also a better ability to withstand the rigors of late pregnancy and labor. Obesity is also associated with increased obstetric complications, such as shoulder dystocia and post-partum thromboembolism.

The case for miscarriage being associated with PCOS is particularly weak based on current evidence, and this is surprising when considering the degree to which this aspect has entered the public consciousness.

Key points

- Several pregnancy-related issues have been reported to have a particular association with PCOS although the strength of the evidence is often weak.
- Hypersecretion of LH, while correlated in early studies with a reduced chance of conception and increased risk of miscarriage, now appears to have an uncertain effect. There have been no prospective studies that have demonstrated a benefit from the suppression of LH during fertility therapy.
- The evidence for an excess risk of miscarriage in women with PCOS is weak, and appears to relate more to obesity than PCOS itself.
- Women with obesity and PCOS have a higher risk of gestational diabetes mellitus and pregnancy-related hypertension.
- Metformin therapy to lower serum insulin concentrations may have a beneficial effect on miscarriage rates and risk of gestational diabetes. Prospective studies are still required.

References

1. Regan L, Owen EJ, Jacobs HS. Hypersecretion of luteinising hormone, infertility, and miscarriage. Lancet 1990; 336:1141–1144.
2. Pettigrew R, Hamilton-Fairley D. Obesity and female reproductive function. Br Med Bull 1997; 53:341–358.
3. Sebire NJ, Jolly M, Harris JP, Wadsworth J et al. Maternal obesity and pregnancy outcome: a study of 287,213 pregnancies in London. Int J Obes Relat Metab Disord 2001; 25:1175–1182.
4. Balen AH, Tan SL, MacDougall J, Jacobs HS. Miscarriage rates following in-vitro fertilization are increased in women with polycystic ovaries and reduced by pituitary desensitization with buserelin. Hum Reprod 1993; 8:959–964.
5. Engmann L, Maconochie N, Sladkevicius P, Bekir J et al. The outcome of in-vitro fertilization treatment in women with sonographic evidence of polycystic ovarian morphology. Hum Reprod 1999; 14:167–171.
6. Wang JX, Davies MJ, Norman RJ. Polycystic ovarian syndrome and the risk of spontaneous abortion following assisted reproductive technology treatment. Hum Reprod 2001; 16:2606–2609.
7. Schieve LA, Tatham L, Peterson HB, Toner J, Jeng G. Spontaneous abortion among pregnancies conceived using assisted reproductive technology in the United States. Obstet Gynecol 2003; 101:959–967.
8. Winter E, Wang J, Davies MJ, Norman R. Early pregnancy loss following assisted reproductive technology treatment. Hum Reprod 2002; 17:3220–3223.
9. Sagle M, Bishop K, Ridley N, Alexander FM et al. Recurrent early miscarriage and polycystic ovaries. Br Med J 1988; 297:1027–1028.
10. Tulppala M, Stenman UH, Cacciatore B, Ylikorkala O. Polycystic ovaries and levels of gonadotrophins and androgens in recurrent miscarriage: prospective study in 50 women. Br J Obstet Gynaecol 1993; 100:348–352.
11. Clifford K, Rai R, Watson H, Regan L. An informative protocol for the investigation of recurrent miscarriage: preliminary experience of 500 consecutive cases. Hum Reprod 1994; 9:1328–1332.
12. Liddell HS, Sowden K, Farquhar CM. Recurrent miscarriage: screening for polycystic ovaries and subsequent pregnancy outcome. Aust NZ J Obstet Gynaecol. 1997; 37:402–406.
13. Nardo LG, Rai R, Backos M, El Gaddal S, Regan L. High serum luteinizing hormone and testosterone concentrations do not predict pregnancy outcome in women with recurrent miscarriage. Fertil Steril 2002; 77:348–352.
14. Polson DW, Adams J, Wadsworth J, Franks S. Polycystic ovaries—a common finding in normal women. Lancet 1988; 1:870–872.
15. Clayton RN, Ogden V, Hodgkinson J, Worswick L et al. How common are polycystic ovaries in normal women and what is their significance for the fertility of the population? Clin Endocrinol (Oxf) 1992; 37:127–134.
16. Farquhar CM, Birdsall M, Manning P, Mitchell JM, France JT. The prevalence of polycystic ovaries on ultrasound scanning in a population of randomly selected women. Aust NZ J Obstet Gynaecol 1994; 34:67–72.
17. Rai R, Backos M, Rushworth F, Regan L. Polycystic ovaries and recurrent miscarriage—a reappraisal. Hum Reprod 2000; 15:612–615.
18. Tsanadis G, Vartholomatos G, Korkontzelos I,

Avgoustatos F et al. Polycystic ovarian syndrome and thrombophilia. Hum Reprod 2002; 17:314–319.

19. Glueck CJ, Wang P, Fontaine RN, Sieve-Smith L et al. Plasminogen activator inhibitor activity: an independent risk factor for the high miscarriage rate during pregnancy in women with polycystic ovary syndrome. Metabolism 1999; 48:1589–1595.

20. Jakubowicz DJ, Iuorno MJ, Jakubowicz S, Roberts KA, Nestler JE. Effects of metformin on early pregnancy loss in the polycystic ovary syndrome. J Clin Endocrinol Metab 2002; 87:524–529.

21. Stanger JD, Yovich JL. Reduced in-vitro fertilization of human oocytes from patients with raised basal luteinizing hormone levels during the follicular phase. Br J Obstet Gynaecol 1985; 92:385–393.

22. Howles CM, Macnamee MC, Edwards RG. Follicular development and early luteal function of conception and non-conceptional cycles after human in-vitro fertilization: endocrine correlates. Hum Reprod 1987; 2:17–21.

23. Homburg R. Adverse effects of luteinizing hormone on fertility: fact or fantasy. Baillieres Clin Obstet Gynaecol 1998; 12:555–563.

24. Homburg R, Armar NA, Eshel A, Adams J, Jacobs HS. Influence of serum luteinising hormone concentrations on ovulation, conception, and early pregnancy loss in polycystic ovary syndrome. Br Med J 1988; 297:1024–1026.

25. Clifford K, Rai R, Regan L. Future pregnancy outcome in unexplained recurrent first trimester miscarriage. Hum Reprod 1997; 12:387–389.

26. Balen AH, Tan SL, Jacobs HS. Hypersecretion of luteinising hormone – a significant cause of subfertility and miscarriage. Br J Obst Gynaecol 1993; 100:1082–1089.

27. Fridstrom M, Nisell H, Sjoblom P, Hillensjo T. Are women with polycystic ovary syndrome at an increased risk of pregnancy-induced hypertension and/or preeclampsia? Hypertens Pregnancy 1999; 18:73–80.

28. Wortsman J, de Angeles S, Futterweit W, Singh KB, Kaufmann RC. Gestational diabetes and neonatal macrosomia in the polycystic ovary syndrome. J Reprod Med 1991; 36:659–661.

29. Vollenhoven B, Clark S, Kovacs G, Burger H, Healy D. Prevalence of gestational diabetes mellitus in polycystic ovarian syndrome (PCOS) patients pregnant after ovulation induction with gonadotrophins. Aust NZ J Obstet Gynaecol 2000; 4:54–58.

30. Haakova L, Cibula D, Rezabek K, Hill M et al. Pregnancy outcome in women with PCOS and in controls matched by age and weight. Hum Reprod 2003; 18:1438–1441.

31. Urman B, Sarac E, Dogan L, Gurgan T. Pregnancy in infertile PCOD patients. Complications and outcome. J Reprod Med 1997; 42:501–505.

32. Turhan NO, Seckin NC, Aybar F, Inegol I. Assessment of glucose tolerance and pregnancy outcome of polycystic ovary patients. Int J Gynaecol Obstet 2003; 81:163–168.

33. McCarthy EA, Walker SP, McLachlan K, Boyle J, Permezel M. Metformin in obstetric and gynecologic practice: a review. Obstet Gynecol Surv 2004; 59:118–127.

34. Lord JM, Flight IH, Norman RJ. Metformin in polycystic ovary syndrome: systematic review and meta-analysis. Br Med J 2003; 327:951–953.

35. Gjonnaess H. The course and outcome of pregnancy after ovarian electrocautery in women with polycystic ovarian syndrome: the influence of body-weight. Br J Obstet Gynaecol 1989; 96:714–719.

36. de Vries MJ, Dekker GA, Schoemaker J. Higher risk of preeclampsia in the polycystic ovary syndrome. A case control study. Eur J Obstet Gynecol Reprod Biol 1998; 76:91–95.

37. Radon PA, McMahon MJ, Meyer WR. Impaired glucose tolerance in pregnant women with polycystic ovary syndrome. Obstet Gynecol 1999; 94:194–197.

38. Kashyap S, Claman P. Polycystic ovary disease and the risk of pregnancy-induced hypertension. J Reprod Med 2000; 45:991–994.

39. Mikola M, Hiilesmaa V, Halttunen M, Suhonen L, Tiitinen A. Obstetric outcome in women with polycystic ovarian syndrome. Hum Reprod 2001; 16:226–229.

Chapter 15

The management of women in the climateric and menopause who have a diagnosis of polycystic ovary syndrome

Introduction

Young women with polycystic ovary syndrome (PCOS) frequently ask the question 'What will happen at the menopause?'. For many, the main issue of concern is not the cardiovascular or diabetes risk, but the natural history of the common PCOS symptoms – hirsutism and menstrual irregularity. The difficulty in providing information to a woman with PCOS approaching the menopause is that very few studies have focused on this age group, and even fewer have longitudinally tracked the natural history over the vital transition time between 45 and 55 years of age. In order to place the sparse literature in context it is useful to review the relevant aspects of normal menopause transition.

Androgens and the menopause transition

Both serum testosterone and serum dehydro-epiandrosterone sulfate (DHEAS) are markers of androgen hypersecretion in PCOS, so it is useful to consider both of these with respect to the menopause. Testosterone is thought to be a better marker of ovarian androgen production and DHEAS reflects the adrenal contribution although this simplistic separation in source is to some degree artificial.[1] Serum testosterone and DHEAS concentrations decline with age, and this negative trend in biochemical markers is paralleled by a generalized reduction in androgen-dependent hair growth in most women. The fall in serum testosterone concentrations is most apparent in pre-menopausal women,[2,3] and less obvious after the menopause.[4,5] In PCOS, one cross-sectional study recorded a fall in mean serum testosterone concentrations of 50% in the 42–47-year-old age group.[6] Therefore, young women with PCOS in whom hirsutism is prominent might find that this symptom becomes less severe in their fourth and fifth decades.

A recent large study of women over the menopause transition years shows no decline in circulating testosterone concentrations synchronous with the last natural period.[7] These data imply that the ovary continues to secrete testosterone after the menopause in similar amounts to those in the pre-menopause. Circulating DHEAS concentrations show a more obvious decline with age, both in pre-menopausal and post-menopausal women. There appears, therefore, to be a divergence of trend between testosterone and DHEAS in the post-menopausal years, with DHEAS continuing to decline and testosterone stabilizing. This divergence between testosterone and DHEAS after the age of 50 may be explained by ovarian testosterone secretion being maintained in the menopause years, with DHEAS reflecting diminished adrenal androgen production. Indeed, post-menopausal women who have had a bilateral oophorectomy have 40% lower bioavailable testosterone compared to intact post-menopausal women – a difference that holds right out to older women over 80 years of age.[5] That the normal menopausal ovary continues to secrete testosterone is made clear by ovarian vein catheterization studies, where the marked fall in estrogen is not paralleled by a fall in androgen precursors.[8] Indeed, a rise in ovarian androgen production has been reported from the menopausal polycystic ovary, compared to the production rate prior to the menopause.[9] In terms of ovarian structure, these concepts can be understood by the fact that the first cell types to disappear at the menopause are germ cells, taking with them surrounding granulosa cells of the primordial follicles. These granulosa cells are the source of estrogen. Theca/interstitial cells, which are the source of ovarian androgen production, are relatively well preserved and may be driven to hypersecrete androgens as serum luteinizing hormone (LH) rises.[10]

The LH drive to menopausal theca cells can result in pathological hypertrophy classified as 'stromal hyperplasia' in a mild form and 'hyperthecosis' in a more severe form. These conditions probably represent the severe end of the spectrum of women presenting with postmenopausal hirsutism.[11] There have been reports that hyperthecosis is associated with hyperinsulinemia,[12] so it may be that both LH and insulin stimulation of the theca cells is required to produce this pathology. In addition, it may be that hair follicles are a target tissue for hyperinsulinemia, and that hair growth is not only androgen but also insulin driven. This notion might explain why oophorectomy is often not effective in reducing hirsutism in PCOS, despite a marked fall in circulating androgen concentrations.

What about women with PCOS – are they going to be at an increased risk of hirsutism after the menopause? The answer to this question is 'probably yes', it might even be exaggerated. We know that the polycystic theca spontaneously hypersecretes androgen,[13] so it seems inevitable that the post-menopausal androgen production will also be elevated. In clinical terms, hirsute women with PCOS may experience postmenopausal hirsutism more often than average and may need continuing anti-androgen cover into the sixth decade of life.

Menstrual cyclicity and the menopause

The well-known pattern of menstrual change in the years leading up to the menopause is of a shortening of the cycle length from an average of 28 to 21 days, with an increase in cycle-to-cycle variability. Several studies have shown that this shortening in menstrual interval holds true in oligomenorrheic women with PCOS.[9,14] That is, women with PCOS may convert from oligomenorrhea to a normal cycle with age. In an interview study of 205 women with PCOS, 40.6% of women in their early 30s had a regular cycle compared with over 80% of women in their early 40s and 100% after the age of 50.[14] Interestingly, in a follow-up study, this group has shown that cardiovascular risk markers are not related to the change in menstrual cycle pattern in PCOS, so this clinical feature has no value in estimating long-term health risk.[15]

The mechanism by which menstrual cyclicity is spontaneously restored in women with PCOS is unclear. It may be that this change simply reflects the fall in serum testosterone concentrations as outlined above. Another proposed mechanism is that the raised inhibin B concentrations in PCOS result in suppression of follicle-stimulating hormone (FSH), and failure of the dominant follicle selection process.[16] With aging, the diminished granulosa cell population secretes less inhibin B, releasing the constraint on FSH secretion, and leading in turn to improved dominant follicle selection and thus cyclicity.[17]

This resolution of cyclicity prior to the menopause is important to recognize and should encourage women to stop treatment at intervals to test whether oligomenorrhea has spontaneously resolved. The timing of the menopause is not altered by the presence of PCOS.[18] Predictably, hysterectomy is more common in women with PCOS compared with controls. Dahlgren et al report hysterectomy in 7/33 (21%) women with PCOS vs 3/132 (2%) controls.[9] The higher hysterectomy rate in PCOS probably reflects persisting menstrual disturbance in a proportion of women, and a higher prevalence of endometrial hyperplasia, particularly in the obese.

Polycystic ovaries and the menopause

Only a few studies have focused on the menopausal years in women with PCOS and it is useful to review the methodologies and conclusions presented in these papers.

Birdsall and Farquhar have made an assessment of the menopausal ovary morphology in en effort to define a post-menopausal diagnosis.[19] This cross-sectional study showed that a polycystic morphology was found in 35/95 post-menopausal women who also had raised testosterone and triglyceride concentrations. It must be noted that this study group were identified through women undergoing coronary angiography, so the relevance to the general population is not clear. In addition, such a cross-sectional study does not help us understand the natural history of a pre-menopausal polycystic ovary; we can only presume that the criteria used in this study equate to a pre-menopausal polycystic ovary. Longitudinal tracking through the menopause is required to clarify the real issues, and only a few small studies have attempted this.

Pasquali et al report one longitudinal study that did not extend to the menopause. Thirty-seven women of mean age 20 years were followed for an average of 10 years.[20] This report is interesting in that women who had used the oral contraceptive in the intervening 10 years appeared to have less progression of the metabolic syndrome than those who took no treatment. Accepting that this is an observational rather than randomized outcome, the possibility arises that effective treatment of PCOS lessens the long-term risks. This is an important point when considering the only other longitudinal studies which do extend into the menopause. The key studies by Dahlgren et al and Wild et al identified their cases by histology from ovarian wedge resection – a fairly effective treatment which may alter the natural history of the condition.[9,18]

Winters et al report a similar follow-up on 84 women with a clinical diagnosis of PCOS, and a follow-up interval of 3–26 years, giving an age at follow up of 20–57 years.[6] Thus, most women in this study were in fact pre-menopausal. In this study the only reported outcome measures were serum testosterone, sex hormone binding globulin (SHBG) and insulin concentrations, in comparison with 57 matched controls. The study confirms raised testosterone and reduced insulin concentrations in the PCOS group, with a decline in testosterone levels with age.

Dahlgren reported on 33 women aged 40–59 years, who had undergone ovarian wedge resection 22 to 31 years earlier.[9] In addition to the cardiovascular risk outcome for which this paper is a landmark, there are also very intriguing endocrine outcome data. Sixty-one per cent of the PCOS women reported hirsutism compared with 11% of controls, but it is unclear how many continued to experience hirsutism after the menopause. However, this study confirms the increased serum testosterone concentrations in the peri- and post-menopause in women with PCOS, compared with the level in controls that is predicted above. Serum testosterone was 2.45 nmol/l in the 14 women with PCOS with raised FSH concentrations, compared with 1.55 nmol/l in 88 controls. Interestingly, serum testosterone was not raised in the nine women with normal FSH concentrations. The key cardiovascular end-points in this paper were a greater prevalence of hypertension, diabetes central adiposity and hyperinsulinemia.

Wild et al performed a similar study expanding the number to 319 women with PCOS and 1060 controls with an age range of 38–98 years, and a follow-up interval of 15–47 years.[18] Once again, the main focus of the study was cardiovascular outcome, and we gain little insight into the natural history of PCOS. Hypertension, diabetes, hypercholesterolemia and central adiposity were more prevalent in the PCOS group. Age of menarche and age of first child were slightly delayed in the PCOS group, but the age of menopause was not altered.

Summary

The symptoms of hirsutism and oligomenorrhea affecting young women with PCOS are likely to improve somewhat in the years leading up to the menopause. Women with PCOS have a greater likelihood of undergoing hysterectomy, but the age of passage through the natural menopause is not altered. After the menopause, women with PCOS who had previously experienced hirsutism may be more likely to proceed to post-menopausal hirsutism even though as a group there had been some improvement in this symptom in the pre-menopausal years.

References

1. Wajchenberg BL, Achando SS, Okada H, Czeresnia CE et al. Determination of the source(s) of androgen overproduction in hirsutism associated with polycystic ovary syndrome by simultaneous adrenal and ovarian venous catheterization. Comparison with the dexamethasone suppression test. J Clin Endocrinol Metab 1986; 63:1204–1210.

2. Zumoff B, Strain GW, Miller LK, Rosner W. Twenty-four-hour mean plasma testosterone concentration declines with age in normal premenopausal women. J Clin Endocrinol Metab 1995; 80:1429–1430.

3. Mushayandebvu T, Castracane VD, Gimpel T, Adel T, Santoro N. Evidence for diminished midcycle ovarian androgen production in older reproductive aged women. Fertil Steril 1996; 65:721–723.

4. Judd HL. Hormonal dynamics associated with the menopause. Clin Obstet Gynecol 1976; 19:775–788.

5. Laughlin GA, Barrett-Connor E, Kritz-Silverstein D, von Muhlen D. Hysterectomy, oophorectomy, and endogenous sex hormone levels in older women: the Rancho Bernardo Study. J Clin Endocrinol Metab 2000; 85:645–651.

6. Winters SJ, Talbott E, Guzick DS, Zborowski J, McHugh KP. Serum testosterone levels decrease in middle age in women with the polycystic ovary syndrome. Fertil Steril 2000; 73:724–729.

7. Burger HG, Dudley EC, Cui J, Dennerstein L, Hopper JL. A prospective longitudinal study of serum testosterone, dehydroepiandrosterone sulfate, and sex hormone-binding globulin levels through the menopause transition. J Clin Endocrinol Metab 2000; 85:2832–2838.

8. Ala-Fossi SL, Maenpaa J, Aine R, Punnonen R. Ovarian testosterone secretion during perimenopause. Maturitas 1998; 29:239–245.

9. Dahlgren E, Johansson S, Lindstedt G, Knutsson F et al. Women with polycystic ovary syndrome wedge resected in 1956 to 1965: a long-term follow-up focusing on natural history and circulating hormones. Fertil Steril 1992; 57:505–513.

10. Sluijmer AV, Heineman MJ, De Jong FH, Evers JL. Endocrine activity of the postmenopausal ovary: the effects of pituitary down-regulation and oophorectomy. J Clin Endocrinol Metab 1995; 80:2163–2167.

11. Rittmaster RS. Polycystic ovary syndrome, hyperthecosis and the menopause. Clin Endocrinol (Oxf) 1997; 46:129–130.

12. Barth JH, Jenkins M, Belchetz PE. Ovarian hyperthecosis, diabetes and hirsuties in postmenopausal women. Clin Endocrinol (Oxf) 1997; 46:123–128.

13. Gilling-Smith C, Willis DS, Beard RW, Franks S. Hypersecretion of androstenedione by isolated thecal cells from polycystic ovaries. J Clin Endocrinol Metab 1994; 79:1158–1165.

14. Elting MW, Korsen TJ, Rekers-Mombarg LT, Schoemaker J. Women with polycystic ovary syndrome gain regular menstrual cycles when ageing. Hum Reprod 2000; 15:24–28.

15. Elting MW, Korsen TJ, Schoemaker J. Obesity, rather than menstrual cycle pattern or follicle cohort size, determines hyperinsulinaemia, dyslipidaemia and hypertension in ageing women with polycystic ovary syndrome. Clin Endocrinol (Oxf) 2001; 55:767–776.

16. Lockwood GM, Muttukrishna S, Groome NP, Matthews DR, Ledger WL. Mid-follicular phase pulses of inhibin B are absent in polycystic ovarian syndrome and are initiated by successful laparoscopic ovarian diathermy: a possible mechanism regulating emergence of the dominant follicle. J Clin Endocrinol Metab 1998; 83:1730–1735.

17. Welt CK, McNicholl DJ, Taylor AE, Hall JE. Female reproductive aging is marked by decreased secretion of dimeric inhibin. J Clin Endocrinol Metab 1999; 84:105–111.

18. Wild S, Pierpoint T, Jacobs H, McKeigue P. Long-term consequences of polycystic ovary syndrome: results of a 31 year follow-up study. Hum Fertil (Camb) 2000; 3:101–105.

19. Birdsall MA, Farquhar CM. Polycystic ovaries in pre and post-menopausal women. Clin Endocrinol (Oxf) 1996; 44:269–276.

20. Pasquali R, Gambineri A, Anconetani B, Vicennati V et al. The natural history of the metabolic syndrome in young women with the polycystic ovary syndrome and the effect of long-term oestrogen-progestagen treatment. Clin Endocrinol (Oxf) 1999; 50:517–527.

Appendix 1

Ultrasound assessment of the polycystic ovary: technical considerations

1 General principles

A pelvic ultrasound scan should be performed by appropriately trained personnel, who have obtained the relevant qualifications and continue to participate in continuing professional development and appraisal programs. Only trained personnel should report on ultrasound scans. Assessment of inter-observer variation should be performed on a regular (e.g. annual) basis and at the start of scientific studies of ovarian function.

State-of-the-art equipment is required. This ideally should be less than five years old and serviced regularly. An appropriate selection of transabdominal and transvaginal probes should be available for all body shapes/sizes.

The ultrasound scan report (2-dimensional)

Name and age of patient
Identifying unique hospital record number
Date of scan
Relation to menstrual cycle
Type of scan (transabdominal (t.a.)/transvaginal (t.v.), etc.)

Ovarian morphology – each ovary recorded separately: volume, number and size range of cysts; stromal echogenicity

Doppler studies (if performed)

Uterine morphology, endometrial thickness

Other features

Grade and signature of person performing scan
Grade and signature of person verifying scan (if relevant)

In addition to a real-time assessment of ovarian and uterine morphology, images should be recorded as either hard copy or electronically.

The scan should be performed with the patient's consent. She should be accompanied by a relative, friend or her partner if she wishes. Due consideration should be taken of her need for privacy when changing. A chaperone should be present and should sign that the procedure has been witnessed.

The scan should be performed in a systematic fashion. Each ovary should be scanned from inner to outer margins, in order to count the total number of cysts/follicles. Appropriate measurements should then be performed of the ovarian and uterine dimensions (see below).

2 Standardize the timing of the scan

Few studies that describe the morphology and endocrinology of polycystic ovary syndrome (PCOS) make reference to timing of the menstrual cycle. The baseline ultrasound scan of the pelvis is best performed in the early follicular phase (days 1–3), when the ovaries are relatively quiescent:

- *Days 1–3 or 1–5?* Days 1–3 most likely to be quiescent.
- *If oligo-/amenorrheic: random or days 1–3/5 after progestogen-induced bleed?* The latter is ideal but for practical use random scans are performed combined with endocrinology (follicle-stimulating hormone (FSH), luteinizing hormone (LH), estradiol (E2)) and be prepared

to repeat for ovarian volume, etc. if evidence of a dominant follicle (>10 mm).

- *Are there any markers that can be used to confirm quiescence and hence timing of the scan (e.g. FSH, LH, estradiol, inhibiting hormone (INH) etc.)?* Probably not reliably.
- *Should time of day be recorded?* Probably not relevant.
- *Should the scan be repeated for validation of the findings and if so after how long?* There is evidence of little change if the scan is repeated one or two times over a 9- to 12-day period,[1] although there is little data from other studies on successive ultrasound scans over time.

3 Type of ultrasound scan

A report of a pelvic ultrasound scan should make reference to the approach to the ovary, whether t.a. or t.v. The type of machine and probe used is not usually recorded on the report but will be seen on the images that are recorded.

- Correlation between t.a., t.v., histology, etc.: highest resolution is obtained with t.v. scan, although t.a. provides adequate assessment of morphology but it may be harder to visualize ovaries in obese individuals.
- Three-dimensional view may provide better correlation with ovarian function; but is still largely used only in research settings rather than routine clinical use (see below).
- The role of other modalities (e.g. Doppler, magnetic resonance imaging (MRI)) is still being established in research settings rather than routine clinical use (see below).

4 Conventions for measurements of the ovaries and uterus

4.1 Ovarian volume

Identify each ovary and measure the maximum diameter in each of three planes (longitudinal, anteroposterior and transverse). It is recognized that because of the irregular shape of the ovary,

any calculation of the volume of a sphere, or prolate ellipse, is at best an estimate.

The left ovary may be harder to measure because of overlying sigmoid colon, particularly if there is distension with gas in the bowel.

Modern ultrasound machines can calculate volume once the calipers have been used to measure the ovary, and an ellipse is drawn around the outline of the ovary. The ultrasound software for this calculation is reported to be quite accurate.

Measuring ovarian volume

Calculation of ovarian volume has been traditionally performed using the formula for a prolate ellipsoid ($\pi/6 \times$ maximal longitudinal, anteroposterior and transverse diameters).[2–4] As $\pi/6 = 0.5233$, a simplified formula for a prolate ellipse is ($0.5 \times$ length $\times$ width $\times$ thickness).[1,5–8]

Nardo et al found good correlations between two-dimensional and three-dimensional ultrasound measurements of ovarian volume and polycystic ovary morphology.[9] A large number of different ultrasound formulae with different weightings for the different diameters were used to calculate ovarian volume, and the prolate spheroid formula ($\pi/6 \times$ anteroposterior diameter^2 $\times$ transverse diameter) was found to correlate well

Table A1.1 Correlation of ultrasound formulaic methods with 3-D ultrasound volume measurements[9]

Method	Correlation coefficient
$\pi/6$ tv $\times$ ap $\times$ long	0.70
$\pi/6$ (tv)^3	0.55
$\pi/6$ (ap)^3	0.61
$\pi/6$ (long)^3	0.10
$\pi/6$ [(tv + ap)/2]^3	0.72
$\pi/6$ [(long + ap)/2]^3	0.49
$\pi/6$ [(tv + long)/2]^3	0.61
$\pi/6$ [(tv + ap + long)/3])^3	0.73
$\pi/6$ (tv)^2(ap)	0.67
$\pi/6$ (ap)^2(tv)	0.73
$\pi/6$ (tv)^2(long)	0.61
$\pi/6$ (ap)^2(long)	0.51
$\pi/6$ (long)^2(tv)	0.49
$\pi/6$ (long)^2(ap)	0.30

ap = anteroposterior diameter, tv = transverse diameter, long = longitudinal diameter with ovarian volume as assessed by 3-D ultra-sound.[9] A similar correlation was found with the spherical volume method ($\pi/6 \times$ ((transverse diameter + anteroposterior diameter + longitudinal diameter)/3))[3]. As polycystic ovaries appear to be more spherical than ovoid it is suggested that the formula should be modified (Table A1.1).[9]

4.2 Uterine size

Uterine dimensions are measured in the sagittal plane: maximum length from cervix to fundus $\times$ maximum anteroposterior diameter, to provide cross-sectional area.[3,10]

5 Definitions of polycystic ovarian morphology (for justifications see Chapter 2)

The characteristic appearances of the polycystic ovary are variable and may be subtle. Ultrasonographers are trained to assess the presence of significant pelvic pathology (e.g. large ovarian cysts, endometriomata), and may not appreciate the finer characteristics of polycystic ovaries or multicystic ovaries.

- *Consider both ovaries.* There is evidence that ovarian volumes, follicle count and stromal echogenicity are similar on the right and left.[1] Unilateral polycystic ovaries have been reported. Ovarian dimensions differ and each should be reported separately. There is no convention for combining and expressing as a mean.
- *Total ovarian volume.* Volume: ≥5.7 cm³;[6] 10 cm³ is considered by many to be diagnostic (see below).
- *Ovarian cross-sectional are (length $\times$ width $\times$ $\pi/4$):* appears to be a poor predictor of ovarian function.[11]
- *Stromal volume/area/echogenicity:*
  - echodensity: subjective, dependent on body habitus and ultrasound settings. Hyperechogenicity correlates well with the presence of PCOS.[11]
  - the myometrium may be used as an index – if stromal echogenicity is greater than that

of the myometrium, this is considered abnormal.
- stromal echogenicity has been described in a semi-quantitative manner with a score for normal (=1), moderately increased (=2) or frankly increased (=3).[1]
- stromal echogenicity has been defined as $(\sum x_i \cdot f_i)/n$, where n = total number of pixels in the measured area, x = intensity level (from 0–63) and f = number of pixels corresponding with the level (see below).[12]
- stromal volume is generally found to correlate weakly with endocrinology, apart from androstenedione on 3-D ultrasound scan.[13]
- The cysts – number, size, total volume:
  - number: per ovary or through a single slice of the ovary in two dimensions (rather than combined total of both ovaries): ≥10,[13] or ≥12,[14] or ≥15;[15] normal ovaries do not have more than 9
  - size: 2–6 mm, 2–8 mm, <10 mm; size is a good discriminator between normal and polycystic ovaries when combined with ovarian volume[16]
  - pattern: circumferential, scattered randomly – does it matter?
- *Ratio of ovarian:uterine volume:* reported to be <1.0 in PCOS,[17] but no longer thought to be useful. Uterine width/ovarian length <1.0 is also a poor predictor.[11] A stromal/area ratio >0.34 was found to be diagnostic of PCOS.[8]
- *Subjective appearance of polycystic ovaries* may be useful, for example in women taking the combined oral contraceptive pill, in whom the volume will be suppressed but the appearance may still be polycystic.[18,19]
- *Blood flow:* increased stromal blood flow correlates with greater stromal volume and also endocrine parameters.

References

1   Pache TD, Hop WC, Wladimiroff JW, Schipper J, Fauser BCJM. Transvaginal sonography and abnormal ovarian appearance in menstrual cycle disturbances. Ultrasound Med Biol 1991; 17:589–593.

2. Sample WF, Lippe BM, Gyepes MT. Grey-scale ultrasonography of the normal female pelvis. Radiology 1977; 125:477–483.

3. Adams J, Polson DW, Abdulwahid N, Morris DV et al. Multifollicular ovaries: clinical and endocrine features and response to pulsatile gonadotropin releasing hormone. Lancet 1985; 2:1375–1379.

4. Orsini LF, Venturoli S, Lorusso R, Pluchinotta V et al. Ultrasonic findings in polycystic ovarian disease. Fertil Steril 1985; 43:709–714.

5. Swanson M, Sauerbrei EE, Cooperberg PL. Medical implications of ultrasonically detected polycystic ovaries. J Clin Ultrasound 1981; 9:219–222.

6. Hann LE, Hall DA, McArdle CR, Seibel M. Polycystic ovarian disease: sonographic spectrum. Radiology 1984; 150:531–534.

7. Saxton DW, Farquhar CM, Rae T, Beard RW, Anderson MC, Wadsworth J. Accuracy of ultrasound measurements of female pelvic organs. Br J Obstet Gynaecol 1990; 97:695–699.

8. Fulghesu AM, Ciampelli M, Belosi C, Apa R et al. A new ultrasound criterion for the diagnosis of polycystic ovary syndrome: the ovarian stroma:total area ratio. Fertil Steril 2001; 76:326–331.

9. Nardo LG, Buckett WM, Khullar V. Determination of the best-fitting ultrasound formulaic method for ovarian volume measurement in women with polycystic ovary syndrome. Fertil Steril 2003; 79:632–633.

10. Balen AH, Conway GS, Kaltsas G, Techatrasak K et al. Polycystic ovary syndrome: the spectrum of the disorder in 1741 patients. Hum Reprod 1995; 10:2107–2111.

11. Ardaens Y, Robert Y, Lemaitre L, Fossati P, Dewailly D. Polycystic ovarian disease: contribution of vaginal endosonography and reassessment of ultrasonic diagnosis. Fertil Steril 1991; 55:1062–1068.

12. Al-Took S, Watkin K, Tulandi T, Tan SL. Ovarian stromal echogenicity in women with clomiphene citrate-sensitive and clomiphene citrate-resistant polycystic ovary syndrome. Fertil Steril 1999; 71:952–954.

13. Kyei-Mensah A, Tan SL, Zaidi J, Jacobs HS. Relationship of ovarian stromal volume to serum androgen concentrations in patients with polycystic ovary syndrome. Hum Reprod 1998; 13:1437–1441.

14. Jonard S, Robert Y, Cortet-Rudelli C, Decanter C, Dewailly D. Ultrasound examination of polycystic ovaries: is it worth counting the follicles? Hum Reprod 2003; 18:598–603.

15. Fox R, Corrigan E, Thomas PA, Hull MG. The diagnosis of polycystic ovaries in women with oligo-amenorrhoea: predictive power of endocrine tests. Clin Endocrinol (Oxf) 1991; 34:127–131.

16. Pache TD, Wladimiroff JW, Hop WC, Fauser BCJM. How to discriminate between normal and polycystic ovaries: Transvaginal ultrasound study. Radiology 1992; 183:421–423.

17. Parisi L, Tramonti M, Casciano S, Zurli A, Gazzarini O. The role of ultrasound in the study of polycystic ovarian disease. J Clin Ultrasound 1982; 10:167–172.

18. Franks S, Adams J, Mason HD, Polson DW. Ovulatory disorders in women with polycystic ovary syndrome. Clin Obstet Gynecol 1985; 12:605–632.

19. Farquhar CM, Birdsall M, Manning P, Mitchell JM, France JT. The prevalence of polycystic ovaries on ultrasound scanning in a population of randomly selected women. Aust NZ J Obstet Gynaecol 1994; 34:67–72.

Appendix 2
Polycystic ovary syndrome history sheet

Name	Date of presentation		Ethnicity

Acne	**Hirsutism (0–4)**	**Menarche**	Birthweight (kg):
Sites:	1 Lip		
	....	**Cycle characteristics:**	Weight (kg):
Grade: 0/1/2/3	2 Face		
	....		Height (m):
	3 Chin		
Alopecia	....		BMI (kg/m²):
	4 Neck		
Grade: 0/1/2/3	....	Oligomenorrhea?	Waist (cm):
	5 Chest		
	....	Longest amenorrhea?	Hip (cm):
Acanthosis nigricans	6 Abdomen		
	....		W:H:
Sites:	7 Arms		
	....		Heaviest weight (kg):
	8 Legs		
	....		
	Total out of 32:		

Age first symptoms	BP (mmHg)

Fertility	**Year and outcome**	**Mode of conception**	**Birthweight**
Outcome:	1		
L,M,E,T, other	2		
Mode of conception:	3		
Sp, CC, Gn, LOD,	4		
IVF, other	5		

Past history	GDM?	**Family history**	
DM		DM	Sisters?
CVS		CVS	
Cancer		Cancer	
Other		Other	

Genetics?

Baseline endocrinology FSH   Total T   A4
                         LH   SHBG   DHEAS
                                      FAI   17-OHP
TSH   U&E   HDL   GTT
T4   LFT   LDL   0'
PRL   FBC   TG   120'

Ultrasound   **Left ovary**   **Right ovary**   Endo (mm)
                        PCO   Y/N   PCO   Y/N   UXA   cm²
                        Vol (cm³)   Vol (cm³)   Other:

Treatments (tick if ever given and state name)
COCP   Metformin   CC   IVF
Spironolactone   Gns   Other

Key

A₄	androstenedione	LFT	liver function tests
COCP	combined oral contraceptive pill	LH	luteinising hormone
CVS	cardiovascular disease	M	miscarriage
DHEAS	dihydroepiandrostenedione sulphate	PRL	prolactin
DM	diabetes mellitus	SHBG	sex hormone binding globulin
E	ectopic pregnancy	T	term birth
FAI	free androgen index	T₄	throxine
FBC	full blood count	TG	triglycerides
FSH	follicle stimulating hormone	Total T	total testosterone
GTT	glucose tolerance test	TSH	thyroid stimulating hormone
HDL	high-density lipoprotein	U&E	urea & electrolytes
L	livebirth	17-OHP	17 hydroxyprogesterone
LDL	low-density lipoprotein		

Appendix 3
Support groups and web sites

1. Websites

1.1 United States

www.androgenexcesssociety.org
The Androgen Excess Society (AES) was consti-
tuted in 2002 to serve as a forum for physicians
and scientists interested in disorders of androgen
excess such as polycystic ovary syndrome,
congenital adrenal, hyperplasia, idiopathic
hirsutism and premature adrenarche. The AES
serves as the premier international organization
that fosters and encourages quality and innova-
tive clinical and basic research related to the etiology, diagnosis, treatment and prevention of
androgen excess disorders. The Executive
Director is Ricardo Azziz, MD. For information on
becoming an AES member or to learn more about
upcoming meetings, please contact Lois Dollar
via email at DollarL@cshs.org.

www.endo-society.org
The Endocrine Society is the world's largest and
most active professional organization of endocrinologists in the world. Founded in 1916, the
society is internationally known as the leading
source of state-of-the-art research and clinical
advancements in endocrinology and metabolism.
The Endocrine Society is dedicated to promoting
excellence in research, education and clinical
practice in the field of endocrinology.

www.asrm.org
The American Society for Reproductive Medicine
(ASRM) was founded by a small group of fertility
experts who met in Chicago in 1944. The ASRM is
an organization devoted to advancing knowledge
and expertise in infertility, reproductive medicine
and biology. The society accomplishes its mission
through the pursuit of excellence in education
and research and through advocacy on behalf of
patients, physicians, and affiliated healthcare
providers.

1.2 Canada

www.cfas.ca/index.asp
The Mission of the Canadian Fertility and
Andrology Society is to promote the study of,
education about, and research on fertility, sterility,
and andrology, respond to social needs in regard
to the complexities of human reproduction,
provide expertise in the accreditation of clinical
and laboratory therapeutics in new reproductive
technologies, and establish valid processes for the
measurement of outcomes of therapy. In 1954 the
society was founded under the name of 'The
Canadian Society for the Study of Fertility'.

1.3 United Kingdom

*www.britishfertilitysociety.org.uk/; bfs@bioscien-
tifica.com*
The British Fertility Society (BFS) was founded in
1972 by a small group with a common interest in
infertility. Since then the burgeoning knowledge in
this exciting area of medicine has resulted in the
development and introduction of many new reproductive technologies and into clinical practice. The
interests of the BFS have broadened to a range
unimaginable 30 years ago. The BFS has grown
alongside the development of our specialty and now
actively promotes the sharing of knowledge, further
education and raising standards of practice. Today,
the society recognizes the multidisciplinary nature of
science and practice of reproductive medicine, and
welcomes andrologists, counselors, embryologists,
endocrinologists, nurses, and other professional
groups working in this field, into its membership.

1.4 Europe

www.eshre.com/
The European Society of Human Reproduction and Embryology held its first Annual meeting in Bonn, 1985. On that occasion the European Society of Human Reproduction and Embryology was officially founded as a result of a broad and lively discussion during the first annual general meeting where delegates from all over Europe participated in the debates. Since that day the society has gradually developed into a well-structured body and is now a non-profit association regulated by the Belgian law. Membership to the society is open to all individuals active in the field of reproductive medicine and science, including medical doctors, scientists, students, and support personnel such as nurses, laboratory technicians, counselors, psychologists, social workers, etc.

1.5 Australia

www.fsa.au.com/
The Fertility Society of Australia is the peak body representing scientists, doctors, researchers, nurses, consumer groups, patients, and counsellors in reproductive medicine in Australia and New Zealand. The Fertility Society of Australia is also at the forefront of research and treatment for disorders relating to contraception, endometriosis, premature menopause, sexually transmitted disease, and cancer.

2 Patient support groups

2.1 United States

www.pcosupport.org
The Polycystic Ovarian Syndrome Association exists to provide comprehensive information, support, and advocacy for women and girls with the condition known as polycystic ovary syndrome.

www.soulcysters.com
This is sponsored by a support group called Soul Cysters. It is not only a reference site, but one where women with PCOS 'speak from the heart' and tell their stories. The SoulCysters Message Board is an online forum for women with PCOS.

www.pcostrategies.org
PCOStrategies, Inc.™ is a national non-profit organization dedicated to fertility enhancement and life management for women with polycystic ovary syndrome.

2.2 United Kingdom

www.verity-pcos.org.uk
Verity is the self-help organization for women whose lives are affected by polycystic ovary syndrome.

2.3 Australia

www.posaa.asn.au
This is the website of the Polycystic Ovarian Syndrome Association of Australia; it is dedicated to the promotion of awareness about PCOS. This site has an Australian focus.

2.4 Ireland

www.obgyn.net
This is a worldwide site dealing with all aspects of infertility and its treatment for medical professionals and lay women alike. The polycystic ovary syndrome site includes a Pavilion section which provides a discussion and medication forum, interviews, and professional powerpoint presentations, as well as much other useful information.

2.5 For Dutch speakers

www.freya.nl
This is the site of the Dutch infertility patients' association which contains a lot of solid information on polycystic ovary syndrome for physicians and patients alike, and also contains opportunities for patients' questions and support.

www.groups.msn.com/PCOSNederland
Run by a lady called Esterella, this is an aesthetically designed site mainly for patients' information but nevertheless containing detailed descriptions. The emphasis is mainly for those who are not presently pursuing a pregnancy.

Appendix 4
Further reading

Balen AH, Jacobs HS. Infertility in Practice, Second Edition. London: Churchill Livingstone/ Harcourt Brace, 2003.
A practical guide to the management of all aspects of infertility.

Craggs-Hinton A, Balen A. Coping with Polycystic Ovary Syndrome – A Patient's Guide. London: Sheldon Press, 2004. Also published in North America as: Craggs-Hinton A & Balen A. Positive Options for Polycystic Ovary Syndrome – Self-Help and Treatment. Hunter House: Berkeley CA, 2004. 131 pages.
A patient's guide to PCOS and how to cope with the condition.

Edwards RG, Brody SA. Principles and practice of assisted human reproduction. London: WB Saunders, 1995.
A detailed scientific analysis of assisted reproduction technology (ART) – science and practice.

Fauser BCJM, Rutherford AJ, Strauss JF, Van Steirteghem A. Molecular biology in reproductive medicine. New York: Parthenon Publishing, 1999.
A detailed overview of molecular biology.

Gardner DK, Weissman A, Howles CM, Shoham Z. Textbook of assisted reproductive techniques – laboratory and clinical perspectives. London: Martin Dunitz, 2001.
A comprehensive text on ART.

Hillier SG, Kitchener HC, Nielson JP. Scientific essentials of reproductive medicine. London: WB Saunders, 1996.
In-depth scientific analysis of reproductive medicine.

Homburg R. Polycystic ovary syndrome. London: Martin Dunitz, 2001.
A multi-author comprehensive overview of polycystic ovary syndrome (PCOS).

Kovacs GT. Polycystic ovary syndrome. Cambridge: Cambridge University Press, 2000.
A multi-author clinically orientated overview of PCOS.

RCOG. The management of infertility in primary, secondary and tertiary care. Three sets of guidelines. London: RCOG Press, 1998 and 2000. Updated in 2004 by The National Institute of Clinical Excellence (NICE).

Shoham Z, Howles CM, Jacobs HS. Female infertility therapy: current practice. London: Martin Dunitz, 1999.
An in-depth overview of infertility therapy in practice.

Templeton A, Cooke I, O'Brien PMS. Evidence-based fertility treatment. London: RCOG Press, 1998.
The proceedings of a RCOG scientific working party on infertility.

Index

T - #0516 - 071024 - C240 - 246/189/11 - PB - 9780367392864 - Gloss Lamination